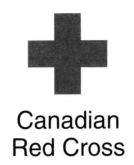

Canadian
Red Cross

# First Responder
## Second Edition

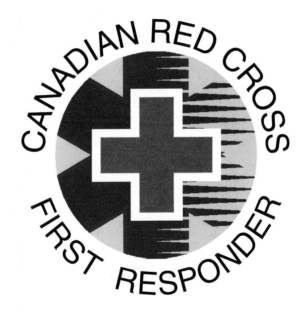

StayWell

# StayWell

**This manual is a reference for the Canadian Red Cross First Responder course.**
**The text material does not constitute comprehensive Red Cross training.**
**Canadian Red Cross certificates can only be issued by certified Canadian Red Cross Instructors.**

**NOTE ON PHOTOS:**
For the most part, the photographs and illustrations in this manual depict appropriate infection control measures through the use of disposable gloves and/or other barrier devices.
However, in cases where the author believed it important to better demonstrate certain procedures or proper artificial respiration procedures, gloves and barrier devices were dispensed with for the sake of clarity.
Please remember that all casualties present an infection risk to the first responder. Infection control procedures should be used whenever there is risk of exposure to a casualty's blood or bodily fluids.

**Copyright © 2002 The Canadian Red Cross Society**

Adaptation of: *Emergency Response*
Copyright © 1993 The American National Red Cross

Printed in Canada

Composition and Color separation by Accu-Color, Inc.
Printing/binding by Transcontinental Printing Inc.

The StayWell Health Company Ltd.
780 Township Line Road
Yardley, PA 19067-4200

**ISBN 1-58480-148-4**

**National Library of CanadaCataloguing in Publication**

Main entry under title:
    First responder/Canadian Red Cross. —2nd ed.
Issued also in French under title: Premier répondant.
Includes index.
ISBN 1-58480-148-4
    1. First aid in illness and injury.    2. CPR (First aid).
I. Canadian Red Cross Society.
RC86.7.F59 2002        616.02'52        C2002-903928-2

02 03 04 05 / 6 5 4 3 2 1

The Basic Life Support skills outlined in this publication are consistent with the Guidelines 2000 for Cardiopulmonary Resuscitation and Emergency Cardiovascular Care.

# Acknowledgments

The original version of this manual *Emergency Response* was developed and produced through a joint effort of the American Red Cross Society and Mosby-Year Book, Inc. Our sister Society kindly authorized us to use their materials and shared with us the success they had with Mosby-Year Book, Inc. The Canadian Red Cross Society wishes to express our appreciation to the volunteers and staff of the American Red Cross Health and Safety Department who made this project possible. The Society also wishes to acknowledge the effort of the many volunteers and staff involved in the Canadian development of this manual. The growth and development of the "First Responder" course and supporting products is a result of the work and dedication of Canadians from across the country. Their commitment to excellence made this training program and its resources possible.

A very special thank you to the members of the Canadian Revision Team: Rick Caissie, Edgar Goulette, Walter Vereschagin, Bruce Cox, John Bessoinette, Gregg Dunn, Conrad Landry, Brenda Pichette.

The Mosby-Year Book editorial and production team included: Claire Merrick, Editor in Chief; Mary Beth Warthen, Senior Assistant Editor; Ross Goldberg, Editorial Project Manager; Shannon Canty, Project Supervisor; Douglas Bruce, Director Editing, Design, Manufacturing, and Production; and Elizabeth Rhone Rudder, Designer.

Special thanks to Veronica Visentin and John Hirst, at the Canadian Office of Mosby Consumer Heath & Safety, for their constant support throughout this project.

The Canadian Red Cross would like to acknowledge the following organizations that reviewed the American Red Cross book, *Emergency Response:*

National Association of Emergency Medical Services Physicians
International Association of Fire Fighters
National Council of State EMS Training Coordinators
National Association of Emergency Medical Technicians

The Canadian Red Cross wishes to thank The Canadian Ski Patrol, The Canadian Hockey Association and Parks Canada for their kind donation of photographs. Thanks go to Edgar Beales for the creation of our First Responder crest.

The Canadian Red Cross gratefully acknowledges the following individuals and organizations for their review of this product:

**Claude Plante (E.M.C.A.)**
Emergency Care Instructor
Lac Mégantic, Estrie, Québec

**D.H. Major, President**
The Paramedic Association of Canada
Winnipeg, Manitoba

**Bonnie Varey RN**
RCMP Medical Office
Training Directorate
Ottawa, Ontario

**Dr. Pierre Fréchette, MD**
Medical Co-ordinator
Pre Hospital Emergency and Trauma Services
Ministry of Health and Social Services Quebec
Associate Director Professional Services
Jésus Children's Hospital
Québec, Québec
Emergency Services Division
Medical Services Branch
Health Canada

**Dr. Brian Weitzman, M.D., C.M., F.R.C.P. (C)**
Medical Advisor
Canadian Red Cross

**Dr. Conrad Watters, M.D., F.R.C.S. (C)**

## First Responder: Revision 2000

*First Responder (Second Edition)* is based on the emergency cardiovascular care (ECC) content revisions outlined in *First Aid: The Vital Link (Second Edition)*. With gratitude we thank the Canadian Red Cross volunteers and employees who participated in the *First Responder* review: Ismael Aquino, Dana Banke, Rick Caissie, Ian Fitzpatrick, Eric Ritterrath, Louis-Philippe Tétreault, and the National Medical Advisory Committee (Dr. Stephen Bolton, MD, Dr. Brendan Hughes, MD, Dr. Andrew MacPherson, MD, Dr. Ernest Prégent, MD). We also want to thank Nathalie Allaire, Yvan Chalifour and Zone First Aid staff (Michael Colpitts, Françoise Filteau, Michèle Mercier, Tannis Nostedt, Elizabeth Ramlogan), and the StayWell production team for their ongoing assistance and support.

# Table of Contents

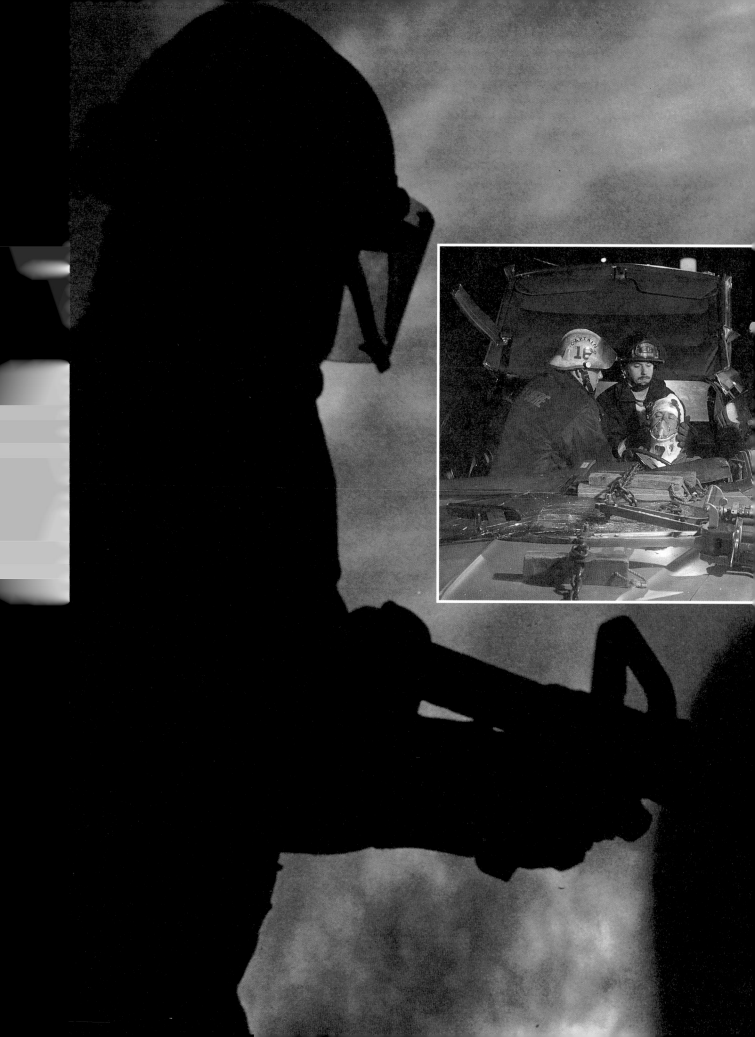

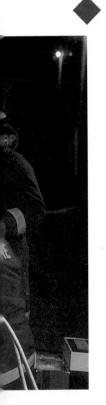

# Part One

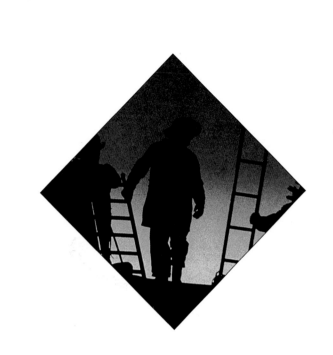

# The First Responder

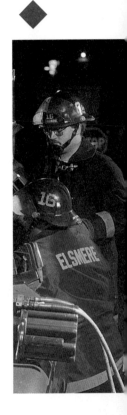

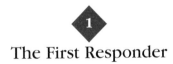

The First Responder

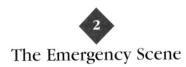

The Emergency Scene

# The First Responder

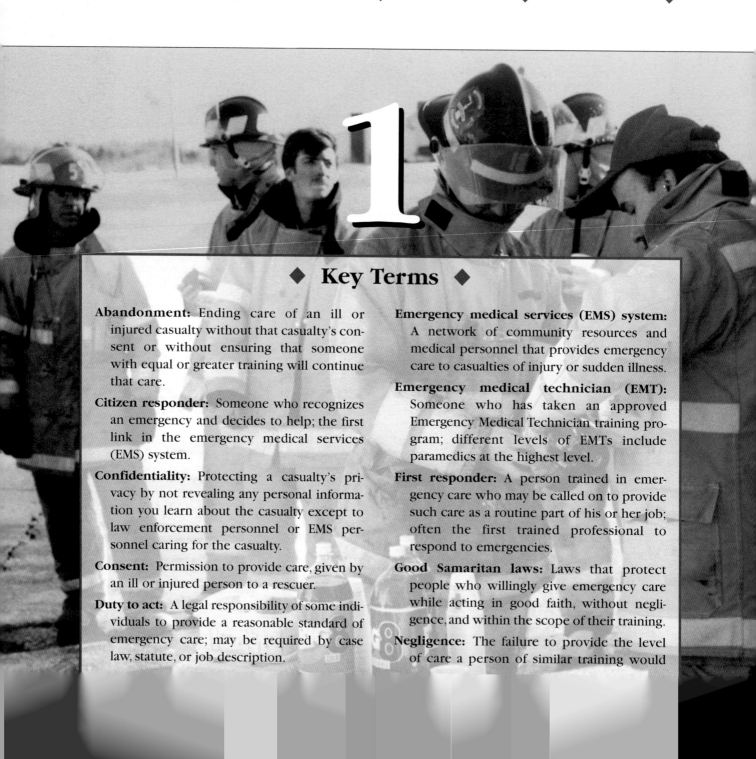

**1**

## ◆ Key Terms ◆

**Abandonment:** Ending care of an ill or injured casualty without that casualty's consent or without ensuring that someone with equal or greater training will continue that care.

**Citizen responder:** Someone who recognizes an emergency and decides to help; the first link in the emergency medical services (EMS) system.

**Confidentiality:** Protecting a casualty's privacy by not revealing any personal information you learn about the casualty except to law enforcement personnel or EMS personnel caring for the casualty.

**Consent:** Permission to provide care, given by an ill or injured person to a rescuer.

**Duty to act:** A legal responsibility of some individuals to provide a reasonable standard of emergency care; may be required by case law, statute, or job description.

**Emergency medical services (EMS) system:** A network of community resources and medical personnel that provides emergency care to casualties of injury or sudden illness.

**Emergency medical technician (EMT):** Someone who has taken an approved Emergency Medical Technician training program; different levels of EMTs include paramedics at the highest level.

**First responder:** A person trained in emergency care who may be called on to provide such care as a routine part of his or her job; often the first trained professional to respond to emergencies.

**Good Samaritan laws:** Laws that protect people who willingly give emergency care while acting in good faith, without negligence, and within the scope of their training.

**Negligence:** The failure to provide the level of care a person of similar training would

## ◆ Key Terms ◆

provide, thereby causing injury or damage to another.

**Refusal of care:** The declining of care by a casualty; a casualty has the right to refuse the care of anyone who responds to an emergency scene.

**Standard of care:** The minimal standard and quality of care expected of an emergency care provider.

## ◆ INTRODUCTION

*A terrified mother pulls her child from the bottom of a pool while a neighbor calls 9-1-1 or the local EMS number for help. You are the first to arrive at the scene to see the neighbor trying to breathe air into the boy's limp body. The mother looks to you helplessly.*

*As a member of your company's emergency response team, you are radioed that a worker's arm is trapped in a piece of machinery. You arrive to find co-workers attempting to free the arm.*

As a first responder, you are a key part of the emergency medical services (EMS) system. You provide a link between the first actions of bystanders and more advanced care. A first responder is a person, paid or volunteer, who is often summoned to provide initial care in an emergency (Fig. 1-1). As the first trained professional on the scene, your actions are often critical. They may determine whether a seriously ill or injured person survives.

By taking this course, you will gain the knowledge, skills, and confidence to give appropriate care when you are called to help a casualty of injury or sudden illness. You will learn how to assess a casualty's condition and how to recognize and care for life-threatening emergencies. You will also learn how to minimize a casualty's discomfort and prevent further complications until more advanced medical personnel take over.

## ◆ THE EMERGENCY MEDICAL SERVICES (EMS) SYSTEM

The first responder is part of the emergency medical services (EMS) system, a network of community resources and medical personnel that provides emergency care to casualties of injury or sudden illness. When bystanders at an emergency scene recognize an emergency and take action, they activate this system. The care provided by more highly trained professionals continues until an ill or injured person receives the level of care that he or she needs. The development of this organized EMS network over the years has led to a higher quality of medical care in our society.

## ◆ THE EMERGENCY RESPONSE— A CHAIN OF SURVIVAL

The EMS system functions as a series of events linked in a chain, a chain of survival (Fig. 1-2). The basic principle is to bring rapid medical care to the casualty rather than the casualty to medical care. From the onset of illness or injury until the casualty receives hospital care, the survival and recovery of critically ill or injured persons depends on this chain of events.

These events include—

1. Recognition of an emergency and initial care by citizen responders.
2. Early activation of the EMS system.

3. First responder care.
4. More advanced prehospital care.
5. Hospital care.
6. Rehabilitation.

## Citizen Response

The first crucial link in the EMS system is the action of the citizen responder. This link depends on a responsible citizen who takes action when an injury or illness occurs. The person must first recognize that what has happened is an emergency. He or she must then activate the EMS system by dialing 9-1-1 or the local EMS number or by notifying a nearby first responder, such as a police officer.

While waiting for more highly trained personnel, the citizen responder can provide basic care to the ill or injured casualty. This initial care may be as simple as applying direct pressure on a bleeding wound or as complex as cardiopulmonary resuscitation (CPR). Often the care provided by citizen responders in these first few minutes is critical. However, their efforts may be futile without the immediate response of more highly trained emergency personnel.

## Rapid Activation of EMS

The next link involves the EMS dispatcher who receives the call for help from either a citizen or a first responder already on the scene. The

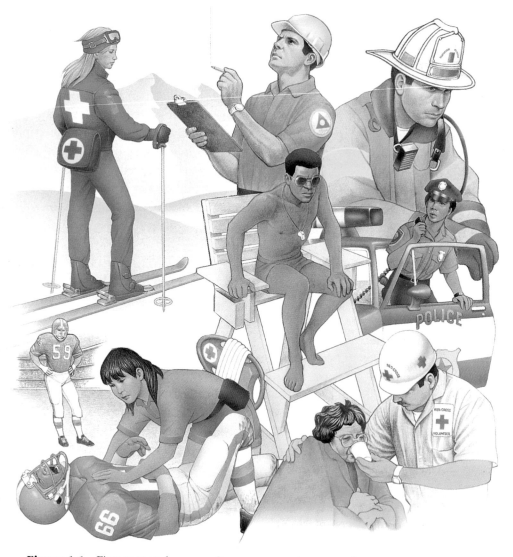

**Figure 1-1** First responders are often summoned to provide care in an emergency.

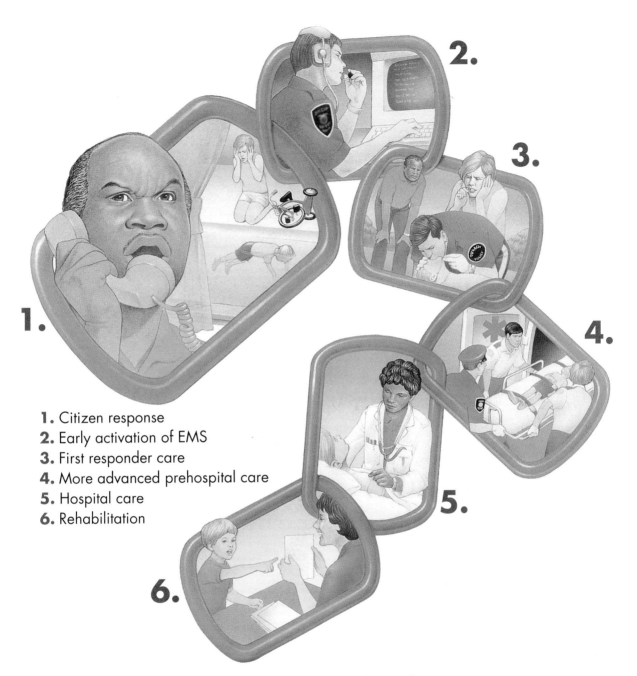

1. Citizen response
2. Early activation of EMS
3. First responder care
4. More advanced prehospital care
5. Hospital care
6. Rehabilitation

**Figure 1-2**  The Chain of Survival.

dispatcher quickly determines what help is needed and sends the appropriate professionals.

## First Responder Care

The first person to arrive on the scene who is trained to provide a higher level of care is often referred to as the first responder (Fig. 1-3). This person has the skills to better assess the casualty's condition and take appropriate actions, which include caring for life-threatening conditions. First responders have traditionally been police officers and fire fighters. Besides these traditional first responders, there are others who also are routinely summoned to emergency situations. These include industrial safety personnel, athletic trainers, and people with similar responsibilities for the safety and well-being of others. Because of the nature of their jobs, first responders are often close to the scene and frequently

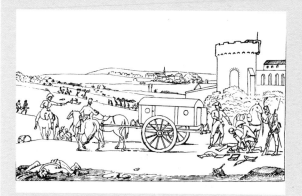

Yesterday's "Flying Ambulance." (Cabanes, Chirurgiens et Blessés a travers l'Histoire, Paris, 1918.)

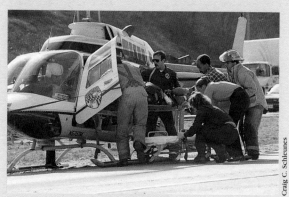

Today's "Flying Ambulance"

# From Horses to Helicopters: A History of Emergency Care

Emergency care originated during the French emperor Napoleon's campaigns in the late 1700s. The surgeon-in-chief for the Grand Army, Dominique Jean Larrey, became the first doctor to try to save the wounded during battles instead of waiting until the fighting was over.[1] Using horse-drawn litters, Larrey and his men dashed onto the battlefield in what became known as "flying ambulances."

By the 1860s, the wartime principles of emergency care were applied to everyday emergencies in some American cities. In 1878, a writer for *Harper's New Monthly Magazine* explained how accidents were reported to the police, who notified the nearest hospitals by a telegraph signal. He described an early hospital ambulance ride in New York City.[2]

"A well-kept horse was quickly harnessed to the ambulance; and as the surgeon took his seat behind, having first put on a jaunty uniform cap with gold lettering, the driver sprang to the box

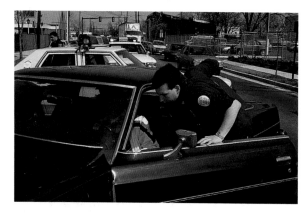

**Figure 1-3** A first responder is often the first person trained to provide a higher level of care to arrive on the scene.

have appropriate supplies and equipment. Your care often provides a critical transition between a citizen's initial actions and the care of more highly trained professionals.

## More Advanced Prehospital Care

The arrival of emergency medical technicians (EMTs) represents the next link in the chain of survival. Depending on the level of training and certification (basic, intermediate, or paramedic), the EMT can provide more advanced care and life-support techniques. An EMT's training requires successful completion of a province-approved

...and with a sharp crack of the whip we rolled off the smooth asphalt of the courtyard and into the street. . . . As we swept around corners and dashed over crossings, both doctor and driver kept up a sharp cry of warning to pedestrians."[2]

While booming industrial cities developed emergency transport systems, rural populations had only rudimentary services. In most small towns, the mortician had the only vehicle large enough to handle the litters, so emergency casualties were just as likely to ride in a hearse to the hospital as in an ambulance.[3]

Cars gave a faster system of transport, but over the next 50 years, car collisions also created the need for more emergency vehicles. In 1966, a major report questioned the quality of emergency services. Dismayed at the rising death toll on the nation's highways, in the 1960s and 1970s laws were passed ordering the improved training of ambulance workers and emergency department staffs, an improved communications network, and the development of regional units with specialized care.

Today, the telegraph signal has been replaced by the 9-1-1 telephone code in many areas, which immediately connects a caller to a dispatcher who can send help. In some areas a computer connected to the enhanced 9-1-1 system displays the caller's name, address, and phone number, even if the caller cannot speak. Ambulance workers have changed from coachmen to trained

medical professionals who can provide lifesaving care at the scene. Horses have been replaced by ambulances and helicopters equipped to provide the most advanced prehospital care available.

The EMS system has expanded in sheer numbers and in services. Today, New York City has 15 times as many hospitals as in the 1870s. Hospitals have also vastly improved their emergency care capabilities. If patients suffer from critical injuries, such as burns, spinal cord injuries, or other traumatic injuries, the EMS system now has developed regional trauma and burn centers where specialists are always available.

In two centuries, the EMS system has gone from horses to helicopters. As technology continues to advance, it is difficult to imagine what changes the next century will bring.

**REFERENCES**

1. Major R, M.D.: *A history of medicine,* Springfield, Ill, 1954, Charles C Thomas.
2. Rideing WH: Hospital life in New York, *Harper's New Monthly Magazine* 57:171, 1878.
3. Division of Medical Sciences, National Academy of Sciences—National Research Council: *Accidental death and disability: the neglected disease of modern society,* Washington, DC, September 1966.

EMT training program, which provides experience in both prehospital and hospital settings. In most parts of Canada, ambulance personnel must be certified at least at the basic EMT level.

Paramedics (EMT-Ps) are highly specialized EMTs. In addition to performing basic EMT skills, paramedics can administer medication and intravenous fluids and deliver advanced care for breathing problems and abnormal heart rhythms. Paramedics provide the highest level of prehospital care. They serve as the field extension of the emergency physician. Regardless of the level of training, the EMT's role is to reassess the casualty's condition and

to begin and continue appropriate care until the injured or ill casualty reaches the hospital.

## Hospital Care

When the casualty arrives at the hospital emergency department, the emergency department staff take over care (Fig. 1-4). Many personnel in this link become involved as needed, including physicians, nurses, and other health-care professionals.

A nurse trained to assess the casualty's condition is usually the first member of the emergency department staff involved. He or she

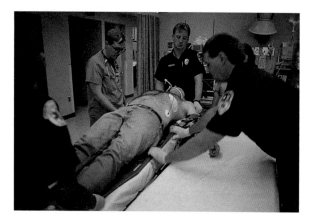

**Figure 1-4**  At the hospital, EMTs turn over care of the casualty to the emergency department staff.

quickly evaluates the casualty and identifies any immediate threats to the casualty's life. Other specially trained emergency department nurses continue to provide needed care.

Most hospital emergency departments are staffed by emergency department physicians trained to care for the acutely ill or injured. They evaluate and provide care that stabilizes a critically ill or injured person. If more specialized care is required, the emergency department physician involves the appropriate medical specialist, such as a cardiologist, orthopedic surgeon, neurosurgeon, or trauma surgeon.

In addition to nurses and physicians, many other allied health personnel may help provide care. These include respiratory technicians, radiology technicians, and laboratory technicians.

## Rehabilitation

The final link in the chain of survival is rehabilitation. The goal of rehabilitation is to return the injured or ill casualty to his or her previous state of health. This phase begins once the person has been moved from the emergency department. Other health care professionals, including family physicians, consulting specialists, social workers, and physical therapists, work together to rehabilitate the casualty.

## ◆ SUPPORTING THE EMS SYSTEM

The chain of survival depends on all persons in the chain performing their roles correctly and promptly to make the EMS system work. Citizens must recognize emergencies and quickly get help by activating the system. They must learn what actions to take in the first critical minutes. They must also learn to prevent emergencies and prepare for them. They need to support the EMS system in their community.

Professionals must respond sensitively, quickly, and effectively to emergencies when they are summoned. They must keep their training current and stay abreast of new issues in emergency response. Each link in the chain working effectively enhances the casualty's chances for a full recovery.

So what happens if one of these links in the chain of survival breaks? Since the casualty's life may depend on each or all of these links, a broken link can cause serious consequences.

For instance, if a citizen responder does not recognize a life-threatening emergency, such as the early signals of a heart attack, and does not quickly call EMS personnel, the casualty may not live. Poor information given to the EMS dispatcher may delay advanced care. Improper care of the ill or injured casualty before more advanced care arrives can result in their condition worsening, possibly leading to permanent disability or death.

In a serious injury or illness, survival and recovery are not a matter of chance. Survival results from a carefully orchestrated chain of events in which all participants fulfill their roles. The EMS system can make the difference between life and death or a partial or full recovery. *You* as a first responder play a critical role in this system.

## ◆ THE FIRST RESPONDER

First responders, unlike lay people, are more likely while on duty to respond to the scene of a medical emergency and to provide emergency medical care to the ill or injured. They should have ready access to supplies and equipment for providing care until more advanced emergency care arrives (Fig. 1-5).

Some occupations, such as law enforcement and fire fighting, require personnel to respond to and assist at the scene of an emergency. These personnel are dispatched through an emergency number, such as 9-1-1 or the local EMS number, and often share common communication networks. When a person dials 9-1-1 or the local EMS number, he or she will contact police, fire, or ambulance personnel. These are typically considered public safety personnel. However, first responders do not necessarily work in public safety agencies. People in many other occupations are called to help in the event of an injury or sudden illness, for example—

- Industrial safety personnel
- Athletic trainers
- Ski patrol members
- Emergency management personnel
- Disaster team members
- First aid station attendants
- Lifeguards

These people are often expected to provide the same minimum standard of care as traditional first responders. As a first responder, you have a duty when called to quickly and safely respond to the scene of an emergency. Your duty also is to assess the casualty's condition and provide necessary care, make sure that any necessary additional help

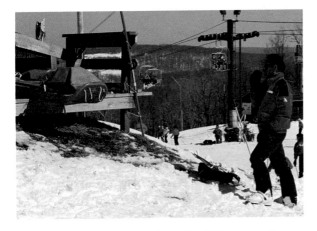

**Figure 1-5** First responders should have ready access to emergency supplies and equipment.

has been summoned, assist other medical personnel at the scene, and document your actions.

## Personal Characteristics

As an emergency care provider who deals with the public, you must be willing to take on responsibilities beyond giving care. These responsibilities require you to demonstrate certain characteristics that include—

- *Maintaining a caring and professional attitude.*
  Ill or injured casualties are sometimes difficult to work with. Be compassionate; try to understand their concerns and fears. Realize that any anger an injured or ill casualty may show is often the result of fear. A citizen who helps at the emergency may also be afraid. Try to be reassuring. Even though citizen responders may not have done everything perfectly, be sure to thank them for taking action. Recognition and praise help to affirm their willingness to act. Also, be careful about what you say. Do not give distressing news about the emergency to the casualty or the casualty's family or friends.
- *Controlling your fears.*
  Try not to reveal your anxieties to the casualty or bystanders. The presence of blood, vomit, unpleasant odors, or torn or burned skin is disturbing to most people. You may need to compose yourself before acting. If you must, turn away for a moment and take a few deep breaths before providing care.
- *Presenting a professional appearance.*
  This helps ease a casualty's fears and inspires confidence.
- *Keeping your skills and knowledge up to date.*
  Involve yourself in continuing education, professional reading, and refresher training.
- *Staying fit with daily exercise and a healthy diet.*
  Job stresses can adversely affect your health. Exercise and diet can help you manage physical, mental, and emotional stress.

◆ *Maintaining a safe and healthy lifestyle.*
As a first responder, it is important to maintain a safe and healthy lifestyle both on and off the job. Identify the risk factors in your life so that you can take steps to reduce them.

## Responsibilities

Since you will often be the first trained professional to arrive in many emergencies, your primary responsibilities center on safety and early emergency care. Your six major responsibilities are to—

1. *Ensure safety for yourself and any bystanders.*
   Your first responsibility is not to make the situation worse by getting hurt yourself or letting bystanders get hurt. By making sure the scene is safe as you approach it, you can avoid unnecessary injuries.
2. *Gain access to the casualty.*
   Carefully approach the casualty unless the scene is too dangerous for you to handle without help. Electrical hazards, unsafe structures, and other dangers may make it difficult to reach the casualty. Recognize when a rescue requires specially trained emergency personnel.
3. *Determine any threats to the casualty's life.*
   Check first for immediate life-threatening conditions and care for any you find. Next, look for other conditions that could eventually threaten the casualty's life or health if not cared for.
4. *Summon more advanced medical personnel as needed.*
   After you quickly assess the casualty, notify more advanced medical personnel of the situation if someone has not already done so.
5. *Provide needed care for the casualty.*
   Remain with the casualty and provide whatever care you can until more advanced personnel take over.
6. *Assist more advanced personnel.*
   Transfer your information about the casualty and the emergency to any more advanced

personnel (Fig. 1-6). Tell them what happened, how you found the casualty, any problems you found, and any care you gave. Assist them as needed, and help with care for any other casualties. When possible, try to anticipate the needs of those giving care.

In addition to these major responsibilities, you have secondary responsibilities that include—

◆ Summoning additional help when needed, such as special rescue teams.
◆ Controlling or directing bystanders or asking them for help.
◆ Taking additional steps, if necessary, to protect bystanders from dangers such as traffic or fire.
◆ Recording what you saw, heard, and did at the scene.
◆ Reassuring the casualty's family or friends.

## ◆ LEGAL CONSIDERATIONS

Many people are concerned about lawsuits. Lawsuits against those who give care at the scene of an emergency, however, are highly unusual and rarely successful. By being aware of some basic legal principles, you may be able to avoid the possibility of legal action in the future (Fig. 1-7).

The following sections address in general terms the legal principles that concern emergency care. Because laws vary from province to

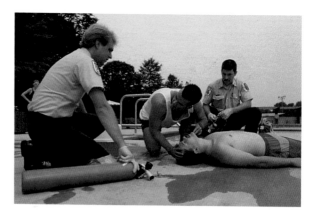

**Figure 1-6** The first responder transfers information about the casualty to more advanced medical personnel.

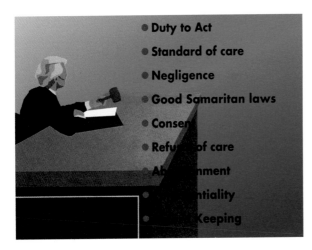

- Duty to Act
- Standard of care
- Negligence
- Good Samaritan laws
- Consen[t]
- Refu[sal] of care
- Ab[ando]nment
- [Confide]ntiality
- [Record] Keeping

**Figure 1-7** First responders should be aware of these basic legal considerations.

province, your instructor may need to update you on the laws in your province that apply to you or tell you where you can find such information.

## Duty to Act

Most first responders, either by case law, statute, or job description, have a duty to act at the scene of an emergency. This duty applies to public safety officers, government employees, licensed and certified professionals, and paraprofessionals while on duty. For instance, members of a volunteer fire department have a duty to act based on their agreement to participate in the fire department. An athletic trainer has a duty to give care to an injured athlete. Failure to adhere to these agreements could result in legal action.

## Standard of Care

The public expects a certain standard of care from personnel summoned to provide emergency care. For instance, the standard of care for first responders may be based on the training guidelines used in different provinces. Provincial laws and other authorities, such as national organizations, may govern the actions of other first responders. If your actions do not meet the standards set for you, you may be successfully sued if your actions harm another person.

## Negligence

Negligence is the failure to follow a reasonable standard of care, thereby causing injury or damage to another. A person could be negligent either by acting wrongly or failing to act at all.

The following scenario is an example of a case in which negligence may be suspected. A car is traveling at a high rate of speed on an icy road. The driver loses control, and the car flips end over end. A passenger is ejected from the car and hurled 10 metres, landing on her back.

The arriving first responder notes the severity of the incident but fails to consider that the passenger may have a spinal injury. The first responder attempts to get the casualty to stand up and move out of the road, even though there is no immediate threat of danger. This movement causes the casualty to experience severe pain, and she suddenly loses feeling in her legs. In this case, the first responder may be negligent because he or she failed to follow a reasonable standard of care.

Four components must be present for a lawsuit charging negligence to be successful:

- Duty
- Breach
- Cause
- Damage

As a first responder, you have a duty to respond in a professional manner, obeying traffic laws and protocols that govern your action. If you fail to act within this duty, then you commit a breach of duty. Sometimes your actions can cause accidental or improper care to be rendered, which can further result in harming a casualty.

## Good Samaritan Laws

Most provinces have enacted Good Samaritan laws, which protect people providing emergency care. These laws, which differ from province to province, will generally protect you from legal liability as a first responder as long as you act in good faith, are not negligent, and act within the scope of your training.

# Consent

An individual has a basic right to decide what can and cannot be done with his or her body. Therefore, to provide care for an ill or injured person, you must first obtain that person's consent. Usually, the person needs to tell you clearly that you have permission to provide care. To obtain consent, you must—

1. Identify yourself to the person.
2. Give your level of training.
3. Explain what you think may be wrong.
4. Explain what you plan to do.

After you have provided this information, the person can decide whether to grant his or her informed (or actual) consent. A person can withdraw consent for care at any time.

Unless an illness or injury is life threatening, a parent or guardian who is present must give consent for a child before care can be given. You may encounter a situation in which a parent or guardian refuses to allow you to give care to a severely injured child. In such cases, a law enforcement officer can help you obtain the necessary legal authority to provide care. This also holds true for adults who are under a legal guardian's care. There is no specific age at which one is old enough to give or reject first aid treatment. In general, the person to receive the treatment must be mature enough to understand the circumstances they are in, the nature of the treatment to be provided, and the consequences of refusal.

A person who is unconscious, confused, or seriously ill or injured may not be able to grant actual or informed consent. In these cases, the law assumes that the person would grant consent for care if he or she were able to do so. This is termed implied consent. Implied consent also applies to minors who obviously need emergency assistance when a parent or guardian is not present.

## Refusal of Care

Some ill or injured people, even those who desperately need care, may refuse the care you offer. Even though the person may be seriously injured, you should honor his or her refusal of care. Try to convince the person of the need for care, but do not argue. Allow more advanced medical personnel to evaluate the situation. If possible, to make it clear that you did not abandon the person, have a witness hear the person's refusal and document it. Many EMS systems have a "Refusal of Care" form that you can use in these situations.

## Abandonment

Just as you must have consent from a person before beginning care, you must also continue to give care once you have begun. Once you have started emergency care, you are legally obligated to continue that care until a person with equal or higher training relieves you. Usually, your obligation for care ends when more advanced medical professionals take over. If you stop your care before that point, you can be legally responsible for the abandonment of a casualty in need.

## Confidentiality

While providing care, you may learn things about the casualty that are generally considered private and confidential. Information, such as previous medical problems, physical problems, and medications being taken, is personal to the casualty. Respect the casualty's privacy by maintaining confidentiality. Television and newspaper reporters may ask you questions. Attorneys may also approach you at the scene. Never discuss the casualty or the care you gave with anyone except law enforcement personnel or other personnel caring for the casualty.

## Record Keeping

Documenting your care is nearly as important as the care itself. Your record will help advanced health-care professionals assess and continue care for the casualty. Because a casualty's condition may change before the casualty arrives at the hospital, a record of the condition immediately after the emergency will provide useful information for EMTs and emergency department staff. They can compare the current condition to what you recorded earlier.

Your record is a legal document and is important if legal action occurs. Should you be called to court for any reason, your record will support what you saw, heard, and did at the scene of the emergency. It is important to write the record as soon as possible after the emergency while all the facts are fresh in your memory (Fig. 1-8). Many systems have printed forms for first responders to use. Your instructor may be able to give you information about the report forms used in your system.

# ◆ SUMMARY

The survival and recovery of a severely ill or injured person depends on all parts of the emergency medical services (EMS) system working together efficiently. Citizen response, rapid EMS response, first responder care, advanced prehospital care, hospital care, and extended care are

the links in this chain of survival. The first responder, the first trained person to arrive on the emergency scene, takes over care of the casualty from any citizen responders present.

After arriving on the scene, the first responder must make sure the scene is safe and then reach the casualty, give care for any life-threatening conditions, and summon more advanced medical personnel if needed. The first responder should give arriving medical personnel any assistance they need.

In your role as an emergency care provider, you are guided by certain legal parameters, such as the duty to act, and professional standards of care. Effective record keeping is important in maintaining the standard of care for a casualty and provides legal protection for you and the organization you represent.

Regardless of your profession, when you are called to help a casualty of injury or sudden illness, you assume the role of an emergency care provider. When an emergency occurs, the people in your care, as well as assisting bystanders, will expect you to know what to do. Be prepared to think and act accordingly. What to do, however, often involves more than giving emergency care. Chapter 2 provides an overview of the first responder's role in assessing and managing emergency scenes.

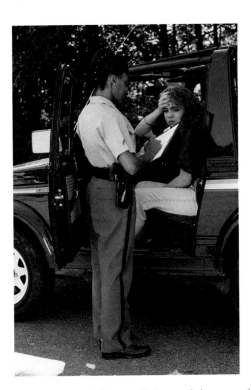

**Figure 1-8** Record the conditions of the casualty at the emergency scene as soon as possible.

## YOU ARE THE RESPONDER

*A 12-year-old elementary school basketball player was temporarily unconscious after hitting his head in a fall during a game. He is now awake, but complaining of dizziness and nausea. You, the first responder, tell the player to go home and rest. At home, the player loses consciousness, and his parents call for an ambulance. Later, in the hospital, the ball player is diagnosed as having a severe head injury that could have been minimized if medical attention had been provided earlier. In your opinion, are there any grounds for legal action against you? State your reasons why or why not.*

# The Emergency Scene

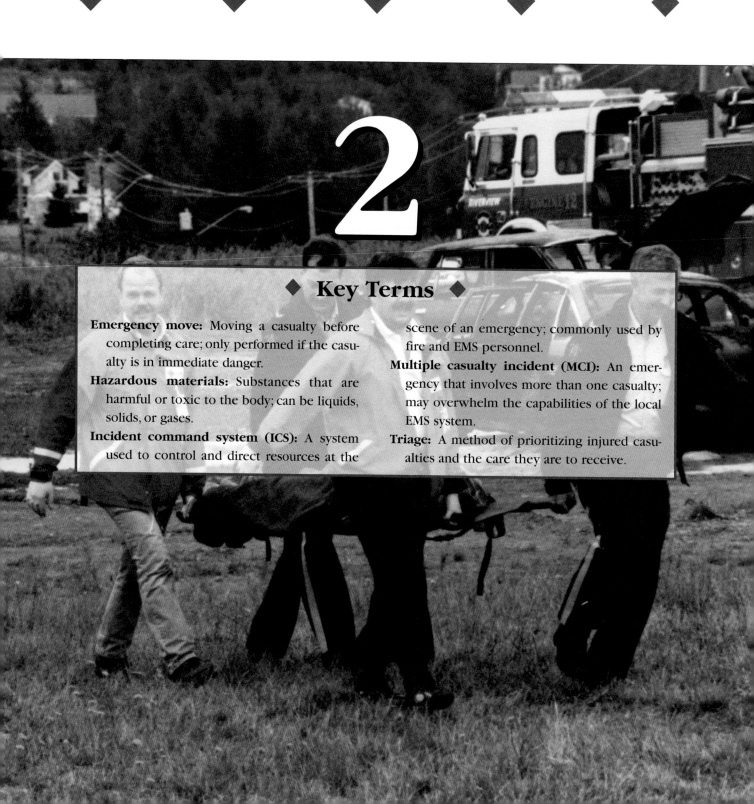

# 2

## ◆ Key Terms ◆

**Emergency move:** Moving a casualty before completing care; only performed if the casualty is in immediate danger.

**Hazardous materials:** Substances that are harmful or toxic to the body; can be liquids, solids, or gases.

**Incident command system (ICS):** A system used to control and direct resources at the scene of an emergency; commonly used by fire and EMS personnel.

**Multiple casualty incident (MCI):** An emergency that involves more than one casualty; may overwhelm the capabilities of the local EMS system.

**Triage:** A method of prioritizing injured casualties and the care they are to receive.

## ◆ For Review ◆

Before reading this chapter, you should be familiar with the primary responsibilities of a first responder (Chapter 1).

## ◆ INTRODUCTION

As a first responder, you have a duty to respond to an emergency when summoned. Although you should immediately proceed to the scene of an emergency when notified, you must do so safely. When you arrive, carefully evaluate the entire scene. Emergency scenes are often dangerous. Never enter a dangerous emergency scene unless you have been trained to do so and have the necessary equipment. Follow your established operating procedures, including when and how to access the EMS system.

This chapter describes the responsibilities for preparing for an emergency response and for identifying and managing initial dangers at an emergency scene.

## ◆ PREPARING FOR THE EMERGENCY RESPONSE

### Equipment and Personnel

The emergency response begins with the preparation of equipment and personnel before an emergency occurs. The first aid kit, or trauma kit, for the first responder should be a standard, available part of your equipment for performing your duties. It should be checked on a regular schedule to ensure that it is well stocked after all shift changes. You should be familiar with the location of all equipment within the kit. Emergency equipment must always be clean and in good working condition. Dressings, bandages, and other supplies kept in kits should be restocked as soon as possible after use. Oxygen cylinders should be kept full. Figure 2-1 shows the supplies and equipment many first responders will have available.

The following is a list of recommended contents for a trauma kit. The quantity of specific items should be determined by individual need.

- ◆ Emergency telephone numbers for EMS and poison centre.
- ◆ Contents checklist.
- ◆ Red Cross manuals.
- ◆ Sterile gauze pads (dressings) in large and small sizes.
- ◆ Large pressure dressings.
- ◆ Adhesive tape.
- ◆ Triangular bandages.
- ◆ Roller bandages.
- ◆ Adhesive bandages in assorted sizes.
- ◆ Bandage scissors.
- ◆ Tweezers.
- ◆ Safety pins.
- ◆ Chemical cold pack.
- ◆ Disposable gloves.
- ◆ Flashlight or penlight with extra batteries in a separate bag.
- ◆ Antiseptic wipes.
- ◆ Pencil or pen and pad or vitals cheatsheet.
- ◆ Emergency blanket.
- ◆ Syrup of ipecac.
- ◆ Sugar, or single-use glucose gel tube.
- ◆ Saline solution or sterile water.
- ◆ Stethoscope.
- ◆ Blood pressure cuff (sphygmomanometer).
- ◆ Properly marked disposable bag for biochemical wastes.
- ◆ Eye protection.
- ◆ Disposable rescue breathing barrier device.
- ◆ Obstetrics kit.
- ◆ Burn kit.

In addition, a first aid kit should be readily available in your home, automobile, work place, and recreation area.

### Plan of Action

To respond most efficiently to certain emergencies, you need a plan of action. A plan of this type is prepared in advance and rehearsed with personnel. Emergency plans should be established

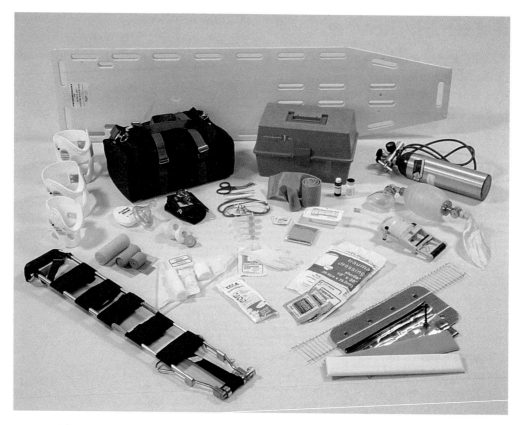

**Figure 2-1** Supplies and equipment first responders may have available.

based on anticipated needs and available resources. All personnel should become familiar with these plans. For example, many businesses and industrial sites have emergency plans that identify trained personnel, locations of supplies and equipment, a communication network, and evacuation routes (Fig. 2-2).

Many fire departments and EMS systems plan responses for large facilities requiring special resources, such as sports stadiums, public buildings, and facilities with hazardous materials. A plan for evacuating a stadium crowded with fans, for example, could save thousands of lives in an emergency. Developing the plan involves inspecting the site, noting potential dangers, and identifying the type of equipment and personnel that will probably be needed. Once developed, plans must be rehearsed, evaluated, and modified periodically.

Learn about the real or potential dangers in your area and familiarize yourself with existing emergency response plans. Evaluate your role and the available local resources. Know the resources in your community for handling special situations, such as a hazardous materials spill, that require specially trained personnel and special equipment.

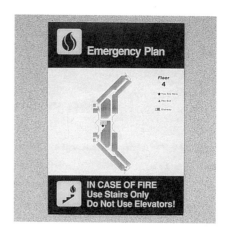

**Figure 2-2** Posted evacuation routes may be part of an emergency plan.

# Communications

Emergency response depends on a reliable and efficient communication system. Make sure you are always able to contact more advanced medical personnel and other special resources. This means having a backup communication system in place. For example, if your system uses a citizens-band radio (CB), have a cellular phone available for backup use. Check communications equipment often to make sure it is working.

Be sure you know how to contact the special resources in your area. Some first responders may use communication networks outside the 9-1-1 or the local EMS number system. Become familiar with your communication networks, and develop an alternative plan in case regular communications fail.

# Training

An important part of being prepared for emergencies is keeping your training current. Continue to practice the skills that you use less often. Pursue activities that will help you perform your job better, including reading appropriate articles and publications and participating in workshops, emergency response exercises, and seminars.

# ◆ RESPONDING TO THE EMERGENCY SCENE
## Mental and Emotional Aspects

Just as it is important to keep equipment ready for emergencies, it is also important for you to be prepared psychologically. You can never predict how the next emergency may affect you. Certain injuries, smells, sights, and sounds can make you feel weak, nauseated, or faint the first time you encounter them. The sight of blood or gaping wounds, cries of pain, the threat of danger, or other factors may so distress any well-intentioned responder that they become barriers to prompt action.

You may never get used to some sights and sounds. With experience and by being prepared, however, you can learn to cope with your feelings. To calm yourself, take a deep breath and look away for a moment. Stay relaxed. Remind yourself that the casualty needs you and you need to be in full control of yourself to give the required care. If you feel nauseated, step back, take several deep breaths, mentally review your task, and then proceed. The casualty's life may depend on you.

The citizen responder may become even more upset than you. Recognizing your emotions and the emotions of others will help you manage the situation in a more understanding and responsive way.

# Notification and Transportation

If you are in a police department, fire department, or rescue squad, for example, you may be notified to go to an emergency by telephone, pager, or radio. Lifeguards, ski patrollers, and athletic trainers may already be near or at the scene when an emergency occurs (Fig. 2-3). If you are at a distance from the scene, you will probably need to use a vehicle to get there. Laws and established procedures govern the use of emergency vehicles and their warning equipment, such as lights and sirens. You must remember that emergency vehicles do not have an absolute right-of-way.

Never drive a private vehicle as if it were an emergency vehicle. Even if you have lights and sirens, people do not always see you, hear you, or yield the right-of-way. People hurrying to an emergency or a hospital sometimes cause vehicle collisions because they fail to drive safely.

# ◆ MANAGING DANGERS AT THE EMERGENCY SCENE

Some emergency scenes are immediately dangerous. Others may become dangerous while you are providing care. Sometimes the dangers are obvious, such as fire or hostile casualties or bystanders. Other dangers may be less obvious, such as the presence of a hazardous material or unstable structures.

## Personal Safety

Of the six primary responsibilities of the first responder discussed in Chapter 1 (box below), safety should always be foremost. You cannot overlook ensuring adequate safety for yourself. Often it requires only simple tasks to make an emergency scene safe.

**Primary Responsibilities of the First Responder**

1. Ensure safety for yourself and any bystanders.
2. Gain access to the casualty.
3. Determine any threats to the casualty's life.
4. Summon more advanced medical personnel as needed.
5. Provide needed care for the casialty.
6. Assist advanced medical personnel as needed.

Approach all emergency scenes cautiously until you can size up the situation. If you arrive at the scene by vehicle, park a safe distance away. If the scene appears safe, continue to evaluate the situation as you approach (Fig. 2-4). Pay particular attention to the—

◆ Location of the emergency.
◆ Extent of the emergency.
◆ Apparent scene dangers.
◆ Apparent number of ill or injured casualties.
◆ Behavior of the casualty(s) and bystanders.

If at any time the scene appears unsafe, retreat to a safe distance. Notify additional personnel and wait for their arrival. This principle cannot be overemphasized. *Never* enter a dangerous scene unless you have the training and equipment to do so safely. Well-meaning rescuers have been injured or killed because they

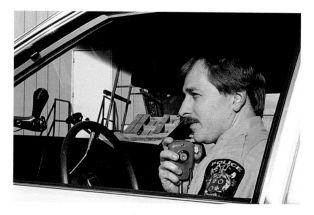

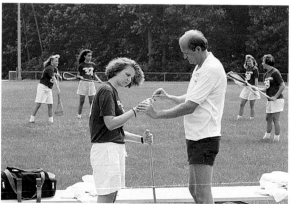

**Figure 2-3** Some first responders are summoned to an emergency; others may be on the scene when an emergency occurs.

forgot to watch for scene hazards. If your training has not prepared you for a specific emergency, such as a fire or an incident involving hazardous materials, notify appropriate personnel.

When arriving on an emergency scene, always follow these four guidelines to ensure your personal safety and that of bystanders:

◆ Take time to evaluate the scene. This will enable you to recognize existing and potential dangers.
◆ Wear appropriate protective gear.
◆ Do *not* attempt to do anything you are not trained to do. Know what resources are available to help.
◆ Get the help you need. If you have not already done so, notify additional personnel. Be able to describe the scene and the type of additional help required.

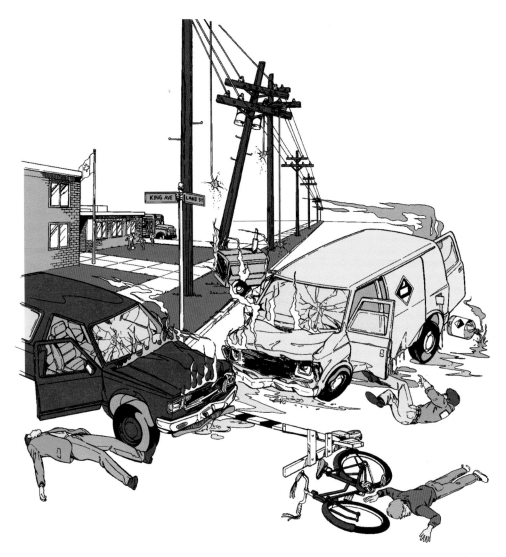

**Figure 2-4** Note the location of the emergency, the dangers, the number of casualties, and other important information while approaching an emergency scene.

## Safety of Others

You have a responsibility for the safety of others at the scene, as well as for your personal safety. Discourage bystanders, family members, or unprepared responders from entering an area that appears unsafe. You can use these well-intentioned individuals to help you keep unauthorized people away from unsafe areas and to summon more appropriate help. Some dangers may require you to take special measures, such as placing physical barriers to prevent onlookers from getting too close. Other situations may require you to act quickly to free someone who is trapped or move a casualty in immediate danger to safety.

Ideally, you should move casualties only after you have assessed and properly cared for them. If, however, immediate dangers threaten a casualty's life, you must decide whether to move him or her. If the situation is dangerous and you cannot move the casualty, retreat to safety yourself. If you can move the casualty, do so quickly and safely.

Situations that may require an emergency move include—

◆ The presence of explosives or other hazardous materials (such as a natural gas leak).
◆ Fire or the danger of fire.

- The inability to make the scene safe (such as a structure about to collapse).
- The need to get to other casualties requiring lifesaving care.

Chapter 22 provides more detailed information about how to move injured or ill casualties safely.

## Specific Emergency Situations

Certain emergency scenes present a special set of problems. These situations include crime scenes, scenes with hazards, and scenes with multiple casualties.

Since every emergency scene has potential dangers, always expect the unexpected. Never attempt a rescue for which you are not properly trained and equipped. Always wear appropriate protective gear, such as gloves and goggles. Be aware that at any time even a seemingly safe emergency scene can turn dangerous. Always take the necessary precautions when you suspect or identify certain dangers. Several of the following situations are also discussed in Chapters 21 through 23.

### Crime

If you arrive at the scene of a crime, do not try to reach any casualty until you are sure the scene is safe. A casualty of a shooting, stabbing, or other violence may have severe injuries, but until the scene is safe, there is nothing you can do to provide care. For the scene to be safe, law enforcement personnel must have made it secure.

Police usually gather evidence at a crime scene, so do not touch anything except what you must to give care. Once you enter a crime scene to give care, make sure that police are aware of your presence and actions.

### Traffic

Traffic is often the most common danger you and other emergency personnel will encounter. If you drive to the collision scene, always try to park where your vehicle will not block other traffic, such as an ambulance, that needs to

reach the scene. The *only* time you should park in a roadway or block traffic is to—

- Protect an injured person.
- Protect any rescuers, including yourself.
- Warn oncoming traffic if the situation is not clearly visible.

Others can help you put reflectors, flares, or lights along the road. These items should be placed well back of the scene to enable oncoming motorists to stop or slow down in time.

Emergency personnel have been injured or killed by traffic at emergency scenes. If you are not a law enforcement officer and dangerous traffic makes the scene unsafe, wait for more help to arrive before giving care.

### Fire

Any fire can be dangerous. Make sure that the local fire department has been summoned. Only fire fighters, who are highly trained and use equipment that protects them against fire and smoke, should approach a fire. Do not let others approach. Gather information to help the responding fire and EMS units. Find out the possible number of people trapped, their location, the fire's cause, and whether any explosives or chemicals are present. Give this information to emergency personnel when they arrive. If you are not trained to fight fires or lack the necessary equipment, follow these basic guidelines:

- Do not approach a burning vehicle.
- Never enter a burning or smoke-filled building.
- If you are in a building that is on fire, always check doors before opening them (Fig. 2-5, *A*). If a door is hot to the touch, *do not* open it.
- Since smoke and fumes rise, stay close to the floor (Fig. 2-5, *B*).
- Never use an elevator in a building that may be burning.

### Electricity

Downed electrical lines also present a major hazard to responders. Always look for downed

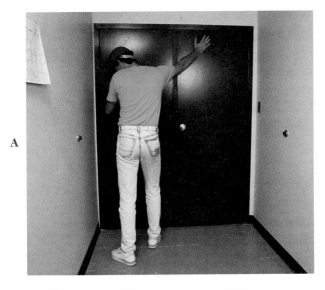

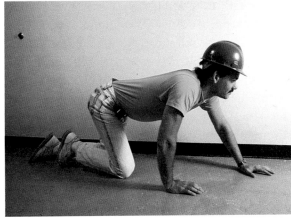

**Figure 2-5**  **A,** If a door in a burning building is hot to the touch, do not open it. **B,** Stay close to the floor to avoid rising smoke and fumes.

wires at a scene, and always treat them as dangerous. If you find downed wires, follow these guidelines:

- Move any crowd back from the danger zone. The safe area should be established at a point twice the length of the span of the wire.
- *Never* attempt to move downed wires.
- Notify the fire department and power company immediately. Always assume that the wires are energized. Even if they are not energized at first, they may become energized later.
- If downed wires contact a vehicle, do *not* touch the vehicle and do not let others touch it. Tell anyone in the vehicle to stay still and

stay inside the vehicle. Never attempt to remove people from a vehicle with downed wires across it, no matter how seriously injured they may seem.
- Do not touch any metal fence, metal structure, or body of water in contact with a downed wire. Wait for the power company to shut off the power source.

## Water and Ice

Water and ice also can be serious hazards. To help a conscious person in the water, always follow the basic rule of "reach, throw, and row." You may reach out to someone in trouble with a branch, a pole, or even your hand, being careful not to be pulled into the water. When the person grasps the object, pull him or her to safety.

If you cannot reach the person, try to throw him or her something nearby that floats. If you have a rope available, attach a floatable object, such as a life jacket, plastic jug, ice chest, or empty gas can, to one end. Never enter a body of water to rescue someone unless you have been trained in water rescue and then only enter as a last resort.

Fast-moving water is extremely dangerous and often occurs with floods, hurricanes, and low head dams. Ice is also treacherous. It can break under your weight, and the cold water beneath can quickly overcome even the best swimmers. *Never* enter fast-moving water or venture out on ice unless you are trained in this type of rescue. Such rescues require careful planning and proper equipment. Wait until trained personnel arrive.

## Hazardous Materials

Hazardous materials are common and are a special risk for responding personnel. When you approach an emergency scene, look for clues that indicate the presence of hazardous materials. These include—

- Signs (placards) on vehicles, storage facilities, or railroad cars identifying the presence of hazardous materials.
- Clouds of vapor.

- Spilled liquids or solids.
- Unusual odors.
- Leaking containers, bottles, or gas cylinders.
- Chemical transport tanks or containers.

Those who transport or store hazardous materials in specific quantities are required to post placards identifying the specific hazardous material, by name or by number, and its dangers (Fig. 2-6). If you do not see a placard but suspect a hazardous material is present, try to get information before you approach the scene.

## Unsafe Structures

Buildings and other structures, such as mines, wells, and unreinforced trenches, can become unsafe because of fire, explosions, natural disasters, deterioration, or other causes. An unsafe building or structure is one in which—

- The air may contain debris or hazardous gases.
- There is a possibility of being trapped or injured by collapsed walls, weakened floors, and other debris.

Try to establish the exact or probable location of anyone in the structure. Gather as much information as you can, call for appropriate help, and wait for the arrival of personnel who are properly trained and equipped.

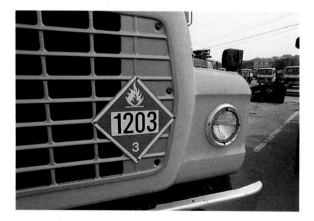

**Figure 2-6**  By law, specific types of placards must indicate the presence of hazardous materials.

## Wreckage

The wreckage of automobiles, aircraft, or machinery may contain hazards, such as sharp pieces of metal or glass, fuel, and moving parts. The wreckage may be unstable. Do not try to rescue someone from wreckage unless you have the proper equipment and training. Rescue is made only after the wreckage has been stabilized. Gather as much information as you can, and be sure advanced medical personnel have been called.

## Natural Disasters

Natural disasters include tornadoes, hurricanes, earthquakes, forest fires, and floods (Fig. 2-7). Rescue efforts after a natural disaster are usually coordinated by local resources until they become overwhelmed. Then the rescue efforts are coordinated by government agencies. Typically, you would report to the person or people in charge at the scene, then work with the disaster response team and follow the rescue plan.

Natural disasters pose more risks than you might be aware of. More injuries and deaths result from electricity, hazardous materials, rising water, and other dangers than from the disaster itself. When responding to a natural disaster, be sure to carefully survey the scene, avoid obvious hazards, and use caution when operating rescue equipment. Never use gasoline-powered equipment, such as chain saws, generators, and pumps, in confined spaces.

## Multiple Casualties

Scenes that involve more than one casualty are referred to as multiple casualty incidents (MCIs). Such scenes make your task more complex, since you must determine who needs immediate care and who can wait for more help to arrive. To make these decisions, you use a process called triage that helps you prioritize the care you give the casualties.

A large multiple-casualty scene, such as a plane or train crash or natural disaster, may overwhelm the capabilities of the local EMS system. To effec-

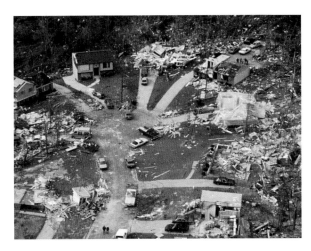

**Figure 2-7** Rescue efforts after large natural disasters are usually coordinated by local resources until they become overwhelmed.

tively handle any emergency involving multiple casualties, the EMS system uses an incident command system (ICS). An incident command system establishes a chain of command at the scene that permits one person to direct all the agencies helping. For example, when police, fire, and EMS personnel are called to a major urban fire, the fire chief takes charge and all other resources report to him or her. These resources may include police evacuating nearby buildings, fire fighters fighting the blaze, and EMS personnel providing emergency care and transportation for casualties. In this way, all available resources will be used effectively and efficiently.

## Hostile Situations

Environmental factors, such as hazardous materials, electricity, and unsafe structures, are not the only dangers you may encounter. You may sometimes encounter a hostile casualty or family member. Any unusual or hostile behavior may be a result of the emergency. A casualty's rage or hostility may be caused by the injury or illness or by fear. Many casualties are afraid of losing control and may show this as anger. Hostile behavior may also result from the use of alcohol or other drugs, lack of oxygen, or an underlying medical condition.

If a person needing care is hostile toward you, try to calmly explain who you are and that you are there to help. Remember that you cannot give care without the person's consent. If the person accepts your offer to help, keep talking to him or her as you assess that person's condition. When the person realizes that you are not a threat, the hostility usually goes away.

If the person refuses your care or threatens you, withdraw from the scene. Never try to restrain, argue with, or force your care on a casualty. If the casualty does not let you provide care, wait for additional help. Sometimes a close friend or a family member will be able to reassure a hostile casualty and convince that person to accept your care.

Family members or friends who are angry or hysterical, however, can make your job more difficult. Sometimes they may not allow you to provide care. At other times, they may try to move the casualty before you have stabilized him or her. A terrified parent may cling to a child and refuse to let you help. When family members act this way, they often feel confused, guilty, and frightened. Be understanding and explain the care you are giving. By remaining calm and professional, you will help calm them.

Hostile crowds are a threat that can develop when you least expect it. As a rule, you cannot reason with a hostile crowd. If you decide the crowd at a scene is hostile, wait at a safe distance until law enforcement and EMS personnel arrive. Approach the scene only when police officers declare it safe and ask you to help. *Never* approach a hostile crowd unless you are trained in crowd management and supported by other trained personnel.

## Suicide

Never enter a suicide scene unless police have made it secure. If the person is obviously dead, be careful not to touch anything at the scene, such as a weapon, medicine bottle, suicide note, or other evidence. If the scene is safe and the person

**Table 2-1   Responding to Specific Emergency Situations**

| Situation | Appropriate behavior |
|---|---|
| Crime | *Do not* enter the scene until summoned by law enforcement personnel. *Do not* touch anything except what you must to give care. |
| Traffic | Leave a path for arriving emergency vehicles. Put up reflectors, flares, or lights to direct dangerous traffic away from the scene. |
| Fire | Never approach a burning vehicle or enter a burning building without proper equipment and training. If in a burning building, *do not* open hot doors or use elevators, and stay close to the floor. |
| Electricity | Assume all downed wires are dangerous. *Do not* attempt to move them. *Do not* touch any metal fence, metal structure, or body of water in contact with a wire. Notify fire department and power company immediately. |
| Water and ice | Follow the rule of reach, throw, and row. Never enter water or go on ice unless you are trained to do so and have proper rescue equipment. |
| Hazardous materials | If you suspect hazardous materials, stay a safe distance away, upwind and uphill. *Do not* create sparks. Notify fire department immediately. |
| Unsafe structures | *Do not* enter structures that you suspect are unsafe. Call for trained and equipped personnel. Gather as much information as possible about the casualty(s). |
| Wreckage | *Do not* attempt a rescue until wreckage has been stabilized. |
| Natural disasters | Report to the person in charge. Follow the rescue plan. Avoid obvious hazards and be cautious when using equipment. |
| Multiple casualties | Report to the person in charge. Care for casualties with the most life-threatening conditions first. |
| Hostile situations | If the casualty or bystanders threaten you, retreat to safety. Never try to restrain, argue with, or force your care on a casualty. Summon law enforcement personnel. |
| Suicide | *Do not* enter until summoned by law enforcement personnel. *Do not* touch anything except what you must to give care. |
| Hostage situations | *Do not* enter until summoned by law enforcement personnel. Gather as much information as possible about the casualties. |

is still alive, give emergency care as needed. Concentrate on your care for the casualty and leave the rest to law enforcement personnel.

Never approach an armed suicidal person unless you are a law enforcement officer trained in crisis intervention. Only approach if you have been summoned to provide care once the scene has been made secure.

If you happen to be on the scene when an unarmed person threatens suicide, try to reassure and calm the person. Make sure that appropriate personnel have been notified. You cannot physically restrain a suicidal person without medical or legal authorization. Listen to him or her, and try to keep the person talking until help arrives. Try to be understanding. Many suicide attempts are an attempt to get help. Do not dare the person to act or trivialize his or her feelings. Unless your personal safety is threatened, *never leave a suicidal person alone.*

## Hostage Situations

If you encounter a hostage situation, your first priority is to not become a hostage yourself. Do not approach the scene unless you are specially trained to handle these situations. Assess the scene from a safe distance and call for law enforcement personnel. A police officer trained in hostage negotiations should take charge.

Try to get any information from bystanders that may help law enforcement personnel. Ask about the number of hostages, any weapons seen, and other possible hazards. Report any information to the first law enforcement official on the scene. Remain at a safe distance until law enforcement personnel summon you.

## ◆ SUMMARY

Emergency scenes by their nature can be dangerous, so never approach a scene until you are sure it is safe. Your personal safety is always your first concern. Potential hazards at emergency scenes include traffic, fire, electricity, water, ice, and unsafe structures. Other dangers include violent or hostile casualties or family members or hostile crowds.

If you have any doubt about the safety of a scene or if you are not trained and equipped to handle the situation, stay back. Be sure appropriate help has been called, and wait for properly trained and equipped personnel.

Once you are sure the scene is safe, you will be expected to provide care to ill or injured casualties. Information on how the human body normally functions, which you will learn in Chapter 3, will help you assess an ill or injured person's condition and provide the appropriate emergency care.

### YOU ARE THE RESPONDER

1. You are the first on the scene of a burning building. Smoke is pouring from the doors and windows. A young girl tells you her brother is still in the building. The fire department is en route, but it will be another five minutes before they arrive. You have no fire protection clothing or equipment and only minimal training. What should you do?

2. While trying to help a pedestrian who has been hit by a car, you are distracted because a noisy crowd has gathered. Should you move the casualty? Why or why not? What should you do?

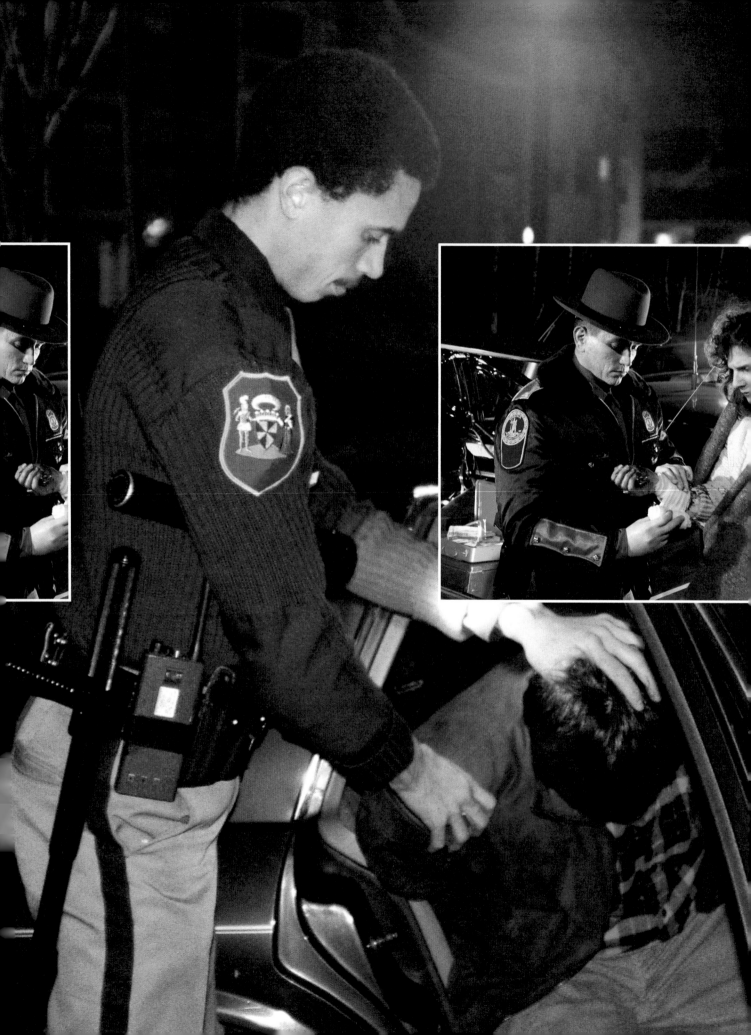

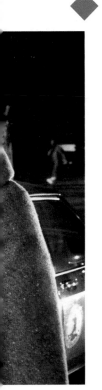

# Part Two

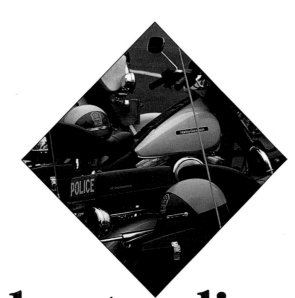

# Understanding the Human Body

# Human Body Systems

## 3

### ◆ Key Terms ◆

**Body system:** A group of organs and other structures working together to carry out specific functions.

**Cells:** The basic units of all living tissue.

**Circulatory (SER ku lah tor e) system:** A group of organs and other structures that carries oxygen-rich blood and other nutrients throughout the body and removes waste.

**Digestive system:** A group of organs and other structures that digests food and eliminates wastes.

**Endocrine (EN do krin) system:** A group of organs and other structures that regulates and coordinates the activities of other systems by producing chemicals that influence the activity of tissues.

**Genitourinary (jen I to U ri ner e) system:** A group of organs and other structures that eliminates waste and enables reproduction.

**Integumentary (in teg u MEN tar e) system:** A group of organs and other structures that

protects the body, retains fluids, and helps to prevent infection.

**Musculoskeletal (mus ku lo SKEL e tal) system:** A group of tissues and other structures that supports the body, protects internal organs, allows movement, stores minerals, manufactures blood cells, and creates heat.

**Nervous system:** A group of organs and other structures that regulates all body functions.

**Organ:** A collection of similar tissues acting together to perform specific body functions.

**Respiratory (re SPI rah to re *or* RES pah rah tor e) system:** A group of organs and other structures that brings air into the body and removes wastes through a process called breathing, or respiration.

**Tissue:** A collection of similar cells acting together to perform specific body functions.

**Vital organs:** Organs whose functions are essential to life, including the brain, heart, and lungs.

# ◆ INTRODUCTION

As a first responder, you need a basic understanding of normal human structure and function. Knowing the body's structures and how they work will help you more easily recognize and understand illnesses and injuries. Body systems do not function independently. Each system depends on other systems to function properly. When your body is healthy, your body systems are working well together. But an injury or illness in one body part or system will often cause problems in others. Knowing the location and function of the major organs and structures within each body system will help you to more accurately assess a casualty's condition and provide the best care.

To remember the location of body structures, it helps to learn to visualize the structures that lie beneath the skin. The structures you can see or feel are reference points for locating the internal structures you cannot see or feel. For example, to locate the pulse on either side of the neck, you can use the Adam's apple on the front of the neck as a reference point. Using reference points will help you describe the location of injuries and other problems you may find. This chapter provides you with an overview of important reference points, terminology, and the functions of eight body systems.

# ◆ ANATOMICAL TERMS

You do not need to be an expert in human body structure and function to provide effective care. Neither should you need a medical dictionary to effectively describe an injury. By knowing a few key structures, their functions, and their location, you can recognize a serious illness or injury and accurately communicate with other emergency care personnel about a casualty's condition.

To learn to use terms that refer to the body, you must first understand the "anatomical position." In this position, the body is standing, arms at the side, palms facing forward (Fig. 3-1, *A*). All medical terms that refer to the body are based on this position. A medical person you are speaking with may not be able to see the casualty's actual position. You will make the situation clearer if you refer to parts of the body as if the body were in the anatomical position. Figure 3-1, *B* and 3-1, *C* shows the basic anatomical terms.

The simplest anatomical terms are based on an imaginary line. It runs down the middle of the body from the head to the ground, dividing the body into two mirror-image right and left halves. This line is called the midline. When you face a casualty, you might tend to refer to that person in terms of what is your right or left. However, in medical terms, right and left *always* refer to the casualty's right and left.

Other terms related to the midline include lateral and medial. Anything away from the midline is called **lateral.** Anything toward the midline is called **medial.** For example, the inner side of the knee is the medial side because it is nearer to the midline. The outer side is the lateral side (Fig. 3-2).

Another reference line can be drawn through the side of the body, dividing it into front and back halves. Anything toward the front of the body is called **anterior;** anything toward the back is called **posterior.**

Other terms that refer to direction can also be useful. When comparing any two structures, such as two body parts, any part toward the casualty's head is described as **superior.** Any part toward the casualty's feet is described as **inferior.** For example, the abdomen is superior to the pelvis but is inferior to the chest. These terms can also be used to describe the location of an injury. For instance, bruising might be described as covering the superior portion of the chest.

Two other terms are generally used when referring to the arms and legs. These terms are proximal and distal. To understand these terms, you must think of the chest, abdomen, and pelvis as those areas that make up the **trunk** of

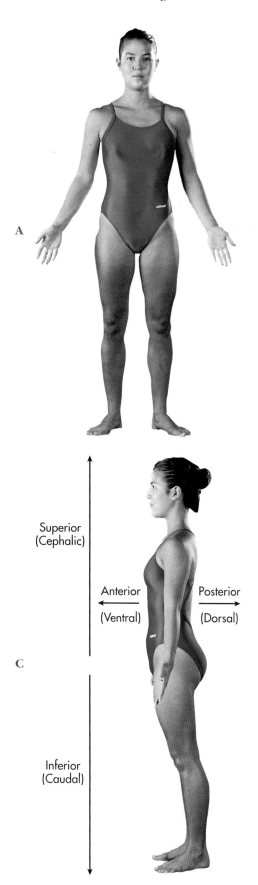

**A**

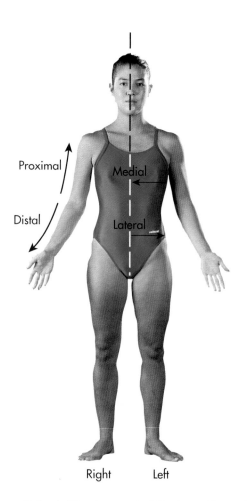

**B**

Proximal

Medial

Distal

Lateral

Right    Left

**Figure 3-1** **A,** The Anatomical Position. **B,** Medical use of the terms *right* and *left* refer to the casualty's right and left. *Medial* refers to anything toward the midline; *lateral* refers to anything away from the midline. *Proximal* and *distal* are usually used to refer to extremities. **C,** *Anterior* refers to the front of the body; *posterior* refers to the back of the body. *Superior* refers to anything toward the head; *inferior* refers to anything toward the feet.

Superior
(Cephalic)

Anterior          Posterior

(Ventral)          (Dorsal)

**C**

Inferior
(Caudal)

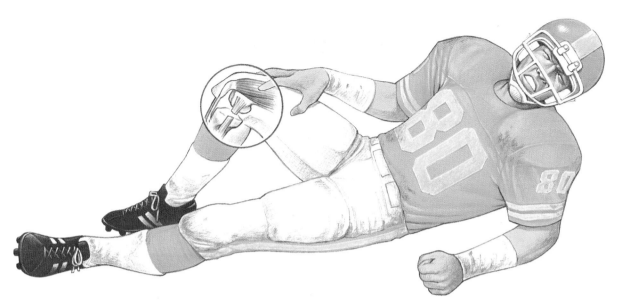

**Figure 3-2**   An Injury to the Medial Side of the Right Knee

the body. The arms and legs are the attachments to the trunk. Points on the body closer to the trunk are described as **proximal.** Points away from the trunk are described as **distal.** For example, the elbow is proximal to the hand because the elbow is closer to the trunk. The hand is distal to the elbow because it is farther from the trunk.

Figure 3-3 shows other basic terms used for body regions and their specific parts. These are all standard terms used by people who provide emergency care. Some terms will be familiar, whereas others may be new to you. Study these terms and learn to use them correctly when describing body parts.

Special anatomical terms are used for the abdomen. The **abdomen** is the part of the trunk below the ribs and above the pelvis. By drawing two imaginary lines, one from the breastbone down through the navel to the lowest point in the pelvis and another line horizontally through the navel, you divide the abdomen into four areas called quadrants. These are the right upper quadrant, the left upper quadrant, the right lower quadrant, and the left lower quadrant. Figure 3-4 shows the abdomen divided into these four quadrants. These terms are important when describing injuries to the

abdomen because different organs may be injured depending on the quadrant involved.

Of all these terms, it is most important to correctly use left and right, lateral and medial, and the basic terms that refer to body parts. Even though you may not use the other terms, you should know what they mean. You may need to understand what other emergency care personnel are saying when they use these terms to refer to injuries.

## ◆ BODY CAVITIES

A **body cavity** is a hollow place in the body that contains organs such as the heart, lungs, and liver. The five major cavities, illustrated in Figure 3-5, are the—

- **Cranial cavity,** located in the head. It contains the brain and is protected by the skull.
- **Spinal cavity,** extending from the bottom of the skull to the lower back. It contains the spinal cord and is protected by the bones of the spine.
- **Thoracic cavity,** also called chest cavity, located in the trunk between the **diaphragm,** a dome-shaped muscle used in breathing, and

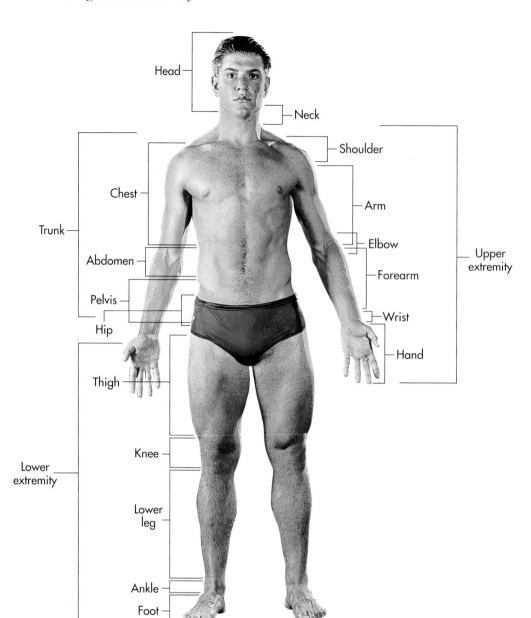

**Figure 3-3** It is important to refer correctly to the parts of the body.

the neck. It contains the heart, the lungs, and other important structures. The thoracic cavity is protected by the rib cage and the upper portion of the spine.

• **Abdominal cavity,** located in the trunk between the diaphragm and the pelvis. It contains many organs, including the liver, pancreas, intestines, stomach, kidneys, and spleen. Because the abdominal cavity is not protected by any bones, the organs in it are vulnerable to injury.

• **Pelvic cavity,** located in the pelvis, is the lowest part of the trunk. It contains the bladder, the rectum, and the reproductive organs. It is protected by the pelvic bones and the lower portion of the spine.

Knowing the general location and relative size of major organs in each cavity will help you assess a casualty's injury or illness. The major organs and their functions are more fully described in the next section of this chapter and in later chapters.

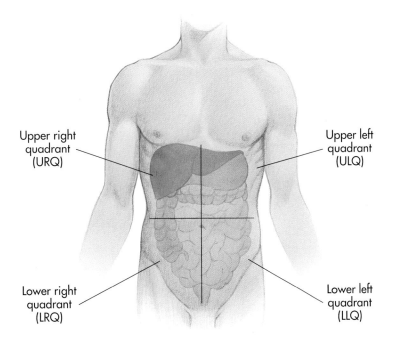

**Figure 3-4** The Abdominal Quadrants

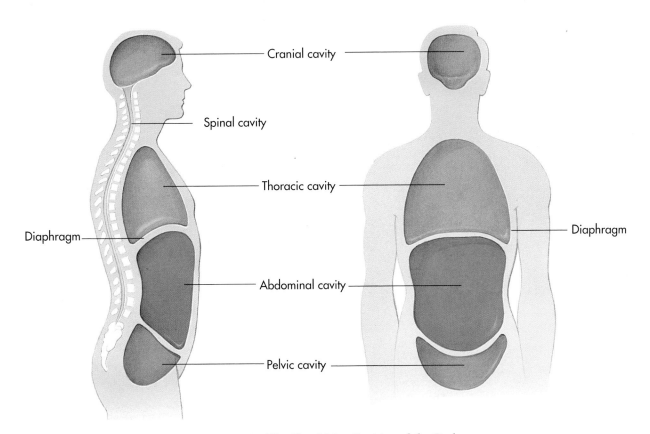

**Figure 3-5** The Five Major Cavities of the Body

## ◆ BODY SYSTEMS

The human body is a miraculous machine. It performs many complex functions, each of which help us live. The body is made up of billions of microscopic *cells,* the basic unit of all living tissue. There are many different types of cells. Each type contributes in a specific way to keep the body functioning normally. Collections of similar cells form *tissues,* which form *organs* (Fig. 3-6). *Vital organs* are organs whose functions are essential for life. They include the brain, heart, and lungs.

A *body system* is a group of organs and other structures that are especially adapted to perform specific body functions. They work together to carry out a function needed for life. For example, the heart, blood, and blood vessels make up the circulatory system. The *circulatory system* keeps all parts of the body supplied with oxygen-rich blood.

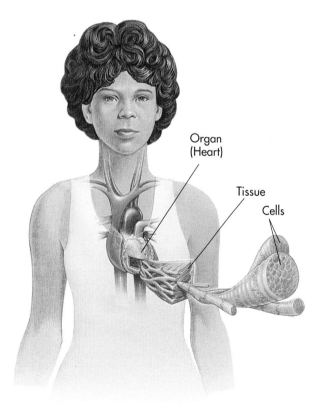

Organ (Heart)

Tissue

Cells

**Figure 3-6** Cells and tissues make up organs.

For the body to work properly, all of the following systems must work well together:

- Respiratory.
- Circulatory.
- Nervous.
- Musculoskeletal.
- Integumentary.
- Endocrine.
- Digestive.
- Genitourinary.

## Respiratory System
### Structure and Function

The body must have a constant supply of oxygen to stay alive. The *respiratory system* supplies the body with oxygen through breathing. When you **inhale**, air fills the lungs, and the **oxygen** in the air is transferred to the blood. The blood carries oxygen to all parts of the body. This same system removes carbon dioxide. Carbon dioxide is transferred from the blood to the lungs. When you **exhale,** air is forced from the lungs, expelling **carbon dioxide** and other waste gases. This breathing process is called **respiration.**

The respiratory system includes the airway and lungs. Figure 3-7 shows the parts of the respiratory system. The **airway,** the passage through which air travels to the lungs, begins at the nose and mouth. The nose and mouth form the upper airway. Air passes through the nose and mouth, through the **pharynx** (the throat), **larynx** (the voice box), and trachea, on its way to the lungs (Fig. 3-8). The **lungs** are a pair of organs in the chest that provide the mechanism for taking in oxygen and removing carbon dioxide during breathing. The **trachea** is also called the windpipe. Behind the trachea is the esophagus. The **esophagus** carries food and liquids from the mouth to the stomach. A small flap of tissue, the **epiglottis,** covers the trachea when you swallow to keep food and liquids out of the lungs.

Air reaches the lungs through two tubes called **bronchi.** The bronchi branch into increasingly smaller tubes (Fig. 3-9, *A*). These eventually end in millions of tiny air sacs called **alveoli** (Fig. 3-9, *B*).

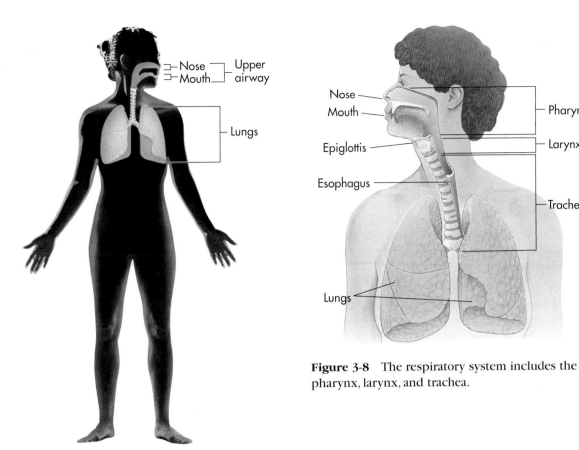

Nose ⟩ Mouth ⟩ Upper airway

Lungs

**Figure 3-7**  The Respiratory System

Nose
Mouth
Epiglottis
Esophagus
Lungs
Pharynx
Larynx
Trachea

**Figure 3-8**  The respiratory system includes the pharynx, larynx, and trachea.

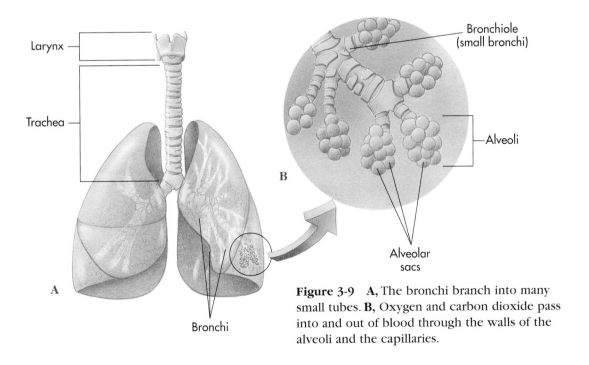

Larynx

Trachea

Bronchi

A

B

Bronchiole (small bronchi)

Alveoli

Alveolar sacs

**Figure 3-9**  **A,** The bronchi branch into many small tubes. **B,** Oxygen and carbon dioxide pass into and out of blood through the walls of the alveoli and the capillaries.

Oxygen and carbon dioxide pass into and out of the blood through the thin cell walls of the alveoli and tiny blood vessels called capillaries.

Air enters the lungs when you inhale and leaves the lungs when you exhale. When you inhale, the chest muscles and the diaphragm contract. This expands the chest and draws air into the lungs. When you exhale, the chest muscles and diaphragm relax, allowing air to exit from the lungs (Fig. 3-10). The average adult breathes about 500 ml (1 pint) of air per breath and breathes about 10 to 20 times per minute. This ongoing breathing process is involuntary and is controlled by the brain.

### Problems That Require Emergency Care

Because of the body's constant need for oxygen, it is important to recognize breathing difficulties and to provide emergency care immediately. Some causes of breathing difficulties include asthma, allergies, and injuries to the chest. Breathing difficulty is referred to as **respiratory distress.**

If a casualty has breathing difficulties, you may hear or see noisy breathing or gasping. The casualty may be conscious or unconscious. The conscious casualty may be anxious or excited or may say that he or she feels short of breath. The casualty's skin, particularly the lips and under the nails, may have a blue tint. This is called cyanosis and occurs when the tissues do not get enough oxygen.

If a person stops breathing, it is called **respiratory arrest.** Respiratory arrest is a life-threatening emergency. Without the oxygen obtained from breathing, other body systems fail to function. For example, if the brain does not receive oxygen, it cannot send messages to the heart to beat. The heart will soon stop.

Respiratory problems require immediate attention. Making sure the airway is open and clear is an important first step. You may have to breathe for a nonbreathing casualty or give abdominal thrusts to someone who is choking. Breathing for the casualty is called **rescue breathing.** These skills are discussed in detail in Chapter 6.

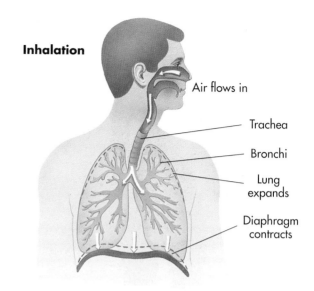

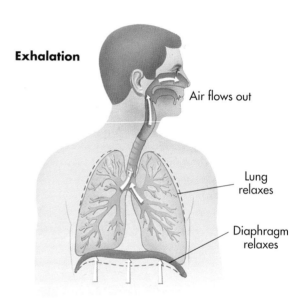

**Figure 3-10**  The chest muscles and the diaphragm contract as you inhale and relax as you exhale.

## Circulatory System

### Structure and Function

The circulatory system works with the respiratory system to carry oxygen to every body cell. It also carries other nutrients throughout the body and removes waste. The circulatory system includes the heart, blood, and blood vessels. Figure 3-11 shows this system.

The **heart** is a muscular organ behind the **sternum,** or breastbone. The heart pumps blood throughout the body through veins and arteries. **Arteries** are large blood vessels that carry oxygen-rich blood from the heart to the rest of the body. The arteries subdivide into smaller blood vessels and ultimately become tiny capillaries. The **capillaries** transport blood to all the cells of the body and nourish them with oxygen.

After the oxygen in the blood is given to the cells, **veins** carry the oxygen-poor blood back to the heart. The heart pumps this oxygen-poor blood to the lungs to pick up more oxygen before pumping it to other parts of the body. This cycle is called the **circulatory cycle.** The cross section of the heart in Figure 3-12 shows how blood moves through the heart to complete the circulatory cycle.

The pumping action of the heart is called a **contraction.** Contractions are controlled by the heart's electrical system, which makes the heart beat regularly. You can feel the heart's contractions in the arteries that are close to the skin, for instance, at the neck or the wrist. The beat you feel with each contraction is called the **pulse.** The heart must beat regularly to deliver oxygen to body cells to keep the body functioning properly.

**Problems That Require Emergency Care**

The following problems threaten the delivery of oxygen to body cells:

- Blood loss caused by severe bleeding (example: a severed artery).
- Impaired circulation (example: a blood clot).
- Failure of the heart to pump adequately (example: a heart attack).

Body tissues that do not receive oxygen die. For example, when an artery supplying the brain with blood is blocked, brain tissue dies. When an artery supplying the heart with blood is blocked, heart muscle tissue dies. This results in a life-threatening emergency, such as a heart attack.

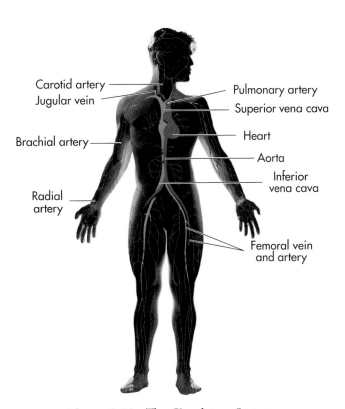

**Figure 3-11** The Circulatory System

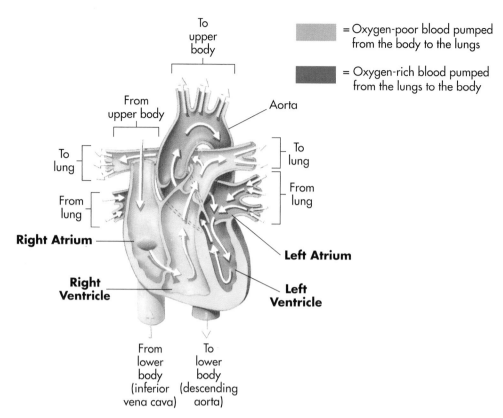

To
upper
body

= Oxygen-poor blood pumped
from the body to the lungs

= Oxygen-rich blood pumped
from the lungs to the body

From
upper body

Aorta

To
lung

To
lung

From
lung

From
lung

**Right Atrium**

**Left Atrium**

**Right
Ventricle**

**Left
Ventricle**

From
lower
body
(inferior
vena cava)

To
lower
body
(descending
aorta)

**Figure 3-12** The heart is a two-sided pump made up of four chambers. A system of one-way valves keeps blood moving in the proper direction to complete the circulatory cycle.

When a person has a heart attack, the heart functions irregularly and may stop. If the heart stops, breathing will also stop. When the heart stops beating, it is called **cardiac arrest.** Casualties of either heart attack or cardiac arrest need emergency care immediately. Cardiac arrest casualties need to have circulation maintained artificially by receiving chest compressions and rescue breathing. This combination of compressions and breaths is called **cardiopulmonary resuscitation,** or **CPR.** You will learn more about the heart and how to perform CPR in Chapter 7.

## Nervous System

### Structure and Function

The *nervous system* is the most complex and delicate of all body systems. The **brain,** the centre of the nervous system, is the master organ of the body. It regulates all body functions, including the respiratory and circulatory systems. The primary functions of the brain can be divided into three categories. These are the sensory functions, the motor functions, and the integrated functions of consciousness, memory, emotions, and use of language.

The brain transmits and receives information through a network of nerves. Figure 3-13 shows the nervous system. The **spinal cord,** a large bundle of nerves, extends from the brain through a canal in the **spine,** or backbone. **Nerves** extend from the brain and spinal cord to every part of the body.

Nerves transmit information as electrical impulses from one area of the body to another. Some nerves conduct impulses from the body to the brain, allowing you to see, hear, smell, taste, and feel. These are the sensory functions. Other nerves conduct impulses from the brain to the muscles to control motor functions, or movement (Fig. 3-14).

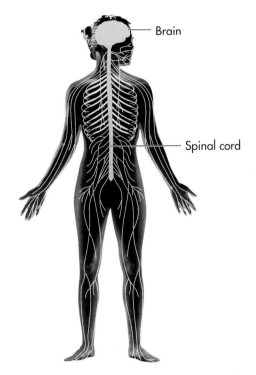

**Figure 3-13**   The Nervous System

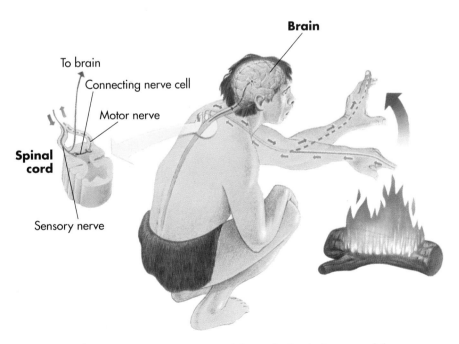

**Figure 3-14**   Messages are sent to and from the brain by way of the nerves.

The integrated functions of the brain are more complex. One of these functions is **consciousness.** Normally, when you are awake, you are conscious. In most cases, being conscious means that you know who you are, where you are, the approximate date and time, and what is happening around you. There are various degrees of consciousness. Your level of consciousness can vary from being highly aware in certain situations to being less aware during periods of relaxation, sleep, illness, or injury.

### Problems That Require Emergency Care
Brain cells, unlike other body cells, cannot regenerate or grow back. Once brain cells die or are damaged, they are not replaced. Brain cells may die from disease or injury. When a particular part of the brain is diseased or injured, a person may lose the body functions controlled by that area of the brain forever. For example, if the part of the brain that regulates breathing is damaged, the person may stop breathing.

Illness or injury may change a person's level of consciousness. Consciousness may be affected by emotions, in which case the casualty may be intensely aware of what is going on. At other times, the casualty's mind may seem to be dull or cloudy. Illness or injury affecting the brain can also alter memory, emotions, and the ability to use language.

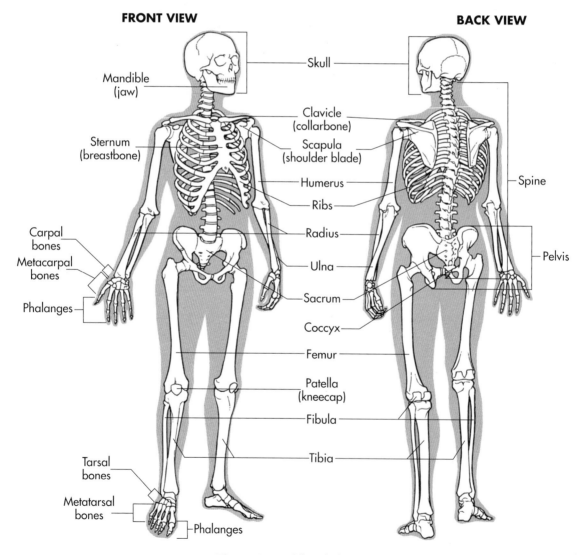

**Figure 3-15** The Skeleton

A head injury can cause a temporary loss of consciousness. Any head injury causing a loss of consciousness can also cause brain injury and must be considered serious. These injuries require evaluation by medical professionals because injury to the brain can cause blood to form pools in the skull. Pooling blood puts pressure on the brain and limits the supply of oxygen to the brain cells.

Injury to the spinal cord or a nerve can result in a permanent loss of feeling and movement below the injury. This condition is called **paralysis.** For example, a lower back injury can result in paralysed legs; a neck injury can result in paralysis of all four limbs. A broken bone or a deep wound can also cause nerve damage, resulting in a loss of sensation or movement. In Chapter 13, you will learn about techniques for caring for head, neck, and back injuries.

## Musculoskeletal System

### Structure and Function

The *musculoskeletal system* consists of the bones, muscles, ligaments, and tendons. This system performs the following functions:

- ♦ Supporting the body.
- ♦ Protecting internal organs.
- ♦ Allowing movement.
- ♦ Storing minerals and producing blood cells.
- ♦ Producing heat.

### Bones and Ligaments

The body has over 200 bones. **Bone** is hard, dense tissue that forms the skeleton. The skeleton forms the framework that supports the body (Fig. 3-15). Where two or more bones join, they form a **joint.** Figure 3-16 shows a typical joint. Bones are usually held together at joints by fibrous bands called **ligaments.** Bones vary in size and shape, allowing them to perform specific functions.

The bones of the skull protect the brain. The spine is made of bones called **vertebrae** that protect the spinal cord. The **ribs** are

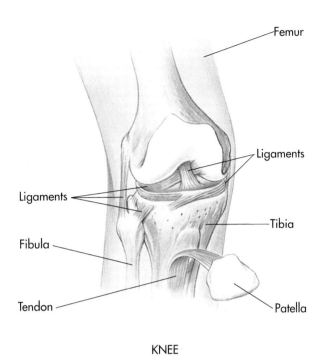

KNEE

**Figure 3-16** A typical joint consists of two or more bones held together by ligaments.

bones that attach to the spine and to the breastbone, forming a protective shell for vital organs, such as the heart and lungs.

In addition to supporting and protecting the body, bones aid movement. The bones of the arms and legs work like a system of levers and pulleys to position the hands and feet so that they can function. Bones of the wrist, hand, and fingers are progressively smaller to allow for fine movements like writing. The small bones of the feet enable you to walk smoothly. Together they work as shock absorbers when you walk, run, or jump. Bones also store minerals and produce certain blood cells.

### Muscles and Tendons

**Muscles** are made of special tissue that can lengthen and shorten, resulting in movement. Figure 3-17 shows the major muscles of the body. **Tendons** are tissues that attach muscles to bones. Muscles band together to form muscle groups. Muscle groups work together

**FRONT VIEW**          **BACK VIEW**

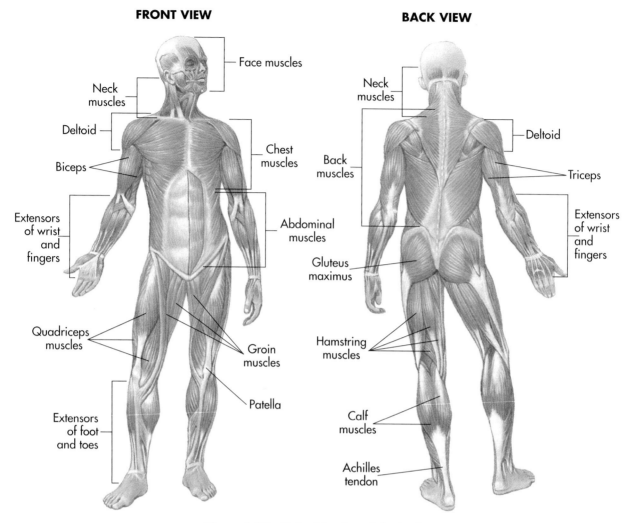

**Figure 3-17**   Major Muscles of the Body

to produce movement (Fig. 3-18). Working muscles also produce heat. Muscles also protect underlying structures, such as bones, nerves, and blood vessels.

Muscle action is controlled by the nervous system. Nerves carry information from the muscles to the brain. The brain takes in this information and directs the muscles through the nerves (Fig. 3-19).

Muscle actions can be voluntary or involuntary. Involuntary muscles, such as the heart and diaphragm, are automatically controlled by the brain. You don't have to think about them to make them work. Voluntary muscles, such as leg and arm muscles, are most often under your conscious control. You are aware of telling them to move.

## Problems That Require Emergency Care

Injuries to bones and muscles include fractures, dislocations, strains, and sprains. A fracture is a broken bone. Dislocations occur when bones of a joint are moved out of place. Strains are injuries to muscles and tendons; sprains are injuries to ligaments. Although injuries to bones and muscles may not look serious, nearby nerves, blood vessels, and other organs may be damaged. Regardless of how they appear, these

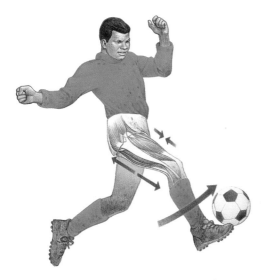

**Figure 3-18** Muscle groups work together to produce movement.

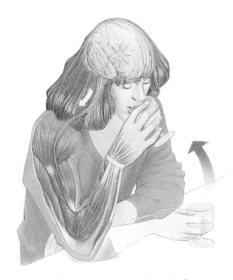

**Figure 3-19** The brain controls muscle movement.

injuries may cause lifelong disabilities or become life-threatening emergencies. For example, torn ligaments in the knee can limit activity, and broken ribs can puncture the lungs and threaten breathing.

When you give emergency care, remember that injuries to muscles and bones often result in additional injuries. You will learn more about musculoskeletal injuries and how to care for them in later chapters.

## Integumentary System

### Structure and Function

The ***integumentary system*** consists of the skin, hair, and nails (Fig. 3-20). Most important among these is the skin because it protects the body. The skin helps keep fluids in. It prevents infection by keeping out disease-producing **microorganisms,** or germs. The **skin** is made of tough, elastic fibres that stretch without easily tearing, protecting it from injury. The skin also helps make vitamin D and stores minerals.

The outer surface of the skin consists of dead cells that are continually rubbed away and replaced by new cells. The skin contains the hair roots, oil glands, and sweat glands. Oil

glands help to keep the skin soft, supple, and waterproof. Sweat glands and pores help regulate body temperature by releasing sweat. The nervous system monitors blood temperature and causes you to sweat if blood temperature rises even slightly. Although you may not see or feel it, sweat is released to the skin's surface.

Blood supplies the skin with nutrients and helps provide its colour. When blood vessels dilate (become wider), the blood circulates close to the skin's surface. This makes some people's skin appear flushed or red and makes the skin feel warm. The reddening may not appear with darker skin. When blood vessels constrict (become narrower), not as much blood is close to the skin's surface, causing the skin to look pale and feel cool.

Nerves in the skin make it very sensitive to sensations such as touch, pain, and temperature. Therefore, the skin is also an important part of the body's communication network.

### Problems That Require Emergency Care

Although the skin is tough, it can be injured. Sharp objects may puncture, cut, or tear the skin. Rough objects can scrape it, and extreme heat or cold may burn or freeze it. Burns and

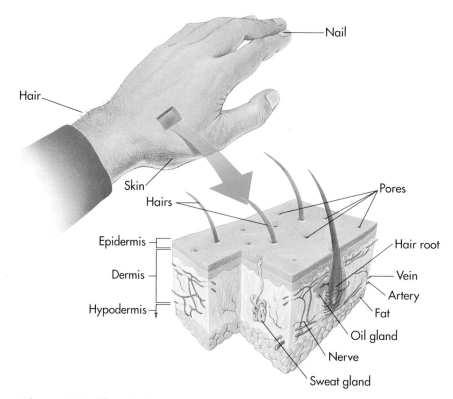

**Figure 3-20**  The skin, hair, and nails make up the integumentary system.

skin injuries that cause bleeding may result in the loss of vital fluids. Germs may enter the body through breaks in the skin, causing potentially serious infection. In later chapters, you will learn how to care for skin injuries such as burns and cuts.

## Endocrine System

### Structure and Function

The ***endocrine system*** is one of the two regulatory systems in the body. Together with the nervous system, it coordinates the activities of other systems. The endocrine system consists of several glands (Fig. 3-21). **Glands** are organs that release fluid and other substances into the blood or onto the skin. Some produce **hormones,** chemical messengers that enter the bloodstream and influence tissue activity in various parts of the body. For example, the thyroid gland makes a hormone that controls **metabolism,** the process by which all cells convert nutrients to energy. Other glands include the sweat and oil glands in the skin.

### Problems That Require Emergency Care

A first responder does not need to know all the glands in the endocrine system or the hormones they produce. Problems in the endocrine system usually develop slowly and are seldom emergencies. Knowing how hormones work in general, however, helps you understand how some illnesses seem to develop suddenly.

For example, an emergency occurs when there is too much or too little of a hormone called insulin in the blood. Without insulin, cells cannot absorb the sugar they need from food. Too much insulin forces blood sugar rapidly into the cells, lowering blood sugar levels and depriving the brain of the blood sugar it needs to function normally. Blood sugar levels that rise or fall can make a person ill, sometimes severely so. You will learn more about this kind of emergency in Chapter 16.

**Table 3-1**    Body Systems

| Systems | Major structures | Primary functions | How the system works with other body systems |
|---|---|---|---|
| Respiratory system | Airway and lungs | Supplies the body with oxygen through breathing | Works with the circulatory system to provide oxygen to cells; is under the control of the nervous system |
| Circulatory system | Heart, blood, and blood vessel | Transports nutrients and oxygen to body cells and removes waste products | Works with the respiratory system to provide oxygen to cells; works in conjunction with the urinary and digestive systems to remove waste products; helps give skin color; is under the control of the nervous system |
| Nervous system | Brain, spinal cord, and nerves | One of two primary regulatory systems in the body; transmits messages to and from the brain | Regulates all body systems through a network of nerves |
| Musculoskeletal system | Bones, ligaments, muscles, and tendons | Provides body's framework; protects internal organs and other underlying structures; allows movement; produces heat; manufactures blood components | Provides protection to organs and structures of other body systems; muscle action is controlled by the nervous system |
| Integumentary system | Skin, hair, and nails | An important part of the body's communication network; helps prevent infection and dehydration; assists with temperature regulation; aids in production of certain vitamins | Helps to protect the body from disease-producing organisms; together with the circulatory system, helps to regulate body temperature under control of the nervous system; communicates sensation to the brain by way of the nerves |
| Endocrine system | Glands | Secretes hormones and other substances into blood and onto skin | Together with the nervous system, coordinates the activities of other systems |
| Digestive system | Mouth, esophagus, stomach, intestines | Breaks down food into a usable form to supply the rest of the body with energy | Works with the circulatory system to transport nutrients to the body |
| Genitourinary system | Uterus and genitalia | Performs the processes of reproduction | |
| | Kidneys, bladder | Removes wastes from the circulatory system and regulates water balance | |

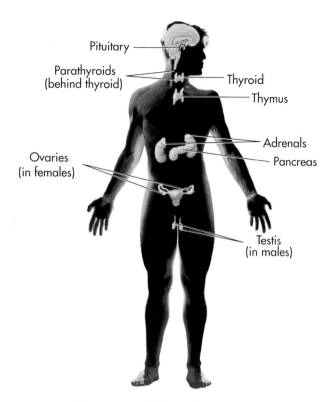

**Figure 3-21** The Endocrine System

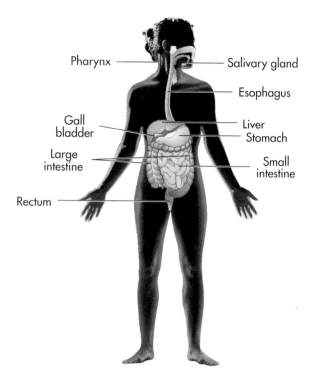

**Figure 3-22** The Digestive System

## Digestive System

### Structure and Function

The *digestive system,* also called the gastrointestinal system, consists of organs that work together to break down food and eliminate waste. Figure 3-22 shows the major organs of the digestive system. Food entering the system is broken down into a form the body can use. As food passes through the system, the body absorbs nutrients that can be converted to use by the cells. The unabsorbed portion continues through the system and is eliminated as waste.

### Problems That Require Emergency Care

Since most digestive system organs are in the unprotected abdominal cavity, they are very vulnerable to injury. Such an injury can occur, for example, if a body strikes a car's steering wheel in a vehicle collision. These organs can also be damaged by a penetrating injury, such as a stab or gunshot wound. Damaged organs may bleed internally, causing severe loss of blood, or spill waste products into the abdominal cavity. This can result in severe infection. Chapter 14 discusses in more detail how to recognize and care for abdominal injuries.

## Genitourinary System

### Structure and Function

The *genitourinary system* is made up of two organ systems: the urinary system and the reproductive system. The **urinary system** consists of organs that eliminate waste products filtered from the blood (Fig. 3-23). The primary organs are the kidneys and the bladder. The **kidneys** are located behind the abdominal cavity just beneath the chest, one on each side. They filter wastes from the circulating blood to form urine. Urine is then stored in the **bladder,** a small muscular sac. The bladder stretches as it fills and then shrinks back when the urine is released.

The male and female **reproductive systems** include the organs for sexual reproduction

# How Does a Person Catch a Frisbee?

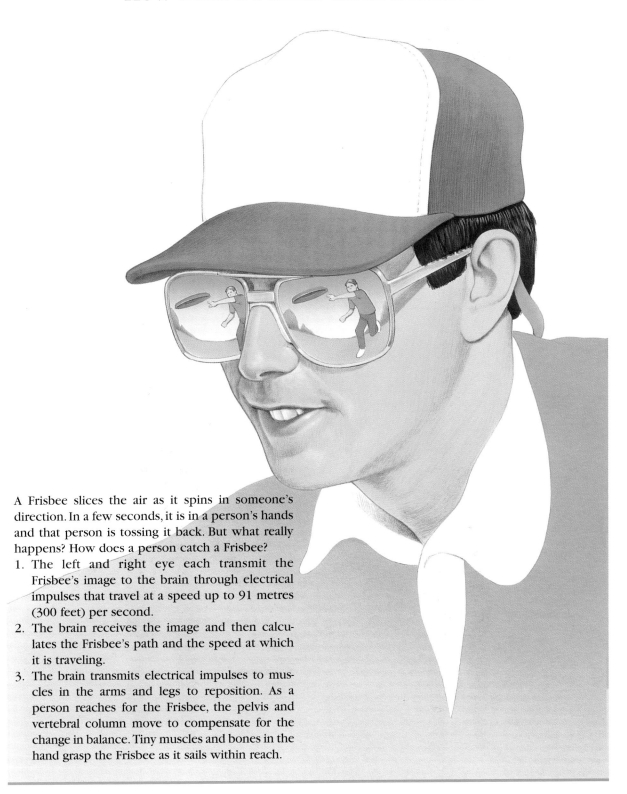

A Frisbee slices the air as it spins in someone's direction. In a few seconds, it is in a person's hands and that person is tossing it back. But what really happens? How does a person catch a Frisbee?

1. The left and right eye each transmit the Frisbee's image to the brain through electrical impulses that travel at a speed up to 91 metres (300 feet) per second.

2. The brain receives the image and then calculates the Frisbee's path and the speed at which it is traveling.

3. The brain transmits electrical impulses to muscles in the arms and legs to reposition. As a person reaches for the Frisbee, the pelvis and vertebral column move to compensate for the change in balance. Tiny muscles and bones in the hand grasp the Frisbee as it sails within reach.

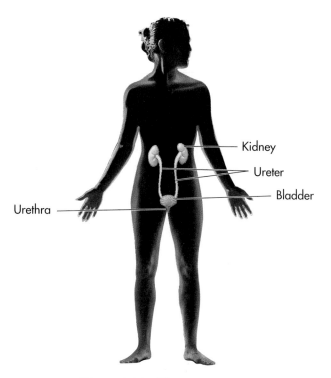

**Figure 3-23** The Urinary System

(Fig. 3-24). Because these organs are close to the urinary system, injuries to the abdominal or pelvic area can injure organs in either system.

The female reproductive organs are smaller than many major organs and are protected by the pelvic bones. The soft tissue external structures are more susceptible to injury, although such injury is uncommon. The male reproductive organs are located outside of the pelvis and are more vulnerable to injury.

## Problems That Require Emergency Care

The frequency of injuries to the organs of the urinary system depends on their vulnerability. Unlike the abdominal organs, the kidneys are partially protected by the lower ribs, making them less vulnerable to injury. But the kidneys may be damaged by a significant blow to the back just below the rib cage or a penetrating wound, such as a stab or gunshot

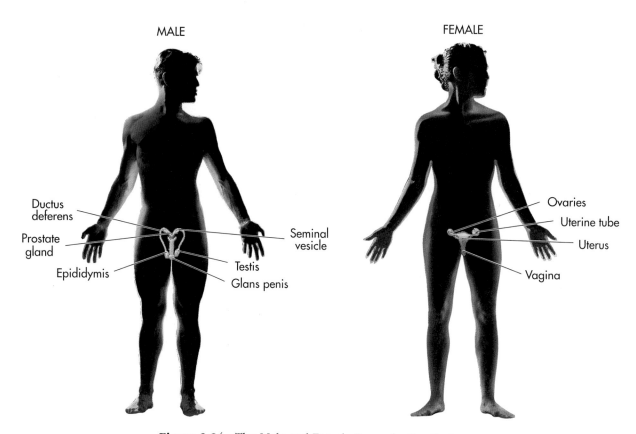

**Figure 3-24** The Male and Female Reproductive Systems

# Did You Know?

A baby is born with 350 bones. Why do adults have fewer bones?

Some bones that are separate at birth fuse together as a person grows. The skull is an excellent example.

We use 17 of our 30 facial muscles when we smile.

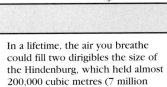

The brain receives about one eighth of the blood the heart pumps each minute. Whereas other body parts receive differing amounts of blood depending on the activity, the brain's portion remains the same.

In a lifetime, the air you breathe could fill two dirigibles the size of the Hindenburg, which held almost 200,000 cubic metres (7 million cubic feet) of gas.

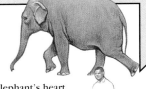

An elephant's heart beats 25 times a minute and weighs 15 kilograms (40 pounds). A man's heart beats about 70 times a minute and weighs about 1/3 kilogram (1 pound). A mouse's heart beats about 700 times a minute and weighs approximately 1/2 gram (.0175 ounces).

In a month, blood will have taken its fantastic journey around the body 43,000 times.

Blood vessels form a branching network of more than almost 100,000 km (60,000 miles), almost 3 times the distance around the earth.

The stomach contains a corrosive acid called hydrochloric acid, which can eat a hole through a carpet. Why doesn't it eat a hole through your stomach? Certain cells that line the stomach produce a substance that neutralizes the acid.

The intestines are 8.5 metres (28 feet) long, the height of a two-story building. Food moves through the intestines at a rate of 2.5 cm (1 inch) per minute.

A nerve impulse can travel 110 metres (360 feet) per second, fast enough to cover the length of a football field in less than a second.

The skin weighs about 2.6 kilograms (7 pounds). If spread out flat, it would cover about 1.9 square metres (20 square feet).

wound. Anyone with an injury to the back below the rib cage may have injured one or both kidneys. Because of the kidney's rich blood supply, such an injury often causes severe bleeding.

The bladder is injured less frequently than the kidneys, but injuries to the abdomen can rupture the bladder, particularly when it is full. Bone fragments from a fracture of the pelvis can also pierce or rupture the bladder.

Injuries to urinary system organs may not be obvious but should be suspected if there are significant injuries to the back just below the rib cage or to the abdomen. Chapter 14 discusses signs and symptoms to watch for and how to provide care.

The external reproductive organs called **genitalia** have a rich supply of blood and nerves. Injuries to these organs may cause heavy bleeding but are rarely life threatening. Injuries to the genitalia are usually caused by a blow to the pelvic area but may be the result of sexual assault or rape. Although such injuries are rarely life threatening, they almost always cause the casualty extreme distress. Such a casualty may refuse care.

## ◆ INTERRELATIONSHIPS OF BODY SYSTEMS

Each body system plays a vital role in survival. Body systems work together to help the body maintain a constant healthy state. When the environment changes, body systems adapt to the new conditions. For example, because your musculoskeletal system works harder when you exercise, your respiratory and circulatory systems must also work harder to meet your body's increased oxygen demands. Your body systems also react to the stresses caused by illness or injury.

Body systems do not work independently of each other. The impact of an injury or a disease is rarely restricted to one body system. For example, a broken bone may result in nerve damage that will impair movement and feeling. Injuries to the ribs can make breathing difficult. If the heart stops beating for any reason, breathing will also stop.

In any significant illness or injury, body systems may be seriously affected. This may result in a progressive failure of body systems called shock. Shock results from the inability of the circulatory system to provide adequate oxygen to all parts of the body, especially the vital organs.

Generally, the more body systems involved in an emergency, the more serious the emergency. Body systems depend on each other for survival. In serious injury or illness, the body may not be able to keep functioning. In these cases, regardless of your best efforts, the casualty may die.

## ◆ SUMMARY

The body includes a number of systems, all of which must work together for the body to function properly. The brain, the center of the nervous system, controls all body functions including those of the other body systems. Knowing a few key structures, their functions, and their locations helps you to understand more about these body systems. Knowing certain anatomical terms helps you to communicate with more advanced medical personnel about any injury or illness you may encounter.

Illness or injury that affects one body system can have a serious impact on other systems. Fortunately, basic care is usually all you need to give to support injured body systems until more advanced care is available. By learning the basic principles of care described in later chapters, you may be able to make the difference between life and death.

### YOU ARE THE RESPONDER

1. *You see a car that has struck a tree. You stop and find the driver not wearing a seat belt and slumped in the front seat. The steering wheel is bent and the windshield is cracked. You see no signs of blood or other obvious injury. The person is breathing fast and does not respond when you speak to her. Which body systems may have been affected by the crash?*
2. *Now that you have identified which body systems could have been affected, what emergency care do you think she might need?*

# Preventing Disease Transmission

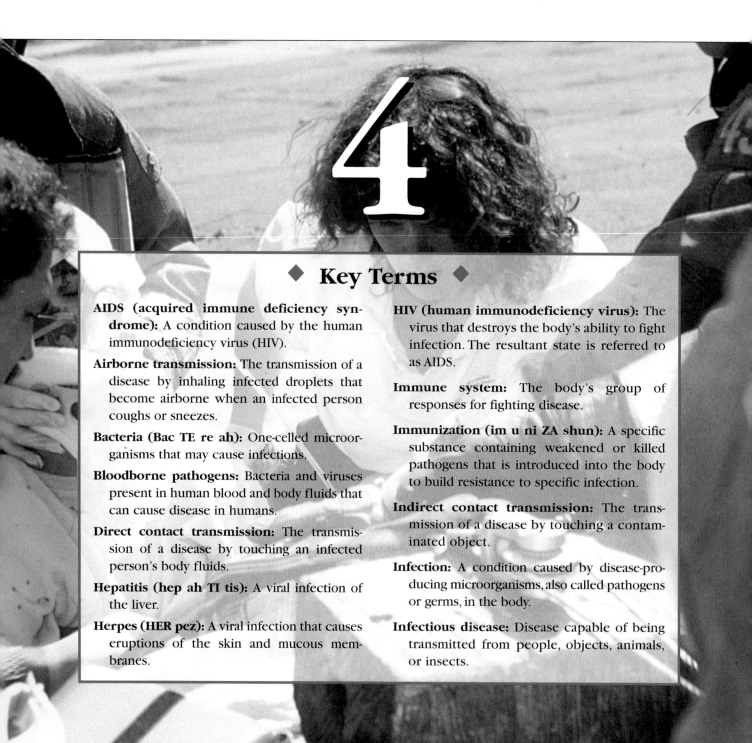

**4**

## ◆ Key Terms ◆

**AIDS (acquired immune deficiency syndrome):** A condition caused by the human immunodeficiency virus (HIV).

**Airborne transmission:** The transmission of a disease by inhaling infected droplets that become airborne when an infected person coughs or sneezes.

**Bacteria (Bac TE re ah):** One-celled microorganisms that may cause infections.

**Bloodborne pathogens:** Bacteria and viruses present in human blood and body fluids that can cause disease in humans.

**Direct contact transmission:** The transmission of a disease by touching an infected person's body fluids.

**Hepatitis (hep ah TI tis):** A viral infection of the liver.

**Herpes (HER pez):** A viral infection that causes eruptions of the skin and mucous membranes.

**HIV (human immunodeficiency virus):** The virus that destroys the body's ability to fight infection. The resultant state is referred to as AIDS.

**Immune system:** The body's group of responses for fighting disease.

**Immunization (im u ni ZA shun):** A specific substance containing weakened or killed pathogens that is introduced into the body to build resistance to specific infection.

**Indirect contact transmission:** The transmission of a disease by touching a contaminated object.

**Infection:** A condition caused by disease-producing microorganisms, also called pathogens or germs, in the body.

**Infectious disease:** Disease capable of being transmitted from people, objects, animals, or insects.

---

## ◆ Key Terms ◆

**Meningitis (men in JI tis):** An inflammation of the brain or spinal cord caused by a viral or bacterial infection.

**Pathogen (PATH o jen):** A disease-causing agent; also called microorganism or germ.

**Tuberculosis (tu ber ku LO sis) (TB):** A respiratory disease caused by a bacterium.

**Vector transmission:** The transmission of a disease by an animal or insect bite through exposure to blood or other body fluids.

**Virus (VI rus):** A disease-causing agent, or pathogen, that requires another organism to live and reproduce.

---

## ◆ For Review ◆

Before reading this chapter, you should have a basic understanding of how the human body systems function (Chapter 3).

## ◆ INTRODUCTION

*A man has collapsed in his office. As the first trained person on the scene, you find the man bleeding from the mouth and face. Vomit and blood are around him. "His face hit the desk when he fell," a bystander says. He is not breathing. How would you respond? Do you have any concerns about contracting disease?*

Someday, you may be in a similar situation in which you are concerned about disease transmission. You may also have concerns about disease transmission that may result from the everyday tasks required of your job or other activities. You need to understand how infections occur, how they are passed from one person to another, and what you can do to protect yourself and others.

Diseases that can be contracted from people, objects, animals, or insects are often called *infectious diseases*. Some diseases can be transmitted more easily than others. During this training, you will learn how to recognize situations that have the potential for **disease transmission** and how to protect yourself and others from contracting disease.

## ◆ HOW INFECTIONS OCCUR

### Disease-Causing Agents

The disease process begins when a *pathogen* (germ) gets into the body. When pathogens enter the body, they can sometimes overpower the body's defence systems and cause illness. This illness is an *infection.* Most infectious diseases are caused by one of the six types of pathogens identified in Table 4-1. The most common pathogens are bacteria and viruses.

*Bacteria* are everywhere (Fig. 4-1). They do not depend on other organisms for life and can live outside the human body. Most bacteria do not infect humans. Those that do may cause serious illness. Meningitis, scarlet fever, and tetanus are examples of disease caused by bacteria. The body has difficulty fighting infections

| Pathogen | Disease they cause |
|----------|-------------------|
| Viruses | Hepatitis, measles, mumps, chicken pox, meningitis, rubella, influenza, warts, colds, herpes, shingles, HIV infection including AIDS, genital warts |
| Bacteria | Tetanus, meningitis, scarlet fever, strep throat, tuberculosis, gonorrhea, syphilis, chlamydia, toxic shock syndrome, Legionnaires' disease, diphtheria, food poisoning |
| Fungi | Athlete's foot and ringworm |
| Protozoa | Malaria and dysentery |
| Rickettsia | Typhus, Rocky Mountain spotted fever |
| Parasitic worms | Abdominal pain, anemia, lymphatic vessel blockage, lowered antibody response, respiratory and circulatory complications |

**Table 4-1**    Disease-Causing Agents

caused by bacteria. Doctors may prescribe medications called **antibiotics** that either kill the bacteria or weaken them enough for the body to get rid of them. Commonly used antibiotics include penicillin, erythromycin, and tetracycline.

Unlike bacteria, *viruses* depend on other organisms to live and reproduce (Fig. 4-2). Viruses cause many diseases, including the common cold. Once they become established within the body, they are difficult to eliminate because very few medications are effective. Antibiotics do not kill or weaken viruses. The body's immune system is the main defence against them.

## The Body's Natural Defences

The body's *immune system* is very good at fighting disease. Its basic tools are the white blood cells. Special white blood cells travel around the body and identify invading pathogens. Once they detect a pathogen, these white blood cells gather around it and release **antibodies** that fight infections.

These antibodies attack the pathogen and weaken or destroy it. Antibodies can usually get rid of pathogens, however, some pathogens can thrive and under ideal conditions overwhelm the immune system. To minimize this possibility,

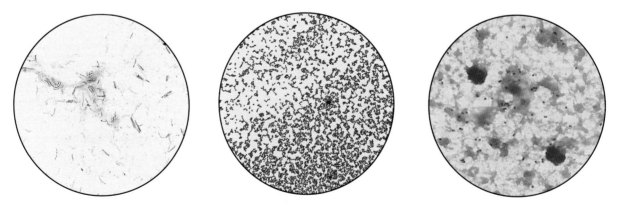

**Figure 4-1**    Common types of bacteria that cause disease. Most bacteria do not infect humans. Those that do may cause serious illness.

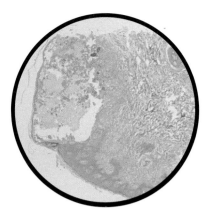

**Figure 4-2** Viruses cause many diseases, such as herpes and the common cold.

the body depends on the skin for protection to keep pathogens out.

This combination of trying to keep pathogens out of the body and destroying them once they get inside is necessary for good health. Sometimes, the body cannot fight off infection. When this occurs, an invading pathogen can become established in the body, causing serious infection. Fever and exhaustion often signal that the body is fighting an infection. Other common signals include headache, nausea, and vomiting.

## How Diseases Spread

For a disease to be transmitted, all four of the following conditions must be met:

◆ A pathogen is present.
◆ There is enough of the pathogen to cause disease.
◆ A person is susceptible to the pathogen.
◆ The pathogen passes through the correct entry site.

You need to understand these four conditions to understand how infections occur. Think of these conditions as the pieces of a puzzle. All the pieces have to be in place for the picture to be complete (Fig. 4-3). If any one of these conditions is missing, an infection cannot occur.

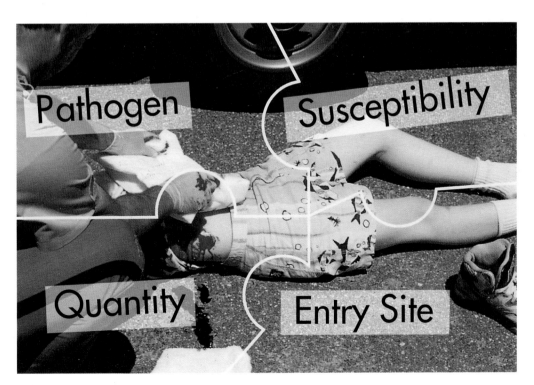

**Figure 4-3** For an infection to occur, all four conditions must be present.

Pathogens enter the body in the following four ways (Fig. 4-4):

◆ Direct contact.
◆ Indirect contact.
◆ Airborne.
◆ Vector-borne.

Not all pathogens can enter the body in all of these ways. For example, certain infections are vector-borne only.

***Direct contact transmission*** (Fig. 4-4, *A*) occurs when a person touches body fluids from an infected person. ***Indirect contact transmission*** (Fig. 4-4, *B*) occurs when a person touches objects that have touched the blood or another body fluid, such as saliva and vomit, of an infected person. These include soiled dressings, equip- ment, and work surfaces with which an infected person comes in contact. Sharp objects present a particular risk. If sharp objects have contacted the blood or body fluids of an infected person and are handled carelessly, they can pierce the skin and transmit infection. ***Airborne transmission*** (Fig. 4-4, *C*) occurs when a person breathes in droplets that become airborne when an infected person coughs or sneezes. Exposure to these droplets is generally too brief for transmission to take place. If a person is coughing heavily, however, avoid face-to-face contact, if possible.

***Vector-borne transmission*** (Fig. 4-4, *D*) occurs when an animal, such as a dog or rac- coon, or an insect, such as a tick, transmits a pathogen into the body through a bite. A bite from an infected human is also a vector-borne

A

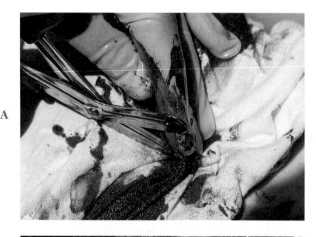

B

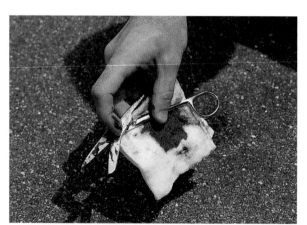

C

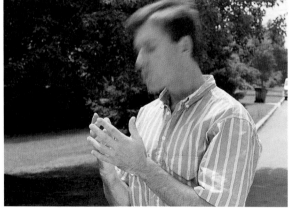

D

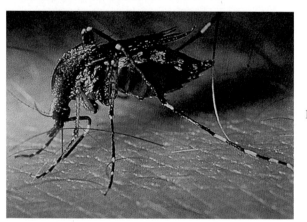

**Figure 4-4**  Ways Pathogens Enter the Body: **A,** Contact—Touching body fluids from an infected person, **B,** Indirect Contact—Touching objects that have touched the blood or another body fluid of an infected person, **C,** Airborne—Breathing in droplets that became airborne when an infected person coughs or sneezes, **D,** Vector-borne—Through a bite from an infected animal or insect.

transmission. The carrier is a vector and passes the infection to another animal or person. Rabies and Lyme disease are transmitted this way.

## ◆ DISEASES THAT CAUSE CONCERN

Some diseases, such as the common cold, are passed from one person to another more easily than others. Although it causes discomfort, the common cold is short-lived and rarely causes serious problems. Other diseases cause more severe problems. Hepatitis B virus, a liver infection, can last many months. The patient is often seriously ill and slow to recover. Another infection, caused by HIV, destroys the body's ability to fight infection. Both infections can cause prolonged illness or death.

You should be familiar with diseases that can have serious consequences if transmitted. These include herpes, meningitis, tuberculosis, hepatitis, and HIV infection, which almost always leads to AIDS (Table 4-2).

## Herpes

There are several viruses that can cause ***herpes*** infections. These viruses cause infections of the skin and mucous membranes. They are very easily passed by direct contact. The herpes virus stays inactive until stimulated. The early stages of herpes may cause headache, sore throat, swelling of the lymph glands, and a general ill feeling. Sometimes swelling occurs around the lips and mouth where small sores like blisters may form (Fig. 4-5). These are commonly called cold sores.

In a more serious form of herpes, sores appear on the face, neck, and shoulders. Another form of herpes causes sores in the genital area. Since antibiotics do not work against viruses, the infection runs its course and becomes inactive for a while. Then it flares up again. Herpes is usually transmitted through direct contact with sores. It enters through an opening in the skin or through mucous membranes, such as in the mouth or eyes. You should avoid unprotected contact with people who have active herpes.

**Table 4-2   How Diseases Are Transmitted**

| Disease | Signs and symptoms | Mode of transmission | Infective material |
|---------|--------------------|----------------------|--------------------|
| Herpes | Lesions, general ill feeling, sore throat | Direct contact | Broken skin, mucous membranes |
| Meningitis | Respiratory illness, sore throat, nausea, vomiting | Airborne, direct and indirect contact | Food and water, mucus |
| Tuberculosis | Weight loss, night sweats, occasional fever, general ill feeling | Airborne, direct and indirect contact | Mucus, broken skin |
| Hepatitis | Flulike, jaundice | Direct and indirect contact | Blood, saliva, semen, feces, food, water, other products |
| HIV/AIDS | Fever, night sweats, weight loss, chronic diarrhea, severe fatigue, shortness of breath, swollen lymph nodes, lesions | Direct and indirect contact | Blood, semen, vaginal fluid |

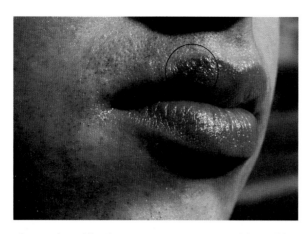

**Figure 4-5** The herpes virus may cause blister-like sores to erupt on or around the lips and mouth.

## Meningitis

*Meningitis* is a severe infection of the covering of the brain and spinal cord. It can be caused by either viruses or bacteria. It is easily transmitted by direct, indirect, and airborne means. You can get the viral form of meningitis from contaminated food and water. Bacterial meningitis can be transmitted through the mucus in the nose and mouth. The germs might be passed if an infected person coughs near your face or if you come in direct contact with the person's mucus. You could get bacterial meningitis from unprotected rescue breathing.

Although meningitis is more common in infants and young children, adults are not immune. The first signals are often respiratory infections, sore throat, stiff neck, rash, nausea, and vomiting. An infected casualty may quickly become seriously ill. In its advanced stages, a casualty may become unconscious. Meningitis, if treated early, is rarely fatal.

## Tuberculosis

*Tuberculosis* most often affects the respiratory system. The bacteria that cause this disease live in the lungs. Infection occurs mainly from inhaling droplets that contain the bacteria. The disease causes weight loss, night sweats, occasional fever, and fatigue. The signals often develop gradually, so people may not notice the early stages. People who do not know they have tuberculosis may even remain in fairly good health for a long time before they rapidly become ill. If the casualty is not coughing and you have no contact with material coughed up by the casualty, you are unlikely to be infected.

## Hepatitis

*Hepatitis* is an inflammation of the liver. The most common forms of hepatitis are caused by alcohol abuse, drugs, or other chemicals and cannot be transmitted. Viruses, however, can also cause hepatitis. The two most common types of viral hepatitis are type A and type B.

**Hepatitis A** is also called infectious hepatitis. It is common in children. It is often transmitted by contact with food or other products soiled by the stool of an infected person. Parents may get the disease from their children by changing diapers. Shellfish and water containing the virus also can transmit hepatitis A. At first, people with hepatitis A feel as if they have the flu. Later, their skin may become a yellowish colour, a condition called jaundice. Hepatitis A usually does not have serious consequences.

**Hepatitis B** is a severe liver infection caused by the hepatitis B virus. Hepatitis B is transmitted by sexual contact and blood-to-blood contact from transfusions, needle sticks, cuts, scrapes, sores, and skin irritations. Hepatitis B has also been found in other body fluids, such as saliva. Hepatitis B is not transmitted by casual contact, such as shaking hands, nor is it transmitted by indirect contact with objects like drinking fountains or telephones. Your risk most often occurs in unprotected direct or indirect contact with infected blood.

The signals of hepatitis B are similar to the flu-like signals of hepatitis A. Hepatitis B infections can be fatal. The disease may be in the body for up to 6 months before signals appear. The person may then not associate the flu-like signals with exposure to hepatitis. Some people can even develop chronic hepatitis after recovering from the early signals.

# HIV and AIDS

Walter is a businessman in a small town in northern California. He has been a respected member of the community for many years, does volunteer work whenever possible, and is a member of the local Rotary Club. A few years ago, Walter had bypass surgery after a heart attack and was transfused with several pints of blood. As a result of those transfusions, Walter became infected with HIV, the virus that causes AIDS.

Walter is like most of us, has similar dreams, hopes, and fears. He may be a personal friend of yours. Seeing him on the street, you would not guess that he has tested positive for HIV. He will most likely develop AIDS someday and most likely he will die as a result.

Walter is fortunate that he has a supportive network of family and friends. Not everyone is this fortunate. Many suffer because of the irrational fears and rejections of family and friends based on incorrect perceptions.

Human tendency is to protect ourselves against any risks we perceive, correctly or incorrectly. Correct perceptions about HIV and AIDS develop as a result of learning the facts about how HIV is transmitted. Incorrect perceptions involve jumping to conclusions without knowing the facts.

Many people tend to associate the risk of HIV infection with specific groups such as drug users, homosexuals, and members of certain ethnic groups. It is not who a person *is* that puts him or her at risk for HIV infection, but rather what that person *does*. Engaging in unsafe sexual practices or using contaminated intravenous needles are examples of risky behavior that increases the chances of HIV infection.

You will rarely know the details of a person's lifestyle and history when you are giving care in an emergency. Value judgments and jumping to conclusions about someone's behavior play no part in what is required of you. Compassion, understanding, and effective care do. The person you are least likely to suspect may be infected; the one who appears to you to be a more obvious risk may not be. The only physical danger to you occurs when you feel so secure in a situation that you neglect to take the safety precautions that prevent disease transmission. The danger to you as a person exists when you allow preconceptions and prejudices to interfere with those qualities that are an important component of being a first responder.

---

**Hepatitis C** is a long-term liver infection that can lead to cirrhosis and liver cancer. These effects may take 10-30 years to develop. The most common means of transmission of the hepatitis C virus is unsanitary injection drug use. Other means of transmission include prolonged sexual exposure and needle sticks.

## HIV

*AIDS (Acquired Immune Deficiency Syndrome)* is a result of HIV-caused infections and a weakened immune system. *HIV (human immunodeficiency virus)* attacks white blood cells and destroys the body's ability to fight infection. The infections that strike people whose immune systems are weakened by HIV or other conditions include severe pneumonia and fungal infections of the mouth and esophagus. HIV-infected people may also develop Kaposi's sarcoma and other unusual cancers (Fig. 4-6).

People infected with HIV may not feel or look sick. A blood test, however, can detect the HIV antibody. When the infected person shows signs of having certain infections or cancers, he or she may be diagnosed as having AIDS. The infections can cause severe fatigue, fever, night sweats, unexplained weight loss, chronic diarrhea, shortness of breath, swollen lymph nodes, and skin lesions. AIDS is a fatal condition. It is important to remember the following points about the transmission of HIV:

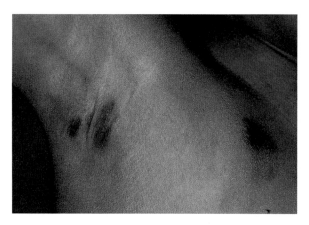

**Figure 4-6** Kaposi's sarcoma is one of the several opportunistic conditions that may strike the HIV-infected person.

- HIV cannot be spread through casual contact.
- The virus that causes HIV infection is easily killed by alcohol, chlorine bleach, and other common disinfectants. You cannot bring a dead virus back to life by adding water.
- HIV is known to be transmitted only through exposure to infected blood, semen, vaginal secretions, or (rarely) breast milk.

Transmission can occur by—

- Having unprotected sex with an infected partner, male or female.
- Being exposed to blood through use of soiled equipment or supplies, needle stick injuries, or blood splashed on mucous membranes or broken skin. (The risk of getting infected through a blood transfusion or blood product has been very low since 1985.)
- Sharing needles or syringes for street drugs, steroids, or ear piercing.
- Being infected as an unborn child or shortly after birth by an infected mother.

## Other Diseases and Immunization

Most people receive immunization as infants against common childhood diseases, such as measles and mumps. *Immunization* is the introduction of a substance that contains specific weakened or killed pathogens into the body. The body's immune system then builds resistance to a specific infection. No immunization exists, however, for chicken pox (varicella). The varicella infection causes fever and "pox" (blister-like sores on the skin). Once you have had chicken pox, it is unlikely that you will contract the disease again.

You should also be immunized against several other diseases. The following immunizations are recommended:

- DPT (Diphtheria, pertussis, tetanus).
- Polio.
- Hepatitis B (HBV).
- MMR (measles, mumps, rubella).
- Influenza.

You might not have been immunized against some of the childhood diseases. If you are not sure about which immunizations you have received or may need to update, contact your doctor or local community health nurse.

## ◆ PROTECTING YOURSELF FROM DISEASE TRANSMISSION

### Precautions

Sometimes we might like to vary the level of protection we use based on what a person looks like, the circumstances surrounding the incident, or where he or she is at the time of the incident. However, the world is not that simple. Often, you will not know the health status of the people you work with or care for. The one time you stop being careful may be the very time that you become infected by someone who does not fit into your notion of people who are likely to be infected. Each time you prepare to provide care, you must follow basic *precautions* (Fig. 4-7).

These precautions include the following four areas:

- Protective clothing and equipment.
- Personal hygiene.
- Engineering and work practice controls.
- Equipment cleaning and disinfecting.

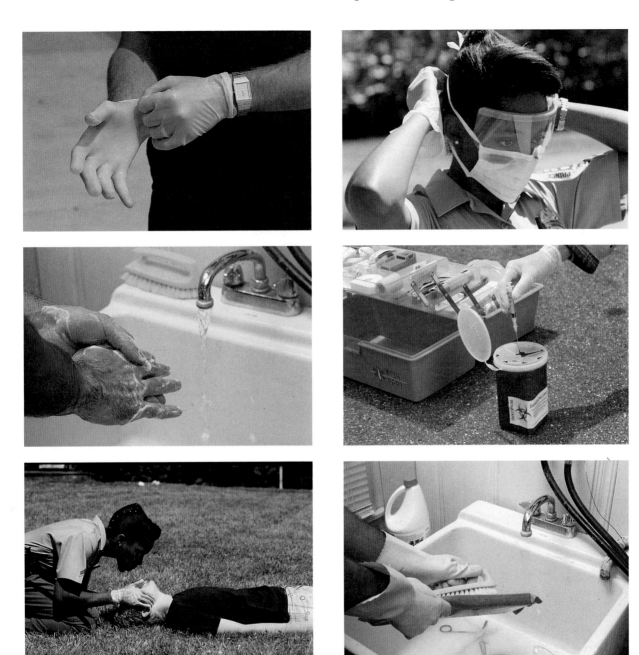

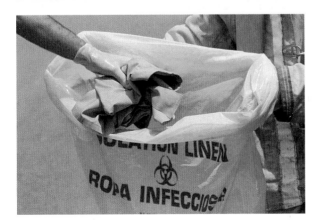

**Figure 4-7** Engineering controls and work practice controls decrease your risk of contracting or transmitting an infection.

**Table 4-3** Recommended Protective Equipment Against HIV and HBV Transmission in Prehospital Settings

| Task or activity | Disposable gloves | Gown | Mask | Protective eyewear |
|---|---|---|---|---|
| Bleeding control with spurting blood | Yes | Yes | Yes | Yes |
| Bleeding control with minimal bleeding | Yes | No | No | No |
| Emergency childbirth | Yes | Yes | Yes, if splashing is likely | Yes, if splashing is likely |
| Helping with an intravenous (IV) line | Yes | No | No | No |
| Oral/nasal suctioning, manually clearing airway | Yes | No | No, unless splashing is likely | No, unless splashing is likely |
| Handling and cleaning contaminated equipment and clothing | Yes | No, unless soiling is likely | No | No |

Excerpt from Department of Health and Human Services, Public Health Services: *A curriculum guide for public-safety and emergency-response workers: prevention of transmission of human immunodeficiency virus and hepatitis B virus,* Atlanta, Ga, February 1989, Dept Health and Human Services, Centers for Disease Control.

Protective clothing and equipment should be used to prevent skin and mucous membrane exposure when contact with blood or other body fluids is anticipated. Protective equipment keeps you from direct contact with infected materials and includes disposable gloves, gowns, masks and shields, protective eye wear, and mouthpieces and resuscitation devices. To minimize your risk of contracting or transmitting an infectious disease, follow these universal precautions.

## Universal Precautions

♦ Handle all blood and other body fluids as if infectious.
♦ Handle all patients in a way that minimizes exposure to blood and other body fluids.
♦ Wear disposable (single-use) gloves when it is possible you will contact blood or body fluids. This may happen directly through contact with a casualty or indirectly through contact with soiled clothing or other personal articles. There is no apparent difference in

barrier effectiveness between intact latex and intact vinyl gloves.
♦ Remove gloves by turning them inside out, beginning at the wrist and peeling them off. When removing the second glove, do not touch the soiled surfaces with your bare hand. Hook the inside of the glove at the wrist and peel the glove off.
♦ Discard gloves that are peeling, discoloured, torn, or punctured.
♦ Do not clean or reuse disposable gloves.
♦ Avoid handling items, such as pens, combs, or radios, yours or another person's, when wearing soiled gloves.
♦ Change gloves when you contact different casualties.
♦ Wear protective coverings, such as a mask, eye wear, and gown, whenever you are likely to contact blood or other body fluids that may splash.
♦ Cover any cuts, scrapes, or skin irritations you may have with protective clothing or bandages.

◆ Use breathing devices, such as disposable resuscitation masks and airway devices. These should be readily available in settings where the need for resuscitation can be anticipated, however, the risk of infection is so slight that no one should hesitate to give mouth-to-mouth resuscitation if such equipment is not available.

Personal hygiene habits, such as frequent hand washing (Fig. 4-8), are as important in preventing infection as any equipment you might use. These habits and practices can prevent any materials that might have gone through the protective equipment from staying in contact with your body.

Engineering controls are controls that isolate or remove the hazard from the workplace. Engineering controls include puncture-resistant containers for sharp equipment and mechanical needle recapping devices. To ensure that they work well, engineering controls should be examined and maintained or replaced on a regular basis. Once put in place, engineering controls should be maintained and replaced periodically.

Work practice controls reduce the likelihood of exposure by changing the way a task is carried out. The protection provided by work practice controls is based on the way people behave rather than on a physical device.

Engineering controls and work practice controls are established to ensure good industrial hygiene. Following certain guidelines for engineering controls and work practice controls can greatly cut down your risk of getting or transmitting an infectious disease.

◆ Ensure that all first aid kits are fully stocked with several pairs of disposable gloves, pocket masks or face shields, and antibacterial hand cleanser.
◆ Ensure that first aid kits are readily available and easily accessible to everyone.

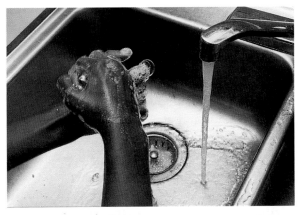

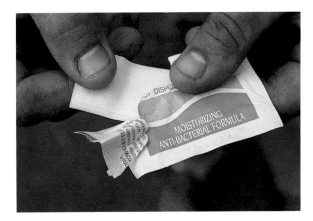

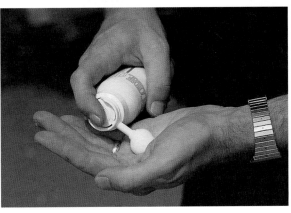

**Figure 4-8** Thorough hand washing after giving care helps protect you against disease.

- Maintain all protective equipment in good working order. Immediately dispose of any protective equipment that is peeling, discoloured, torn, or punctured.
- Check and restock first aid kits on a regular basis.
- Use dressings and tissues to minimize direct contact with blood, other body fluids, and wounds. If possible, have the casualty wash the wound first and assist you, e.g. holding a dressing in place, applying pressure if necessary.
- Avoid needle stick injuries by not trying to bend or recap any needles.
- If a procedure requires the recapping of a needle, use mechanical devices or one-handed techniques to recap or remove contaminated needles.
- Place sharp items (e.g., needles, scalpel blades) in puncture-resistant, leak-proof, labeled containers.
- Prohibit mouth pipetting or suctioning of blood or other potentially infectious materials.
- Perform all procedures in such a way that cuts down on splashing, spraying, splattering, and producing droplets of blood or other potentially infectious materials.
- Remove soiled protective clothing as soon as possible.
- Avoid eating, drinking, smoking, applying cosmetics or lip balm, handling contact lenses, and touching the mouth, nose, or eyes in work areas where exposure to infectious materials may occur.
- Clean and disinfect equipment and work surfaces possibly soiled by blood or other body fluids to prevent infections. Handle all soiled equipment, supplies, or other materials with great care until they are properly cleaned and disinfected. Place all disposable items that are contaminated in labeled containers. Place all soiled clothing in properly marked plastic bags for disposal or washing.
- Wash your hands thoroughly with soap and water immediately after providing care. Use a utility or restroom sink, not one in a food preparation area.

- For cleaning equipment and surfaces, general-purpose household gloves (neoprene, rubber) are appropriate. These can be decontaminated and reused but should be discarded when they become peeled, cracked, or discoloured, even though they may not become punctured or torn.
- Surfaces such as floors, woodwork, ambulance and automobile seats, and countertops, must be cleaned with soap and water first, using disposable towels, then disinfected. To disinfect equipment soiled with blood or body fluids, wash thoroughly with a solution of common household chlorine bleach and water. Approximately 60 ml ($^1/_4$ cup) of bleach per 4 litres (1 gallon) of water is enough.
- Wash and dry protective clothing and work uniforms according to the manufacturer's instructions. Scrub soiled boots, leather shoes, and other leather goods, such as belts, with soap, a brush, and hot water.
- If something occurs that creates disposable waste or soiled laundry, the materials should be stored in appropriate containers until they are disposed of or laundered. The containers must have warning labels or signs, such as "biohazard," to eliminate or minimize exposure of individuals. In addition, training should be provided to ensure that everyone understands and avoids the hazard.
- Work areas should be kept in clean and sanitary conditions based on a written schedule for cleaning and decontamination. The schedule should be based on the location in the facility, the type of surface to be cleaned, the type of soil present, and the tasks or procedures being done.

In addition, there should be a plan in place to deal with any spill that might occur. The plan should include a system to report a spill and the action taken to resolve the spill. It should also include a list of people responsible for containment, instructions for clean-up, and the final disposition of the spill. The first step in dealing with a spill is containment. Spill containment units designed for hazardous materials are sold and work very well. However, any absorbent material, such as paper towels, can be used if the material is disposed of properly.

The steps for spill management are as follows:

◆ Wear gloves and other appropriate personal protective equipment when cleaning spills.
◆ Clean up spills immediately or as soon as possible after the spill occurs.
◆ If the spill is mixed with sharp objects, such as broken glass and needles, do not pick these up with your hands. Use tongs, broom and dust pan, or two pieces of cardboard.
◆ Dispose of the absorbent material used to collect the spill in a labeled biohazard container.
◆ Flood the area with disinfectant solution, and allow it to stand for at least 20 minutes.
◆ Use paper towels to absorb the solution, and put the towels in the biohazard container.

Following these precautions will usually remove at least one of the four conditions necessary for disease transmission. Remember, if only one condition is missing, infection will not occur (see Fig. 4-3).

## The Exposure Control Plan

Preventing infectious disease begins with preparation and planning. An exposure control plan is an important step in removing or reducing exposure to blood and other possibly infectious materials. The exposure control plan is a system to protect people in a given environment from infection and should be placed where it can easily be used. The plan should be updated each year or more often if changes in exposure occur.

An exposure control plan should contain the following elements:

◆ Exposure determination
◆ Identification of who will receive training, protective equipment, and vaccination
◆ Procedures for evaluating details of an exposure incident

Exposure determination is one of the key elements of an exposure control plan. It includes identifying and making a written record of tasks in which exposure to blood can occur. The determination should be made without regard to using personal protective equipment.

The following Health Canada recommendations for health-care professionals can be applied to individuals at risk in any environment:

◆ Initial orientation and continuing education on modes of transmission and prevention of HIV and other bloodborne infections and the need for routine use of universal blood and body-fluid precautions for all patients.
◆ Provision of equipment and supplies necessary to minimize the risk of infection with HIV and other ***bloodborne pathogens.***
◆ Monitoring adherence to recommended protective measures. When monitoring reveals a failure to follow recommended precautions, counseling, education, or retraining should be provided.
◆ Health Canada also recommends that hepatitis B vaccinations be offered to all susceptible health-care workers, particularly those who work in high-risk areas.
◆ The exposure control plan should include reporting procedures for any first aid incidents. The procedures must ensure that incidents are reported before the end of the shift in which they occur.
◆ Reports of first aid incidents should include the names of all first aiders involved and the details of the incident. The report should also include the date and time of the incident and if an exposure incident has occurred.
◆ Exposure reports should be included on lists of first aid incidents.
◆ First aid providers should be trained in reporting procedure specifics.
◆ All first aiders who provide assistance in any incident involving blood or other potentially infectious materials, regardless of whether a specific exposure incident occurs, should be offered the full hepatitis B vaccination series. The immunization should be offered as soon as possible but in no event later than 24 hours after exposure. If an exposure incident occurs, other post-exposure follow-up procedures should be initiated immediately.

# ◆ IF AN EXPOSURE OCCURS

If you suspect you have been exposed to an infectious disease, wash any area of contact as quickly as possible and write down what happened. Exposures usually involve contact with potentially infectious blood or other fluids through a needle stick, broken or scraped skin, or the mucous membranes of the eyes, nose, or mouth. Inhaling potentially infected airborne droplets also may be an exposure. Most organizations have **protocols** (standardized procedures) for reporting infectious disease exposure.

The procedures should include the following elements:

- Be easy to access and user-friendly.
- Assurance of confidentiality.
- List of events covered by the procedure.
- List of immediate actions to be taken by exposed individual to reduce the chances of infection.
- When or how quickly the individual should report the exposure incident.
- Where and to whom the individual should report the exposure incident.
- Which forms the individual should complete.
- Directions for investigating the incident.
- List of information required from health-care workers.
- Medical follow-up including post-exposure vaccination.
- Instill confidence in the exposed worker.

If you think you have been exposed to an infectious disease, you should report the exposure immediately. A test may be done to see if the material was infected. Even before a disease is confirmed, you should receive medical evaluation, counseling, and post-exposure care, such as the hepatitis B vaccine. Your medical personnel or supervisor is responsible for notifying any other personnel who might have been exposed. If your system does not have a designated physician or nurse at a local hospital for follow-up care, see your personal physician.

# ◆ SUMMARY

Although the body's natural defence system defends well against disease, pathogens can still enter the body and sometimes cause infection. These pathogens can be transmitted in four ways:

- By direct contact with an infected person.
- By indirect contact with a soiled object.
- By inhaling air exhaled by an infected person.
- By vector-borne contact, through a bite from an infected animal, insect, or even a person.

Infectious diseases that you should be aware of include hepatitis, herpes, meningitis, tuberculosis, and HIV infections, including AIDS. You should know how the diseases are transmitted and take appropriate measures to protect yourself from them. Remember that the four conditions of infection must be present for a disease to be transmitted.

- A pathogen is present.
- There is enough of the pathogen to cause disease.
- A person is susceptible to the pathogen.
- The pathogen passes through the correct entry site.

It has been determined that individuals face a significant risk as a result of exposure to blood and other potentially infectious materials because they may contain bloodborne pathogens. This hazard can be reduced or removed using a combination of engineering and work practice controls, personal protective clothing and equipment, training, medical surveillance, hepatitis B vaccination, signs and labels, and other provisions.

Organizations have responsibilities that include—

- Identifying positions or tasks potentially at risk.
- Developing an annual training system for all at-risk individuals.

♦ Offering the opportunity for individuals to get counselling and medical care, such as the hepatitis B vaccination, at no cost.

♦ Using work practices, such as following universal and other precautions, to minimize the possibility of infection.

♦ Using engineering controls, such as puncture-resistant containers for sharp objects, to minimize the possibility of infection.

♦ Creating a system for easy identification of soiled material and its disposal.

♦ Creating an exposure control plan to minimize the possibility of exposure.

♦ Establishing clear procedures to follow for reporting an exposure.

♦ Creating a system of record keeping that includes updates in protocols and exposure control plans, training, medical records, and follow-up.

Following these guidelines, especially the precautions, greatly decreases your risk of contracting or transmitting an infectious disease. If you suspect you have been exposed to such a disease, always document it and notify appropriate personnel. Seek medical help and participate in any follow-up procedures.

## YOU ARE THE RESPONDER

1. You are called to check on a woman having difficulty breathing. The woman is kneeling on the ground. She has a cough and looks very ill. What are your concerns regarding disease transmission?

2. You stop to assist with an automobile crash. The casualty has a large amount of blood on her head. She continues to bleed from a large cut on her face. What are your concerns regarding disease transmission? How would you protect yourself?

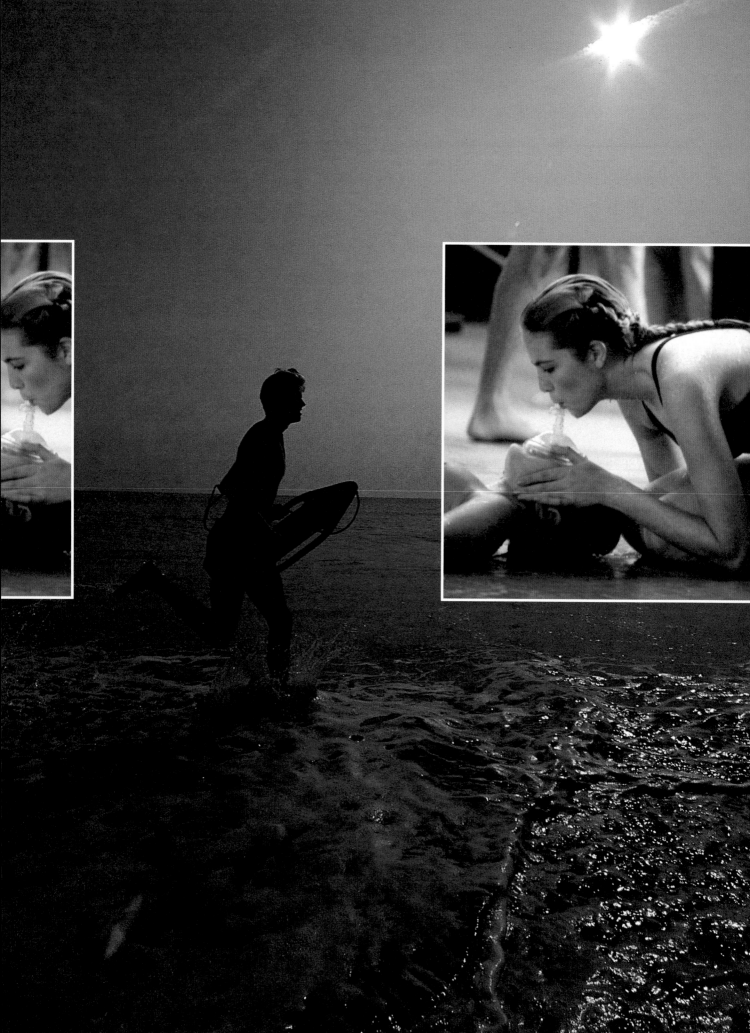

# Part Three

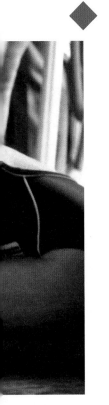

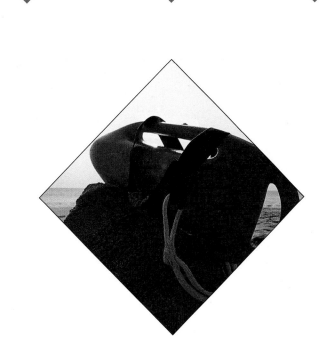

# Establishing Priorities of Care

# Primary and Secondary Survey

**5**

## Key Terms

**Blood pressure (BP):** The force exerted by blood against the blood vessel walls as it travels throughout the body.

**Brachial (BRA ke al) artery:** A large artery located in the upper arm.

**Carotid arteries:** Arteries located in the neck that supply blood to the head and neck.

**Emergency action principles (EAPs):** Six steps to guide a person's actions in any emergency.

**Level of consciousness (LOC):** A person's state of awareness, ranging from being fully alert to unconscious.

**Mechanism of injury:** The event or forces that caused the casualty's injury.

**Primary survey:** A check for conditions that are an immediate threat to a casualty's life.

**Secondary survey:** A check for injuries or conditions that could become life threatening if not cared for.

**Signs:** Any observable evidence of injury or illness, such as bleeding or an unusually pale skin colour.

**Symptoms:** Something the casualty tells you about his or her condition, such as, "my head hurts," or "I am dizzy."

**Vital signs:** Important information about the casualty's condition, obtained by checking level of consciousness, pulse, breathing, skin characteristics, and blood pressure.

## ♦ For Review ♦

Before reading this chapter, you should have a basic understanding of how the respiratory and circulatory systems function and how body systems interrelate (Chapter 3).

## ♦ INTRODUCTION

In previous chapters, you learned how to prepare for an emergency, the precautions to take when approaching the scene, and how to recognize a dangerous situation. You also learned about your roles and responsibilities as a first responder. You learned that you can make a difference in an emergency—you may even save a life. But to do this, you must learn how to provide care for an ill or injured casualty. More important, you need to learn how to set priorities for the care you provide.

In this chapter, you will learn a plan of action to guide you through any emergency. When an emergency occurs, you may at first feel confused. But you can train yourself to remain calm and to think before you act. Ask yourself, "What do I need to do? How can I help most effectively?" The six *emergency action principles (EAPs)* answer these questions. They are your plan of action for any emergency.

## ♦ EMERGENCY ACTION PRINCIPLES

The emergency action principles (EAPs) are—

1. Survey the scene.
2. Check the casualty for unresponsiveness and call more advanced medical personnel when needed.
3. Do a *primary survey* to identify and care for life-threatening problems.
4. Do a *secondary survey* to identify and care for any additional problems.
5. Keep monitoring the casualty's condition for life-threatening problems while waiting for advanced medical personnel to arrive.
6. Help the casualty rest in the most comfortable position and give reassurance.

These principles, conducted in this order, can ensure your safety and that of the casualty and bystanders. They will also increase the casualty's chance of survival if he or she has a serious illness or injury.

## Step One: Survey the Scene

Once you recognize that an emergency has occurred and decide to act, you must make sure the emergency scene is safe for you, the casualty(s), and any bystanders. Take time to survey the scene and answer these questions:

1. Is the scene safe?
2. What was the mechanism of the casualty's injury?
3. How many casualties are there?
4. Can bystanders help?

### Before You Approach the Casualty

When you survey the scene, look for anything that may threaten your safety and that of the casualty and bystanders. Examples of dangers that may be present are given in Chapter 2. They include downed power lines, traffic, fire, unstable structures, and deep or swift-moving water. Take the necessary precautions when working in a dangerous environment. If you are not properly trained and do not have the necessary equipment, do not approach the casualty. Summon the necessary personnel.

Nothing is gained by risking your safety. An emergency that begins with one casualty could end up with two if you are hurt. If you suspect the scene is unsafe, wait and watch until the necessary personnel and equipment arrive. If conditions change, you may then be able to approach the casualty.

## As You Approach the Casualty

Try to find out what happened. Look around the scene for clues to what caused the emergency (the mechanism of injury) and the extent of the damage. Doing this will cause you to think about the possible type and extent of the casualty's injuries. You may discover a situation that requires you to act immediately. As you approach the casualty, take in the whole picture. Nearby objects, such as shattered glass, a fallen ladder, or a spilled medicine container, may suggest what happened (Fig. 5-1). If the casualty is unconscious, surveying the scene may be the only way you can determine what happened.

When you survey the scene, look carefully for more than one casualty. You may not see everyone at first. For example, in a vehicle collision, an open door may be a clue that a casualty has left the car or was thrown from it. If one casualty is bleeding or screaming loudly, you may overlook another casualty who is unconscious. It is also easy in any emergency situation to overlook an infant or small child. Always look for more than one casualty. Ask anyone present how many people may be involved. If you find more than one casualty, ask bystanders to help you provide care.

Look for bystanders who can help. Bystanders may be able to tell you what happened or help in other ways. A bystander who knows the casualty may know whether he or she has any medical conditions or allergies. Bystanders can meet and direct the ambulance to your location, help keep the area free of unnecessary traffic, and help you provide care.

## Once You Reach the Casualty

Once you reach the casualty, quickly survey the scene again to see if it is still safe. At this point, you may see other dangers, clues to what happened, casualties or bystanders that you did not notice before.

You respond to an automobile crash. A car has veered off the road and landed in a ditch.

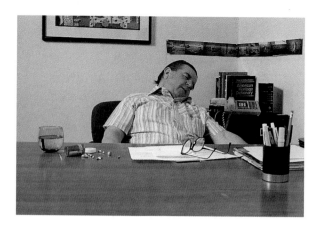

**Figure 5-1** If the casualty is unconscious, nearby objects may be your only clue to what has happened.

After surveying the scene and deciding it is safe to approach, you move to the car. As you come closer, you see a woman lying motionless on the ground near the car. But you also smell gasoline. What should you do? Is there a danger? Should you move her away from the car or try to care for her there?

As a rule, do not move a casualty unless there is an immediate danger, such as a fire, poisonous fumes, or an unstable structure. The odour of gasoline by itself is not sufficient cause to move the casualty. If the area is dangerous and the casualty does not seem to be seriously injured, ask the casualty to move to safety where you can help him or her. If the area is dangerous and the casualty cannot move, you may try to move the casualty as quickly as possible without making his or her condition worse. If there is no immediate danger, tell the casualty not to move. If the casualty suffers from trauma, stabilize the cervical spine immediately as you begin to check the airway.

When you reach the casualty, try not to alarm him or her. Try to position yourself close to the casualty's eye level (Fig. 5-2). Speak in a calm and positive manner. Identify yourself to the casualty. Ask if you can help. This lets a conscious casualty know that a caring and skilled person will be giving care.

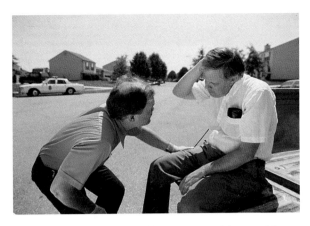

**Figure 5-2** When talking to the casualty, position yourself close to the casualty's eye level and speak in a calm and positive manner.

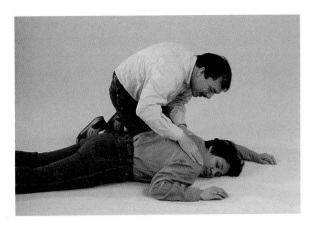

**Figure 5-3** Determine if the person is conscious by gently tapping and asking, "Are you okay?"

## Step Two: Check the Casualty for Unresponsiveness and Call More Advanced Medical Personnel

First, determine if the casualty is conscious. Do this by gently tapping him or her and asking, "Are you okay?" (Fig. 5-3). Do not jostle or move the casualty. A casualty who can speak or cry is conscious, breathing, and has a pulse.

If the casualty is unable to respond, he or she may be unconscious. Unconsciousness can indicate a life-threatening condition. When a person is unconscious, the tongue relaxes and may fall to the back of the throat, blocking the airway. This can cause breathing to stop. Soon after, the heart will stop beating. With an unconscious casualty, always call for more advanced medical personnel.

You then proceed to the next step, the primary survey, to check for life-threatening conditions, and call for more advanced medical personnel if such a condition is found.

If your communication network is not directly linked to advanced medical personnel, you will need to use a telephone to call. If possible, ask another first responder or a bystander to call the emergency number for you. Sending someone else to make the call will enable you to stay with the casualty to provide care.

Whether placing the call yourself or sending someone to call, the following should be done:

1. Dial the local emergency number. This number is 9-1-1 in many communities. Dial "O" (the operator) only if you do not know the emergency number for the area. Sometimes the emergency number is on the inside front cover of telephone directories and on pay phones.

2. Provide the dispatcher with the necessary information:

    a. *Where the emergency is located.* Give the exact address or location and the name of the city or town. It is helpful to give the names of nearby intersecting streets (cross streets), landmarks, the name of the building, the floor, and the room number.

    b. *Telephone number from which the call is being made.*

    c. *Caller's name.*

    d. *What happened*—for example, a motor vehicle collision, fall, fire.

    e. *The number of people involved.*

    f. *Condition of the casualty(s)*—for example, chest pain, difficulty breathing, no pulse, bleeding.

    g. *Care being given.*

3. *Do not hang up until the dispatcher has finished gathering information. It is important to make sure the dispatcher has all the information needed to send the appropriate help immediately.*

| Table 5-1 | When to Summon More Advanced Medical Personnel |

| Condition | Signs and symptoms |
| --- | --- |
| Unconscious, or not easily aroused | Casualty does not respond to tapping, loud voices, or other attempts to arouse |
| Difficulty breathing | Noisy breathing, such as wheezing or gasping<br>Casualty feels short of breath<br>Skin has a flushed, pale, or bluish appearance |
| No breathing | You cannot see the casualty's chest rise and fall<br>You cannot hear and feel air escaping from the nose and mouth |
| No circulation | You cannot feel the carotid pulse in the neck or the radial and brachial pulses in the arms and legs |
| Severe bleeding | Casualty has bleeding that spurts or gushes from the wound |
| Persistent pain in the chest or abdomen | Casualty has persistent pain or pressure in the chest or abdomen that is not relieved by resting or changing positions |
| Vomiting blood or passing blood | You can see blood in vomit, urine, or feces |
| Poisoning | Casualty shows evidence of swallowed, inhaled, or injected poison, such as presence of drugs, medications, or cleaning agents<br>Mouth or lips may be burned |
| Sudden illness requiring assistance | Casualty has seizures, severe headaches, changes in level of consciousness, unusually high or low blood pressure, or a known diabetic problem |
| Head, neck, or back injuries | How the injury happened; for example, a fall, severe blow, or collision suggests a head injury<br>Casualty complains of severe headaches, neck or back pain<br>Casualty is unconscious<br>Bleeding, clear fluid, or deformity of the scalp, face, or neck |
| Possible broken bones | How the injury happened; for example, a fall, severe blow, or collision suggests a fracture<br>Evidence of damage to blood vessels or nerves, for example, slow capillary refill, no pulse below the injury, loss of sensation in the affected part<br>Inability to move body part without pain or discomfort<br>Fractures associated with open wounds |

## Step Three: Do a Primary Survey and Care for Life-Threatening Conditions

In every emergency situation, you first must find out if there are conditions that are an immediate threat to the casualty's life. You will discover these conditions by looking for *signs,* evidence of injury or illness that you can observe. You discover the signs of life-threatening conditions in the primary survey step. In the primary survey, you check to see if the casualty—

◆ Has an open airway.
◆ Is breathing.
◆ Has a heartbeat.
◆ Is not bleeding severely.

The primary survey takes only seconds to perform.

Remembering these steps is easy. The three steps of the primary survey are called the ABCs.

| A = AIRWAY/C-SPINE |
| B = BREATHING |
| C = CIRCULATION |

If you can, try to check the ABCs in whatever position you find the casualty, especially if you suspect the casualty has a head or spine injury. Sometimes, however, the casualty's position prevents you from checking the ABCs. In this case, you may roll the casualty gently onto his or her back, keeping the head and spine in as straight a line as possible (Fig. 5-4).

## Check the Airway

Be sure the casualty has an open airway, the pathway for air from the mouth and nose to the lungs. Without an open airway, the casualty cannot breathe. Remember, a casualty who can speak or cry is conscious, has an open airway, is breathing, and has a pulse.

It is more difficult to tell if an unconscious casualty has an open airway. To open an unconscious casualty's airway, tilt the head back and lift the chin (Fig. 5-5). This moves the tongue away from the back of the throat, allowing air to enter the lungs. For someone you suspect has a head or spine injury, modify this technique, as you will read in Chapter 6. After opening the airway, check for breathing.

Sometimes, opening the airway does not result in a free passage of air. This happens when a casualty's airway is blocked by liquid, food, or other objects. In this case, you will need to remove the obstruction. Chapter 6 describes how to care for an obstructed airway.

## Check Breathing

If the casualty is breathing, the chest will rise and fall. However, chest movement by itself does not mean air is reaching the lungs. You must also listen and feel for signs of breathing. Position yourself so that you can hear and feel air as it escapes from the casualty's nose and mouth. At the same time, watch the chest rise and fall. Look, listen, and feel for breathing for no more than 10 seconds (Fig. 5-6). A casualty

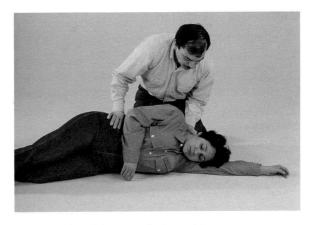

**Figure 5-4** If the casualty's position prevents you from checking the ABCs, roll the casualty gently onto his or her back.

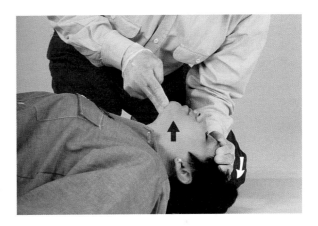

**Figure 5-5** Tilt the head and lift the chin to open the airway.

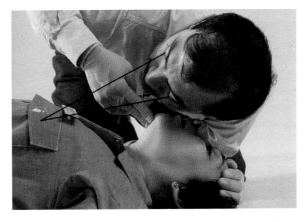

**Figure 5-6** To check breathing, look, listen, and feel for breathing for no more than 10 seconds.

with breathing difficulty needs oxygen immediately (see Chapter 8). By assessing the quality of respirations you can determine if this is needed.

If the casualty is not breathing, you must breathe for him or her. Begin by giving 2 slow breaths, each lasting 2 full seconds. Each breath should be given until the chest gently rises. This will get air into the casualty's lungs. The longer a casualty goes without oxygen, the more likely he or she is to die. This process of breathing for the casualty is called **rescue breathing.** You will learn how to give rescue breathing in Chapter 6.

### Check Circulation

The last step in the primary survey is checking for blood circulation. If the heart has stopped, blood will not circulate throughout the body. If blood does not circulate, the casualty will die in just a few minutes because the brain will not get any oxygen.

If a person is breathing, his or her heart is beating and is circulating blood. If the casualty is not breathing, you must check for signs of circulation and find out if the heart is beating. To check for circulation, look for movement of the casualty, effective breathing (more than an occasional gasp), coughing, appropriate colour of the skin and presence of a carotid pulse. In the primary survey, you feel for an adult's or child's pulse at either of the **carotid arteries** located in the neck (Fig. 5-7).

To find the pulse, feel for the Adam's apple at the front of the neck, then slide your fingers into the groove at the side of the neck. Sometimes the pulse may be difficult to find, since it may be slow or weak. If at first you do not find a pulse, relocate the Adam's apple and again slide your fingers into place. When you think you are in the right spot, keep feeling for no more than 10 seconds. To find an infant's pulse, you place your fingers over the **brachial artery,** located on the inside of the upper arm, midway between the shoulder and elbow (Fig. 5-8).

If you do not observe the presence of the signs of circulation, you need to keep oxygen-rich blood circulating. This involves doing rescue breathing to get oxygen into the casualty's lungs and chest compressions to circulate the oxygen to the brain. This procedure is called cardiopulmonary resuscitation (CPR) and is described in Chapter 7.

Checking circulation also means looking for severe bleeding. Bleeding is severe when blood spurts from the wound or cannot be controlled. It is life threatening. Check for severe bleeding by looking from head to toe for signs of external bleeding (Fig. 5-9). Severe bleeding must be controlled before you provide any further care. Techniques for controlling severe bleeding are described in Chapter 9.

If you must leave the casualty for any reason, such as to call your emergency number, place

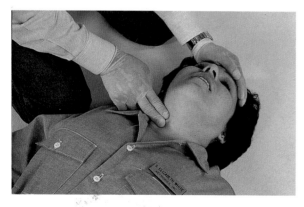

**Figure 5-7**  Determine if the heart is beating by checking for signs of circulation and feeling for a carotid pulse at either side of the neck.

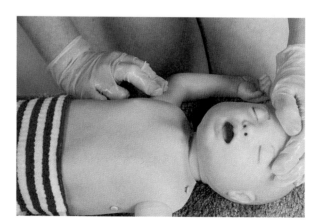

**Figure 5-8**  To find an infant's pulse, feel for the brachial artery in the upper arm.

him or her in the recovery position to help keep the airway open (Fig. 5-10). Place the casualty on one side, bend the top leg, and move it forward to hold the casualty in that position. Support the head so that it is angled toward the ground. In this position, if the casualty vomits, the airway will stay clear.

Call for more advanced medical personnel if the primary survey determines a life-threatening condition and if you have not already called for help. Your standard procedures will tell you when and whom to call. The EMS system works more effectively if you can provide information about the casualty's condition as soon as possible. The information you provide will help to ensure that the casualty receives proper medical care as quickly as possible.

With your training, you can do two important things that can make a difference in the outcome of a seriously ill or injured person:

(1) Give care for life-threatening conditions.

(2) Summon more advanced medical personnel as quickly as possible.

At times, you may be unsure if more advanced medical personnel are needed. For example, the casualty may say not to call an ambulance because he or she is embarrassed about creating a scene. Sometimes you may be unsure if the casualty's condition is severe enough to require more advanced care. Your training as a first responder will help you make the decision.

As a general rule, summon more advanced medical personnel for any of the following conditions:

- Unconsciousness or altered level of consciousness.
- Breathing problems (difficulty or no breathing).
- Persistent chest or abdominal pain or pressure.
- No pulse or signs of circulation.
- Severe bleeding.
- Vomiting or passing blood.
- Suspected poisoning.
- Seizures, severe headache, slurred speech.
- Suspected or obvious injuries to head or spine.
- Suspected broken bones.

These conditions are by no means a complete list. It is impossible to provide a definitive list, since there are always exceptions. Trust your instincts. If you think there is an emergency, there probably is. It is better to have personnel respond to a non-emergency than arrive at an emergency too late to help.

## Step Four: Do a Secondary Survey

Once you are certain that the casualty has no life-threatening conditions, you can begin the fourth EAP, the secondary survey. If, however, you find life-threatening conditions, such as unconsciousness, no breathing, no pulse, or severe bleeding, during the primary survey, do *not* waste time with a secondary survey. Instead, provide care only for the life-threatening conditions.

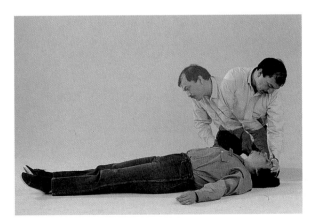

**Figure 5-9** Visually check for signs of severe bleeding by looking from head to toe.

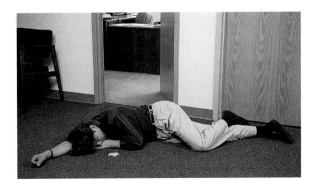

**Figure 5-10** Place an unconscious casualty in the recovery position if you must leave him alone.

The secondary survey is a systematic method of gathering additional information about injuries or conditions that may need care. These injuries or conditions are not immediately life threatening but could become so if not cared for. For example, you might find possible broken bones, minor bleeding, or a specific medical condition, such as diabetes. The secondary survey has the following three steps:

1.  Interview the casualty and bystanders.
2.  Check vital signs.
3.  Do a head-to-toe examination.

When possible, write down the information you find during the secondary survey and the time the information was noted. Sometimes you may need to have someone else write down the information or help you remember it. You can give this information to more advanced medical personnel when they arrive. Your information may help determine what type of medical care the casualty will receive later.

As you do the secondary survey, try not to move the casualty. Most injured people will find the most comfortable position for themselves. For example, a person with a chest injury who is having trouble breathing may be sitting up and supporting the injured area. Let the casualty continue to do this. Do not ask him or her to change positions.

## Interview the Casualty and Bystanders

Begin by asking the casualty and bystanders simple questions to learn more about what happened and the casualty's condition. This should not take much time. You are looking not only for signs of the casualty's condition but also for symptoms. A *symptom* is something the casualty tells you about his or her condition, such as "I am dizzy" or "my head hurts." A sign is any evidence you can see of injury or illness, such as bleeding or unusually pale skin color.

If you have not done so already, remember to identify yourself and to get the casualty's consent before helping. Begin the interview by asking the casualty's name. Using his or her

name will make the casualty more comfortable. First ask what happened and whether the casualty feels any pain. Use the acronym **AMPLE** to remember to ask the following questions:

A = Allergies (Do you have any allergies?)
M = Medications (Are you taking any medications?)
P = Past medical history (Do you have any medical conditions?)
L = Last meal (When did you last eat?)
E = Events before the incident (What happened to cause the problem?)

If the casualty has pain, ask him or her to describe it. You may use the abbreviation PQRST to remember the questions to ask (Table 5-2). You can expect to get descriptions such as burning, throbbing, aching, or sharp pain. Ask when the pain started. Ask how bad the pain is.

Sometimes the casualty will be unable to give you the information. This is often the case with a child or with an adult who momentarily lost consciousness and may not be able to recall what happened or is disoriented. These casualties may be frightened. Be calm and patient. Speak normally and in simple terms. Offer reassurance. Ask family members, friends, or bystanders what happened. They may be able to give you helpful information, such as telling you if a casualty has a medical condition you

| Table 5-2 | Questions About Pain: PQRST |
| --- | --- |
| **Acronym** | **Question to ask** |
| Provoke | What provokes the pain or causes it to get worse? |
| Quality | What does the pain feel like? (sharp, dull, stabbing, moving, etc.) |
| Region (or Radiate) | Where exactly is the pain located? Does it radiate to other areas? |
| Severity | How bad is the pain? |
| Time | When did the pain begin? |

should be aware of. They may also be able to help calm the casualty if necessary.

## Check Vital Signs

A person's level of consciousness, pulse, breathing, skin characteristics, and blood pressure are *vital signs.* These vital signs can tell you how the body is responding to injury or illness. Look for changes in vital signs. Note anything unusual. Recheck vital signs about every 5 minutes.

### Level of consciousness

One of the most important indicators of a person's condition is his or her *level of consciousness (LOC).* A person's level of consciousness can range from being fully alert to being unconscious. In describing a person's LOC, a four-level scale is used. The letters *A, V, P,* and *U* each refer to a stage of awareness.

A = Alert: This implies that the person is aware of his or her surroundings and is able to respond appropriately to your questions, such as—

◆ What happened?
◆ What is your name?
◆ Where are you?
◆ What day of the week is it?

A person who is able to answer these questions is considered alert and oriented. Someone who is unable to answer these questions correctly or who may be unusually slow to respond is said to be **disoriented.**

V = Verbal: Sometimes a person only reacts to sounds, such as your voice. This person may appear to be lapsing into unconsciousness. A person who has to be stimulated by sound is described as responding to verbal stimuli.

P = Pain: If a person only responds when someone inflicts pain, then he or she is described as responding to painful stimuli. Pinching the earlobe or the skin above the collarbone are examples of painful stimuli used to try to get a response (Fig. 5-11).

U = Unresponsive: A person who does not respond to any stimuli is described as unconscious, or unresponsive to stimuli.

| Table 5-3 | Levels of Consciousness |
| --- | --- |
| **Level** | **Characteristic behavior** |
| *A*lert | Able to respond appropriately to questions |
| *V*erbal | Responds appropriately to verbal stimuli |
| *P*ainful | Only responds appropriately to painful stimuli |
| *U*nresponsive | Does not respond |

Observe the person's LOC as you conduct your interview. Note the time you arrived and the person's LOC at that time. Continue to note any changes that occur while you complete the secondary survey and provide care. Record your findings. For example, you might note, "At 5:15 PM casualty was responsive to verbal stimuli. At 5:20 PM casualty was responsive only to painful stimuli."

### Pulse

With every heartbeat, a wave of blood moves through the blood vessels. This creates a beat called the **pulse.** You can feel it with your fingertips in arteries near the skin. In the primary survey, you are only concerned with whether a pulse is present. To determine this, you check the

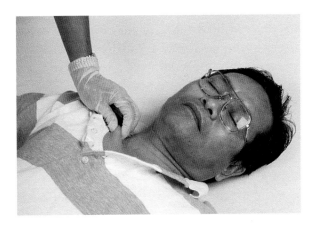

**Figure 5-11**  Pinching the skin above the collarbone is an example of a painful stimulus used to get a response.

carotid arteries. In the secondary survey, you are trying to determine pulse rate and quality. This is most often done by checking the **radial pulse** located on the thumb side of the casualty's wrist.

When the heart is healthy, it beats with a steady rhythm. This beat creates a regular pulse. A normal pulse for an adult is between 60 and 100 beats per minute. A well-conditioned athlete may have a pulse of 50 beats per minute or lower. Table 5-4 lists average pulses at different ages. If the heartbeat changes, so does the pulse. An abnormal pulse may be a sign of a potential problem. These signs include—

◆ Irregular pulse.
◆ Weak and hard-to-find pulse.
◆ Excessively fast or slow pulse.

When severely injured or not healthy, the heart may beat unevenly, producing an irregular pulse. The rate at which the heart beats can also change. The pulse speeds up when a person is excited, anxious, in pain, losing blood, or under stress. It slows down when a person is relaxed. Some heart conditions can also speed up or slow down the pulse rate. Sometimes changes may be very subtle and difficult for you to detect. The most important change to note is a pulse that changes from being present to no pulse at all.

Checking a pulse is a simple procedure. It merely involves placing two fingers on top of a major artery where it is located close to the skin's surface. Pulse sites that are easy to locate are the carotid arteries in the neck, the radial artery in the wrist, and, for infants, the brachial artery in the upper arm (Fig. 5-12). There are other pulse sites you may use. Figure 5-13 shows these sites. To check the pulse rate, count the number of beats in 15 seconds and multiply that number by 4. The number you get is the number of heartbeats per minute.

A sick or injured person's pulse may be hard to find. If you have trouble finding a pulse, keep checking for one periodically. Take your time. Remember, if a person is breathing, his or her heart is also beating. However, there may be a loss in circulation to the injured area, causing a loss of pulse. If you cannot find the pulse in one place, check it in another major artery, such as in the other wrist.

In later chapters, you will learn more about what any changes in pulse may mean and what care to provide.

### Breathing

A healthy person breathes regularly, quietly, and effortlessly. The normal breathing rate for an adult is between 12 and 20 breaths per minute (see Table 5-4). However, some people breathe slightly slower or faster. Excitement, fear, or exercise will cause breathing to increase and become deeper. Certain injuries or illnesses can also cause both the breathing rate and quality to change.

During the secondary survey, watch and listen for any changes in breathing. Abnormal breathing may indicate a potential problem. The signs and symbols of abnormal breathing include—

◆ Gasping for air.
◆ Noisy breathing, including whistling sounds, crowing, gurgling, or snoring.

**Table 5-4    Average\* Vital Signs by Age**

| Age | Pulse | Respirations | Blood pressure |
|-----|-------|--------------|----------------|
| Newborn | 120-160 | 40-60 | 80/40 |
| Infant (0-1 years) | 100-120 | 30-40 | 80/40 |
| Child (1-8 years) | 80-120 | 16-24 | 90/50 |
| Adult (over age 8) | 60-100 | 12-20 | 120/80 |

\*These values vary among individuals and should not be considered "normal" values. They are averages for each age group.

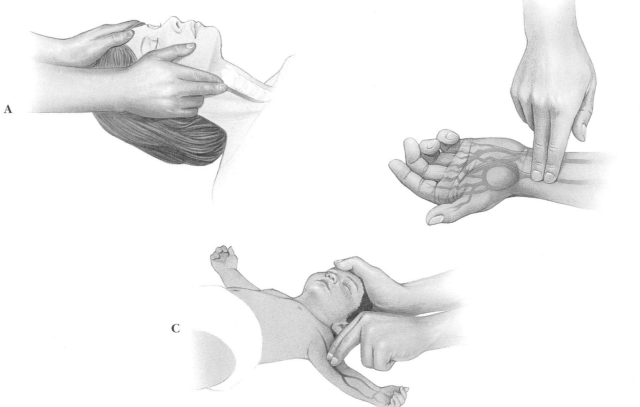

**Figure 5-12** A pulse can be checked in arteries that circulate close to the surface, such as **A,** the carotid artery, **B,** the radial artery, and, **C,** for infants, the brachial artery.

◆ Excessively fast or slow breathing.
◆ Painful breathing.

Unlike the primary survey, in which you are concerned with whether a person is breathing at all, in the secondary survey, you are concerned with the rate and the quality of breathing. Look, listen, and feel again for breathing. Look for the rise and fall of the casualty's chest or abdomen. Listen for sounds as the person inhales and exhales. Count the number of times a person breathes (inhales or exhales) in 15 seconds and multiply that number by 4 (Fig. 5-14). This is the number of breaths per minute. As you check for the rate and quality of breathing, try to do it without the casualty's knowledge. If a casualty realizes that you are checking his or her breathing, the casualty may attempt to change his or her breathing pattern without being aware of doing so. Maintain the same position you were in when checking the pulse. In later chapters, you will learn more about what changes in breathing may mean and what specific care to provide.

**Skin appearance and temperature**

The appearance of the skin and its temperature often indicate something about the casualty's condition. For example, a casualty with a breathing problem may have a flushed or pale face.

The skin looks red when the body is forced to work harder. The heart pumps faster to get more blood to the tissues. This increased blood flow causes reddened skin and makes the skin feel warm. In contrast, the skin may look pale or bluish and feel cool and moist if the blood flow is directed away from the skin's surface. When a person with darker skin becomes pale, the skin

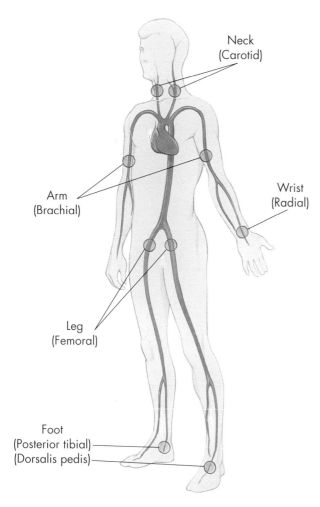

**Figure 5-13** Easily located pulse sites.

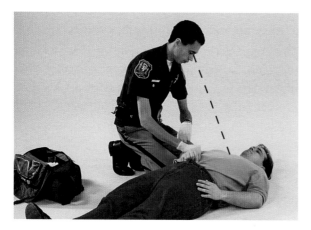

**Figure 5-14** Determine the rate and quality of breathing.

turns **ashen,** a grayish color. Any of these skin conditions may indicate a problem.

One technique for estimating how the body is reacting to illness or injury is to check the capillaries ability to refill with blood. **Capillary refill** is an estimate of the amount of blood flowing through the capillary beds, such as those in the fingertips. The capillary beds in the fingertips are normally rich with blood, which causes the pink color under the fingernails. When a serious illness or injury occurs, the body attempts to conserve blood in the vital organs. As a result, capillaries in the fingertips are among the first blood vessels to constrict, thereby limiting their blood supply.

To check capillary refill, squeeze the casualty's fingernail for about 2 seconds and then release. In a healthy person, the normal response is for the area beneath the fingernail to turn pale as you press it and immediately turn pink again as you release and it refills with blood (Fig. 5-15). If the area does not return to pink within 2 seconds (the time it takes to say "capillary refill"), this indicates insufficient circulation and a potentially serious illness or injury.

### Blood pressure

Another vital sign that helps to indicate a person's condition is blood pressure. ***Blood pressure (BP)*** is the force exerted by the blood against the blood vessel walls as it travels throughout the body. Blood pressure is necessary to move the oxygen and nutrients in the blood to the body's organs and muscles. It is also necessary to move waste products, such as carbon dioxide, to various parts of the body for removal. Blood pressure is a good indicator of how the circulatory system is functioning. If a person's circulatory system is working normally, blood pressure remains constant and within a normal range. If the circulatory system is failing, blood pressure drops.

Blood pressure is created by the pumping action of the heart. The pumping action involves two phases: the working (contracting) phase and the resting (refilling) phase. During the working phase, the **ventricles** (lower chambers) of the heart contract. This causes blood to be pumped

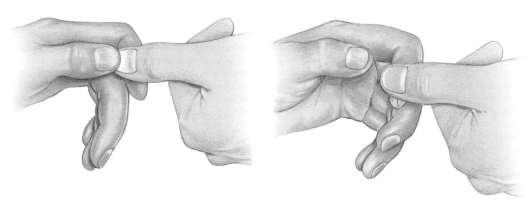

**Figure 5-15** Checking capillary refill is one technique used to estimate whether blood is circulating properly in the extremities.

through the arteries to all parts of the body. During the resting phase, the ventricles relax and refill with blood before the next contraction.

Because a person's blood pressure can vary greatly, blood pressure is only one of several factors that give you an overall picture of a person's condition. Stress, excitement, illness, or injury often affect blood pressure. When a casualty is ill or injured, a single blood pressure measurement is often of little value. A more accurate picture of a casualty's condition immediately following an injury or the onset of an illness is whether his or her blood pressure changes over time while you provide care. For example, a casualty's initial blood pressure reading could be uncommonly high due to the stress of the emergency. Providing care, however, usually relieves some of the fear, and blood pressure may return to a normal range. At other times, blood pressure will remain unusually high or low. For example, an injury resulting in severe blood loss may cause blood pressure to remain unusually low. You should be concerned about unusually high or low blood pressure whenever symptoms of injury or illness are present.

To accurately assess a person's blood pressure, you need a **blood pressure cuff.** The cuff is a strip of fabric that is wrapped around the arm. Cuffs come in sizes for small, average, and large arms (Fig. 5-16). Inside the cuff is a rubber bladder, similar to an inner tube, that can be inflated. A pressure gauge, inflation bulb, and regulating valve are connected to the bladder by rubber tubing.

Blood pressure is measured in units called millimetres of mercury (mm Hg). These units, written on the blood pressure gauge, range from 20 mm Hg to 300 mm Hg. In measuring blood pressure, two different numbers are usually recorded. The first number reflects the pressure in the arteries when the heart is working, or contracting. This pressure is called the **systolic** blood pressure. The second number reflects the pressure in the arteries when the heart is at rest and refilling. This is called the **diastolic** blood pressure.

You report blood pressure by giving the systolic number first, then the diastolic (S/D). Write this as: BP 120/80. When reporting 120/80, you would say "one twenty over eighty."

To determine both the systolic and diastolic pressure, you need a **stethoscope.** The stetho-

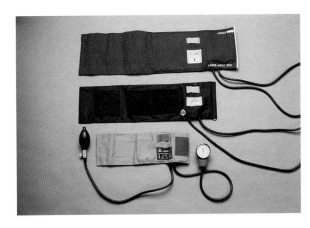

**Figure 5-16** Blood pressure cuffs come in sizes for small, average, and large arms.

scope enables you to hear the pulsating sounds of blood moving through the arteries with each contraction of the heart. Sometimes you may not have a stethoscope or, because of noise, are unable to use one. You can still determine the systolic blood pressure through a method known as palpation. **Palpation** requires you to feel (palpate) the radial artery as you inflate the blood pressure cuff (Fig. 5-17).

To determine blood pressure by palpation, begin by having the person sit or lie down. Wrap the blood pressure cuff around the person's arm so that the lower edge is about 1" above the crease at the elbow. The centre of the cuff should be over the brachial artery, the major artery of

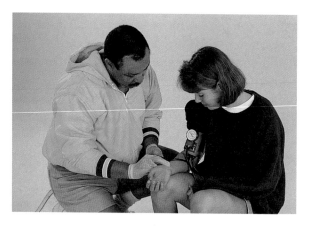

**Figure 5-17** Estimating a systolic blood pressure requires you to feel for the radial pulse.

the arm (Fig. 5-18). Next, locate the radial pulse. Close the regulating valve by turning the valve clockwise, and begin to inflate the cuff. Inflate the cuff until you can no longer feel the radial pulse. Note the number on the gauge.

Continue to inflate the cuff for another 20 mm Hg beyond this point. Slowly release the pressure in the cuff by turning the regulating valve counterclockwise (Fig. 5-19). Allow the cuff to deflate at a rate of about 2 mm Hg per second. Continue to feel for the radial pulse as the cuff deflates. The point at which the pulse returns is the approximate systolic blood pressure by palpation. This blood pressure reading is expressed as one number only, such as 130/P. The systolic pressure is 130, and *P* refers to palpation. Once you know the approximate systolic pressure, quickly deflate the cuff. Record the systolic pressure and whether the person was sitting or lying down when the blood pressure was taken.

The process of using a blood pressure cuff and stethoscope to listen for characteristic sounds is called **auscultation.** To auscultate means to listen. This method allows you to get accurate systolic and diastolic pressures. To auscultate blood pressure, begin by determining the systolic pressure using the palpation method. Next, locate the brachial pulse. Place the earpieces of the stethoscope in your ears and the other end, the diaphragm, over the spot

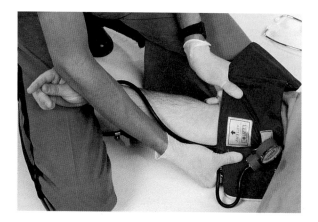

**Figure 5-18** To obtain an accurate blood pressure reading, centre the cuff over the brachial artery, about 2.5 cm (1 inch) above the crease of the elbow.

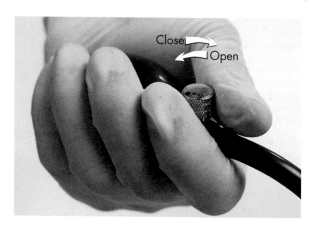

**Figure 5-19** To close the regulating valve, turn the valve clockwise. To open the regulating valve, turn it counterclockwise.

where you found the brachial pulse (Fig. 5-20). Close the valve and begin to inflate the cuff. Inflate the cuff to 20 mm Hg above the approximate systolic blood pressure.

Slowly deflate the cuff at a rate of about 2 mm Hg per second. As you deflate the cuff, listen carefully for the pulse. In some instances, it may sound like a tapping sound. The point at which the pulse is first heard is the systolic pressure.

As the cuff deflates, the pulse sound will fade. The point at which the sound disappears is the diastolic pressure. Release the remaining air quickly. Record the blood pressure as two numbers, such as 130/80. Also record whether the person was sitting or lying down.

## Do a Head-to-Toe Examination

The last step of the secondary survey is the head-to-toe examination. This examination helps you gather more information about the casualty's condition. When you do the head-to-toe examination, use your senses—sight, sound, smell, and touch—tone detect anything abnormal. For example, you may smell an unusual odour that could indicate a casualty has been poisoned. You may see a bruise or feel a deformed body part.

Begin the head-to-toe examination by telling the casualty what you are going to do. Ask the casualty to remain still. Though a casualty may be moving around in pain, he or she usually will not move a body part that is injured. Ask the casualty to tell you if any areas hurt. *Avoid touching any painful areas or having the casualty move any area in which there is discomfort.* Watch facial expressions; listen for a tone of voice that may reveal pain. Look for a medical alert tag on a necklace or bracelet (Fig. 5-21). This tag may help you determine what is wrong, whom to call for help, and what care to give.

As you do the head-to-toe examination, think about how the body normally looks and feels. Be alert for any sign of injuries—anything that looks or feels unusual. If you are uncertain whether your finding is unusual, check the other side of the body.

To do a head-to-toe examination, inspect the entire body, starting with the head (Fig. 5-22). You might see abnormal skin colour from bruising, a body fluid such as blood, or an unusual position of body parts. You may see and feel odd bumps or depressions. The casualty may seem groggy or faint.

Check the head. Look for blood or clear fluid in or around the ears, nose, and mouth. Blood or clear fluid can indicate a serious head injury. Check the level of consciousness again and note any change. Look closely at the pupils to determine whether they are of equal size. If possible, check to see how each pupil responds to light. You can do this by shading each eye

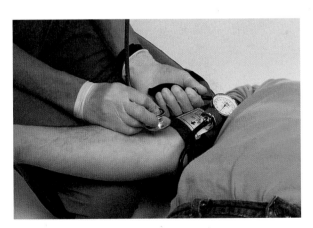

**Figure 5-20** To auscultate blood pressure, position the cuff, find the brachial pulse, and position the stethoscope over it.

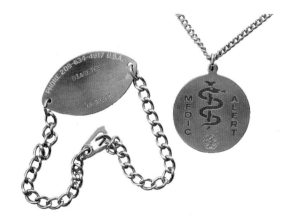

**Figure 5-21** Medical alert tags can provide important medical information about the casualty.

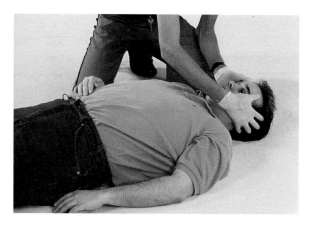

**Figure 5-22** During the head-to-toe examination, inspect the entire body, starting with the head.

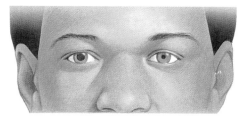

Unequal

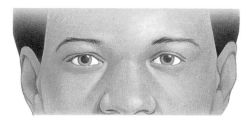

Dilated

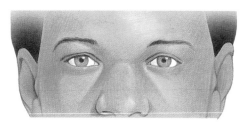

Constricted

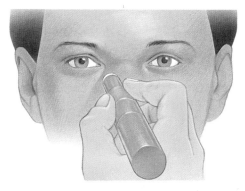

Unresponsive to light

**Figure 5-23** Pupils that are unequal, fully dilated, fully constricted, or unresponsive to light may indicate a serious injury or illness.

and then allowing light to enter. You can also check by shining a light into each eye and then removing the light. Pupils that are unequal, fully dilated or constricted, or unresponsive to light indicate a serious injury or illness (Fig. 5-23).

To check the neck, look and feel for any abnormalities (Fig. 5-24). If the casualty has not suffered an injury involving the head or trunk and does not have any pain or discomfort in the head, neck, or back, then there is little likelihood of spinal injury. You should proceed to check other body parts. If, however, you suspect a possible head or spine injury because of the ***mechanism of injury,*** such as a motor vehicle collision or a fall from a height, minimize movement to the casualty's head and spine. If you suspect head or spine injuries, take care of them first. Do not be concerned about finishing the secondary survey. You will learn techniques for stabilizing and immobilizing the head and spine in Chapter 13.

**If you do not suspect injury,** check the collarbones and shoulders by feeling for deformity (Fig. 5-25). Ask the casualty to shrug his or her shoulders. Check the chest by asking the casualty to take a deep breath and then blow the air out. Look and listen for signs of difficulty breathing. Feel the ribs for deformity (Fig. 5-26). Ask the casualty if he or she is experiencing pain.

Next, ask if the casualty has any pain in the abdomen. Apply slight pressure to each side of the abdomen, high and low (Fig. 5-27). The abdomen should be soft. If it is rigid, this indi-

cates a problem. Check the hips, asking the casualty if he or she has any pain. Place your hands on both sides of the pelvis and push down and in (Fig. 5-28).

Next, look and feel each leg for any deformity (Fig. 5-29). If there is no apparent sign of injury, ask the casualty to move his or her toes, foot, and leg. Then, check the back by gently reaching

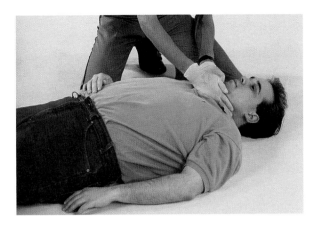

**Figure 5-24** To check the neck, look and feel for any abnormalities.

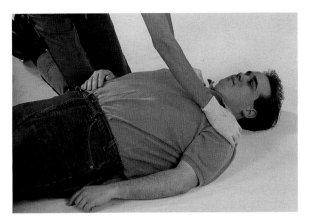

**Figure 5-25** Check the shoulders by looking and feeling for deformity. Ask the casualty to shrug his shoulders.

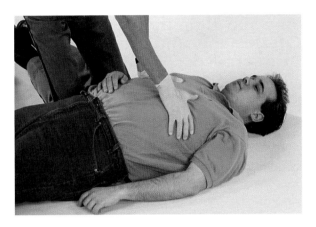

**Figure 5-26** Check the chest by feeling the ribs for deformity. Ask the casualty to take a deep breath and exhale.

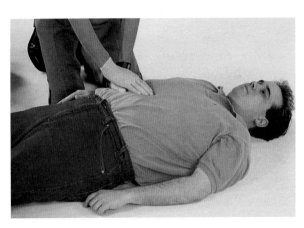

**Figure 5-27** Apply slight pressure to the abdomen to see if it is soft or rigid.

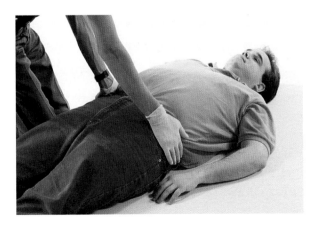

**Figure 5-28** To check the hips, place your hands on both sides of the pelvis and push down and in, asking the casualty if he or she feels any pain.

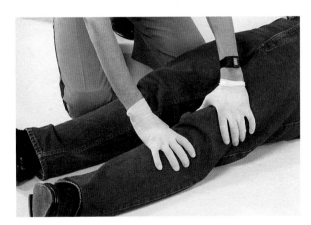

**Figure 5-29** Check the legs by feeling for any deformity. If there is no apparent sign of injury, ask the casualty to bend the legs and move the feet and toes.

under the casualty (Fig. 5-30). Finally, determine if the casualty has any pain in the arms or hands. Feel the arms for any deformity (Fig. 5-31). It is best to check only one extremity at a time. If there is no apparent sign of injury, ask the casualty if he or she can move the fingers, hand, and arm. Repeat this procedure on the other arm.

If the casualty can move all of the body parts without pain or discomfort and there are no other apparent signs or symptoms of injury, have him or her attempt to rest for a few minutes in a sitting position. If more advanced help is not needed, continue to check the signs and symptoms and monitor the ABCs.

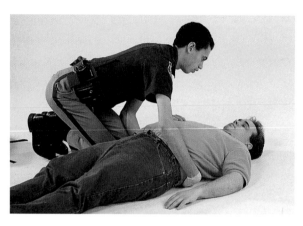

**Figure 5-30** Gently reach under the casualty to check the back.

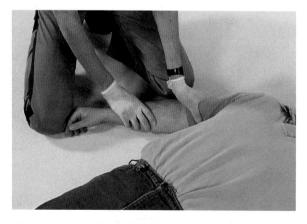

**Figure 5-31** Check the arms by feeling for any deformity. If there is no apparent sign of injury, ask the casualty to bend the arms and move the hands and fingers.

## Step Five: Keep Monitoring the Casualty's ABCs

If you have completed the secondary survey and have given care for any injuries and illness, continue to monitor the ABCs while you wait for advanced medical personnel to arrive. The casualty's condition can gradually worsen, or a life-threatening condition, such as respiratory or cardiac arrest, can occur suddenly. Do not assume that the casualty is out of danger just because there were no serious problems at first. Keep watching the casualty's level of consciousness, breathing, and skin colour. If any life-threatening conditions develop, *stop* whatever you are doing and provide care *immediately*.

## Step Six: Help the Casualty Rest Comfortably and Provide Reassurance

While waiting for advanced medical personnel, help the casualty stay calm and as comfortable as possible. Tell the casualty help is on the way and try to relieve the casualty's anxiety. Anxiety can actually make a casualty's condition worse. To prevent shock, maintain normal body temperature by protecting the casualty from cold or shading the casualty from excess heat.

## ♦ SUMMARY

When you respond to an emergency, remember to follow the six emergency action principles (EAPs). These principles guide your actions in any emergency. They remind you of what to do and when to do it. They ensure your safety and the safety of others. They also ensure that necessary or urgent care is provided for life-threatening emergencies. By following the EAPs, you will give the casualty of a serious illness or injury the best chance of survival.

Remember the EAPs:

♦ First, survey the scene. Make sure there are no dangers to you, the casualty, and bystanders.

◆ Second, check for responsiveness and call more advanced medical personnel if the casualty is unresponsive.

◆ Third, do a primary survey. Determine if there are any life-threatening conditions with the airway, breathing, or circulation, and care for them right away. Immediate care is essential for the casualty's survival. If needed, summon more advanced medical personnel now if they have not already been called. Provide necessary information about the casualty's condition.

◆ Fourth, if you find no life-threatening conditions, do a secondary survey to find and care for any other injuries. Problems that are not an immediate threat to life can become serious if you do not recognize them and provide care.

◆ Fifth, keep monitoring the casualty's ABCs while waiting for advanced medical personnel to arrive.

◆ Sixth, help the casualty rest comfortably and provide reassurance while waiting for advanced medical personnel.

Although the EAPs help you decide what care to give in any emergency, providing care is not an exact science. Because each emergency and each casualty is unique, an emergency may not occur exactly as it did in a classroom setting. Even within a single emergency, the care needed may change from one moment to the next. For example, the primary survey may indicate the casualty is conscious, breathing, has a pulse, and has no severe bleeding. However, during your secondary survey, you may notice the casualty beginning to experience difficulty breathing. At this point, you need to summon more advanced medical personnel if this has not already been done and provide appropriate care.

Many variables exist when dealing with emergencies. You do not need to "diagnose" what is wrong with the casualty to provide appropriate care. Use the EAPs as a tool to help you assess the casualty's condition. The EAPs ensure that you recognize life-threatening emergencies immediately. As you read the following chapters, remember the EAPs. They form the basis for providing care in any emergency (Fig. 5-32).

| Survey the scene | • Is it safe?<br>• What happened? |
|---|---|
| Assess unresponsiveness and phone EMS | If person is unresponsive:<br>• Send someone to call EMS.<br>• If alone call EMS before beginning a primary survey "CALL FIRST." |
| Begin a primary survey | • Is the casualty conscious?<br>• Does the casualty have an open airway?<br>• Is the casualty breathing?<br>• Are there signs of circulation—major bleeding?<br>• Is the person in shock? |
| Do a secondary survey | • Interview the casualty.<br>• Check vital signs.<br>• Perform a head-to-toe survey. |
| Monitor casualty's condition | • Continue checking vital signs. |
| Rest and reassure the casualty | • Treat for shock.<br>• Help casualty rest in the most comfortable position and give reassurance. |

**Figure 5-32** Use the EAPs to make care decisions in any emergency.

### YOU ARE THE RESPONDER

1. *During a basketball game, two players collide while diving for a loose ball. Both players fall to the floor. One player is holding her knee, screaming in pain. The second player is lying still but is moaning. No head or spinal injury is suspected. What would you do?*
2. *Which player are you inclined to check first and why?*

◆ **NOTES:**

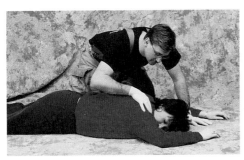

1. Check for responsiveness and call for help. If alone, "CALL FIRST."

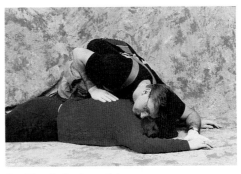

2. Check for breathing.

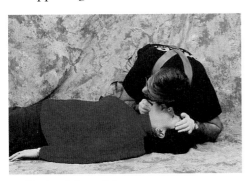

3. If uncertain whether casualty is breathing, roll casualty onto back, supporting head.

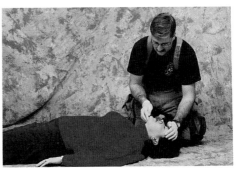

4. Tilt head back, lift chin, and open airway.

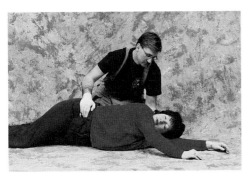

5. Recheck breathing.

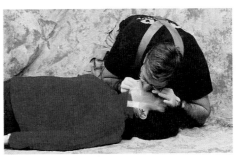

6. If not breathing, give 2 slow breaths.

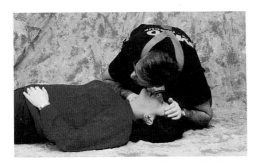

7. Check for signs of circulation (and pulse).

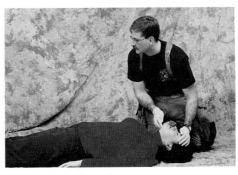

8. Check for bleeding.

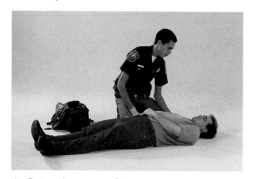

**1.** Interview casualty.

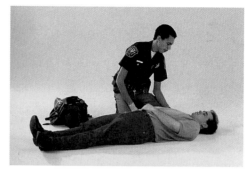

**2.** Check vital signs, beginning with level of consciousness.

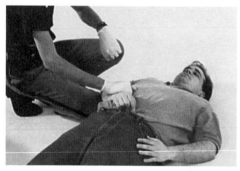

Check pulse.

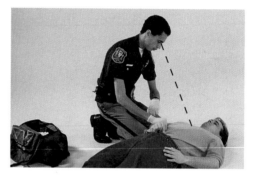

Check breathing.

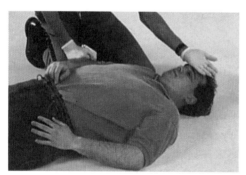

Check skin.

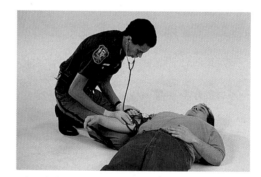

Check blood pressure.

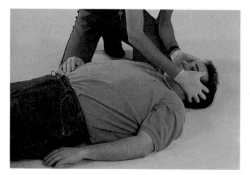

**3.** Do head-to-toe examination, beginning with head and neck.

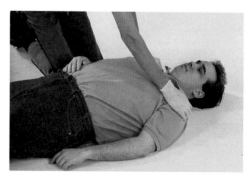

Check shoulders.

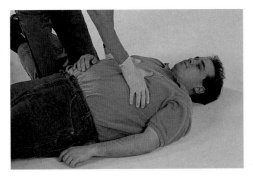

Check chest.

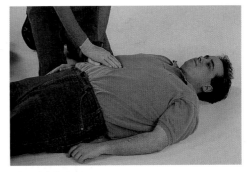

Check abdomen.

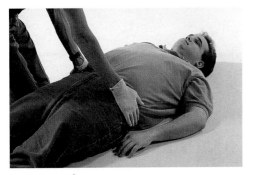

Check hips.

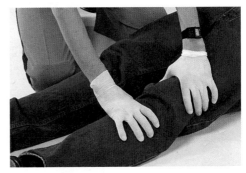

Check legs and feet.

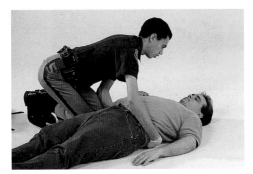

Check back.

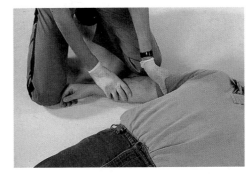

Check arms and hands.

# Measuring Blood Pressure (Palpation)

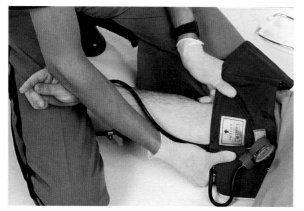

**1.** Position cuff.

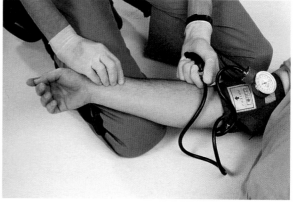

**2.** Locate radial pulse.

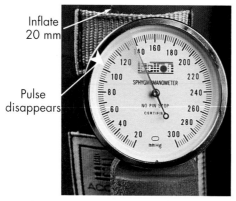

Inflate 20 mm

Pulse disappears

**3.** Inflate cuff beyond point where pulse disappears.

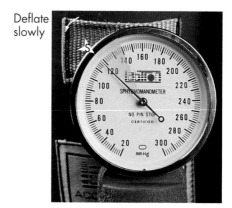

Deflate slowly

**4.** Deflate cuff slowly until pulse returns. This is approximate systolic blood pressure.

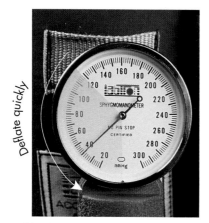

Deflate quickly

**5.** Quickly deflate cuff by opening valve.

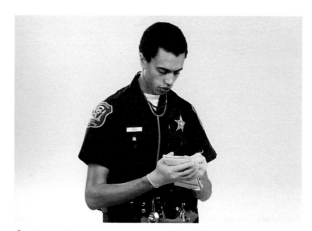

**6.** Record approximate systolic blood pressure.

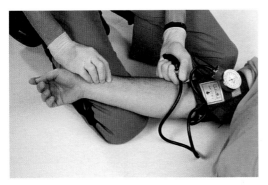

1. Approximate systolic blood pressure.

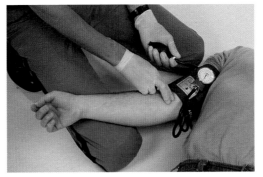

2. Locate brachial pulse.

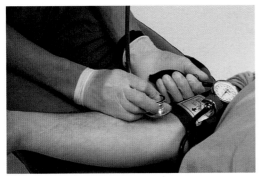

3. Position stethoscope.

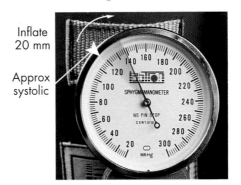

4. Inflate cuff 20 mm Hg beyond approximate systolic blood pressure.

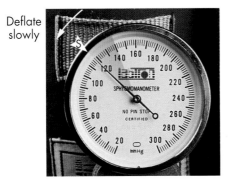

5. Deflate cuff slowly until pulse is heard (systolic).

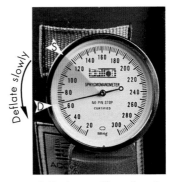

6. Continue deflating cuff until pulse disappears (diastolic).

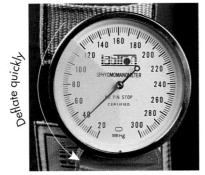

7. Quickly deflate cuff.

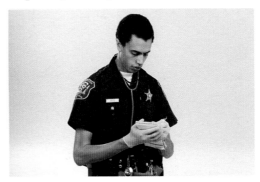

8. Record blood pressure (S/D).

95

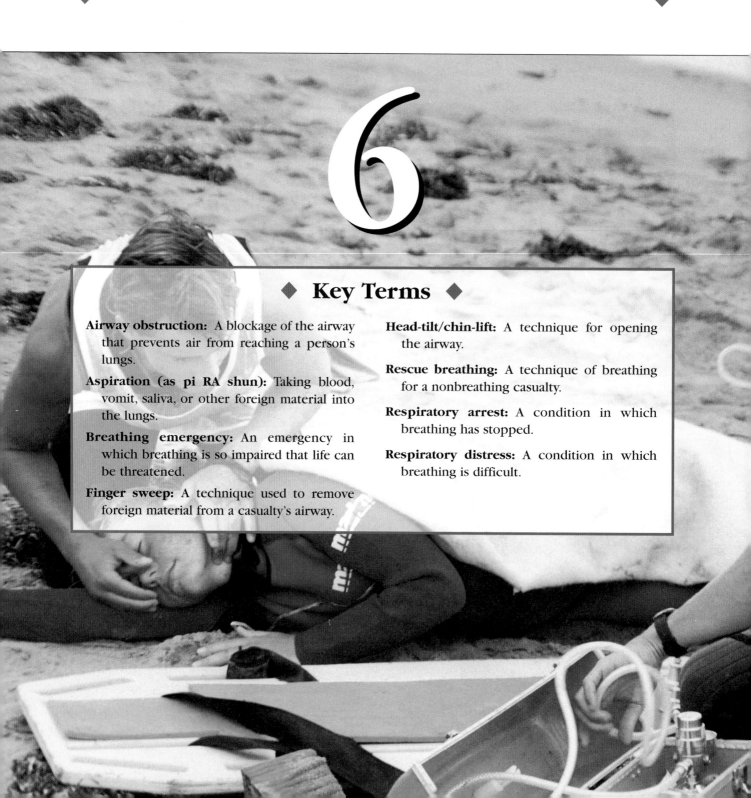

# Respiratory Emergencies

# 6

## ◆ Key Terms ◆

**Airway obstruction:** A blockage of the airway that prevents air from reaching a person's lungs.

**Aspiration (as pi RA shun):** Taking blood, vomit, saliva, or other foreign material into the lungs.

**Breathing emergency:** An emergency in which breathing is so impaired that life can be threatened.

**Finger sweep:** A technique used to remove foreign material from a casualty's airway.

**Head-tilt/chin-lift:** A technique for opening the airway.

**Rescue breathing:** A technique of breathing for a nonbreathing casualty.

**Respiratory arrest:** A condition in which breathing has stopped.

**Respiratory distress:** A condition in which breathing is difficult.

## ◆ For Review ◆

Before reading this chapter, you should have a basic understanding of the parts of the airway and how the respiratory and circulatory systems function (Chapter 3). You should also know the steps of the primary survey (Chapter 5).

## ◆ INTRODUCTION

In Chapter 3, you learned the parts of the airway and how the respiratory system functions. In Chapter 5, you learned that once you are sure the scene is safe, you begin a primary survey of the casualty. The primary survey detects any life-threatening conditions. First, check to see if the casualty is conscious. Then complete the primary survey by checking the ABCs.

> A = Airway/C-spine
> B = Breathing
> C = Circulation

In this chapter, you will learn how to care for breathing emergencies. Because oxygen is vital to life, you must always ensure that the casualty has an open airway and is breathing. You will often detect a breathing emergency during the primary survey. In a ***breathing emergency,*** a casualty's breathing is so impaired that life is threatened. This kind of emergency can occur in two ways—breathing becomes difficult or breathing stops. A person who is having difficulty breathing is in ***respiratory distress.*** A person who has stopped breathing is in ***respiratory arrest.***

## ◆ THE BREATHING PROCESS

Air enters the respiratory system through the nose and mouth and passes through the pharynx (Fig. 6-1). The pharynx divides into two

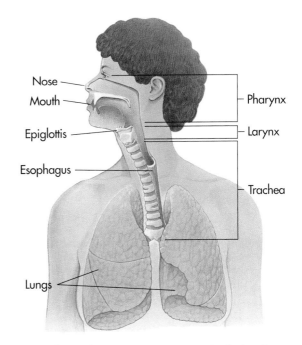

**Figure 6-1**  The respiratory system includes the pharynx, larynx, and trachea.

passageways: one for food, the esophagus, and one for air, the trachea. The epiglottis protects the opening of the trachea when a person swallows so that food and liquid do not enter the lungs.

The body requires a constant supply of oxygen for survival. When a person breathes oxygen into the lungs, the oxygen is transferred to the blood. The blood transports the oxygen to the brain, organs, muscles, and other parts of the body where it is used to provide energy. This energy allows the body to perform its many functions, such as breathing, walking, talking, digesting food, and maintaining body temperature. Different functions require different levels of energy and, therefore, different amounts of oxygen. For example, sitting in a chair requires less energy and less oxygen than jogging around the block. A body fighting off an illness, even the common cold, uses more energy and oxygen than a body in its healthy state. With illness, the body must carry out all regular functions and also fight the illness. Some tissues, such as brain tissue, are very sensitive to oxygen starvation. Without oxygen, brain cells begin to die in as few as 4 to 6 minutes (Fig. 6-2). Other vital

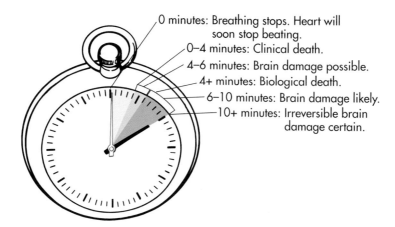

0 minutes: Breathing stops. Heart will soon stop beating.
0–4 minutes: Clinical death.
4–6 minutes: Brain damage possible.
4+ minutes: Biological death.
6–10 minutes: Brain damage likely.
10+ minutes: Irreversible brain damage certain.

**Figure 6-2**  In clinical death the heart and breathing stop. Clinical death can lead to biological death, which is the irreversible death of brain cells.

organs will also be affected unless oxygen supplies are restored.

The brain is the control centre for breathing. It adjusts the rate and depth of breaths according to the oxygen and carbon dioxide levels in the body. Breathing requires the respiratory, circulatory, nervous, and musculoskeletal systems to work together. As you read in Chapter 3, injuries or illnesses that affect any of these systems may cause breathing emergencies. For example, if the heart stops beating, the casualty will stop breathing. Injury or disease in areas of the brain that control breathing may impair breathing or stop it entirely. Damage to muscles or bones of the chest and back can make breathing difficult or painful.

Breathing emergencies can be caused by the following:

- An obstructed airway (choking).
- Illness, such as pneumonia.
- Respiratory conditions, such as emphysema and asthma.
- Electrocution.
- Shock.
- Drowning.
- Heart attack or heart disease.
- Injury to the chest or lungs.
- Allergic reactions, such as to food or to insect stings.
- Drugs.

- Poisoning, such as inhaling or ingesting toxic substances.

Other causes of breathing emergencies are discussed in later chapters.

## ◆ PREVENTION OF CHOKING

Choking can usually be prevented, if you are careful when eating. Follow these guidelines:

- Chew food well before swallowing; eat slowly and calmly. Be especially careful if you have dentures. Avoid talking or laughing with food in your mouth.
- Minimize alcohol consumption before and during meals.
- Avoid walking or other physical activity with food in your mouth.
- Keep other objects out of the mouth. For example, do not hold a pen cap or nails in your mouth when your hands are busy.

Infants and young are particularly at risk for choking. Parents and other supervisors should follow these guidelines:

- Feed children only when they are seated in a high chair or a secure seat. Do not let young children move about with food in their hands or mouth.

- Feed an infant or young child appropriate soft food in small pieces. Constantly watch the child when eating.
- Check the environment and all toys to be sure no small objects or parts are present that the infant or young child may put in the mouth.
- Keep young children away from balloons, which can burst into small pieces that can be easily inhaled.

## ◆ RESPIRATORY DISTRESS

Respiratory distress is the most common breathing emergency. It is not always caused by injuries or illnesses. It may also result from excitement or anxiety. Learn to recognize the signs and symptoms of respiratory distress.

## Signs and Symptoms of Respiratory Distress

The signs and symptoms of respiratory distress are usually obvious. Casualties may look as if they cannot catch their breath, or they may gasp for air. Their breaths may be unusually fast, slow, deep, or shallow. They may make unusual noises, such as wheezing or gurgling or high-pitched, shrill sounds.

The casualty's skin may also signal respiratory distress. At first, the skin may be unusually moist and appear flushed. Later, it may appear pale or bluish as the oxygen level in the blood falls. When the casualty's skin or the nail beds of the fingers or toes appear blue, the condition is called cyanosis.

Casualties may say they feel dizzy or light-headed. They may feel pain in the chest and tingling in the hands and feet. They may be apprehensive or fearful. Any of these symptoms is a clue that the casualty may be in respiratory distress. Table 6-1 lists the signs and symptoms of respiratory distress.

## Specific Types of Respiratory Distress

Although respiratory distress is often caused by injury, several other conditions also can cause it. These include asthma, bronchitis, emphysema, hyperventilation, and anaphylactic shock.

### Asthma

**Asthma** is a condition that narrows the air passages and makes breathing difficult. During an asthma attack, the air passages become constricted, or narrowed, by a spasm of the muscles lining the bronchi or by swelling of the bronchi themselves. Casualties may become anxious or frightened because breathing is difficult.

Asthma is more common in children and young adults. It may be triggered by an allergic reaction to food, pollen, a drug, or an insect sting. Emotional stress may also trigger it. For

---

**Table 6-1** Signs and Symptoms of Respiratory Distress

| Conditions | Signs and symptoms |
|---|---|
| Abnormal breathing | Breathing is unusually slow, rapid, deep, or shallow<br>Casualty is gasping for breath<br>Casualty is wheezing or gurgling or making high-pitched shrill noises |
| Abnormal skin appearance | Skin is unusually moist<br>Skin has a flushed, pale or ashen, or bluish appearance |
| How the casualty feels | Short of breath<br>Dizzy or lightheaded<br>Pain in the chest or tingling in hands and feet |

some people, physical activity induces asthma. Normally, someone with asthma easily controls attacks with medication. These medications stop the muscle spasm, opening the airway and making breathing easier.

A characteristic sign of asthma is wheezing when exhaling, which occurs because air becomes trapped in the lungs. This trapped air may also make the casualty's chest appear larger than normal, particularly in small children.

## Bronchitis

**Bronchitis** is a disease causing excessive mucous secretions and inflammatory changes to the bronchi. These secretions make breathing difficult. Bronchitis is often caused from prolonged exposure to irritants (most commonly, cigarette smoke). Casualties suffer from shortness of breath and the presence of cough with sputum. This disease will get worse over time.

## Emphysema

**Emphysema** is a disease in which the lungs lose their ability to exchange carbon dioxide and oxygen effectively. Emphysema is often caused by smoking and usually develops over many years.

Casualties suffer from shortness of breath. Exhaling is extremely difficult. They may cough and may have cyanosis or fever. Casualties with advanced cases may be restless, confused, and weak and can go into respiratory or cardiac arrest. People with chronic (long-lasting or frequently recurring) emphysema will get worse over time.

## Hyperventilation

**Hyperventilation** occurs when someone breathes faster than normal. This rapid breathing upsets the body's balance of oxygen and carbon dioxide. Hyperventilation is often the result of fear or anxiety and is more likely to occur in people who are tense and nervous. But it is also caused by injuries such as head injuries, by severe bleeding, or by conditions such as high fever, heart failure, lung disease, or diabetic emergencies. It can be triggered by asthma or exercise.

A characteristic sign of hyperventilation is shallow, rapid breathing. Despite their breathing efforts, casualties say that they cannot get enough air or that they are suffocating. Therefore, they are often fearful and apprehensive or may appear confused. They may say they feel dizzy or that their fingers and toes feel numb or tingly.

## Anaphylactic Shock

*While at a company picnic, a co-worker is stung by a hornet. You provide care for the sting and she returns to her activity. A few minutes later, she develops a rash and begins to feel tightness in her chest and throat. She is having difficulty breathing. She states that she feels her neck, face, and tongue begin to swell. She is a casualty of a life-threatening condition known as anaphylactic shock.*

**Anaphylactic shock,** also known as **anaphylaxis,** is a severe allergic reaction. The air passages may swell and restrict the casualty's breathing. Anaphylaxis may be caused by insect stings, food, or medications such as penicillin. Some people know that they have a severe allergic reaction to certain substances. They may therefore have learned to avoid these substances and may carry medication to reverse an allergic reaction. Medication may be carried in an **anaphylaxis kit.**

The signs and symptoms of anaphylaxis can include a rash, a feeling of tightness in the chest and throat, and swelling of the face, neck, and tongue. The person may also feel dizzy or confused. Anaphylactic shock is a life-threatening emergency requiring advanced medical care.

# Care for Respiratory Distress

Recognizing the signs and symptoms of respiratory distress and providing emergency care are often the keys to preventing other emergencies. Respiratory distress may signal the beginning of a life-threatening condition. For example, it can be the first signal of a more serious breathing emergency or even a heart attack. Respiratory distress can lead to respiratory arrest, which, if not cared for, will result in death.

Many of the signs and symptoms of different kinds of respiratory distress are similar. You do not need to know the specific cause to provide care. If the casualty is breathing, you know the heart is beating. Make sure the casualty is not bleeding severely. Help him or her rest in a comfortable position. Usually, sitting is more comfortable than lying down because breathing is easier. Open a window to provide more air if necessary. Reassure and comfort the casualty. Have bystanders move back. Make sure that more advanced medical personnel have been summoned.

When you are able, do a secondary survey. Remember that a casualty experiencing breathing difficulty may have trouble talking. Talk to any bystanders who may know about the casualty's problem. The casualty can confirm answers or answer yes-or-no questions by nodding. If possible, try to help reduce any anxiety; it may contribute to the casualty's breathing difficulty. Help the casualty take any prescribed medication for the condition if it is available. This may be oxygen or an inhalant (bronchial dilator) (Fig. 6-3). Continue to look and listen for any changes in the casualty's vital signs. Calm and reassure the casualty. Help maintain normal body temperature by preventing chilling or overheating.

If the casualty's breathing is rapid and there are signs of an injury or an underlying illness, call for more advanced help immediately. If the casualty's breathing is rapid and you suspect that it is caused by emotion, such as excitement, try to calm the casualty to slow his or her breathing. Reassurance is often enough to correct hyperventilation. But you can also ask the casualty to try to breathe with you. Breathe at a normal rate, emphasizing inhaling and exhaling.

If the condition does not improve, the casualty may become unconscious. Summon more advanced medical personnel if this has not already been done. Keep the casualty's airway open and monitor breathing. In many cases, hyperventilation caused by emotion will correct itself after the casualty becomes unconscious.

## ◆ RESPIRATORY ARREST

Respiratory arrest is the condition in which breathing stops. It may be caused by illness, injury, or an obstructed airway. The causes of respiratory distress can also lead to respiratory arrest. In respiratory arrest, the person gets no oxygen. The body can function for only a few minutes without oxygen before body systems begin to fail. Without oxygen, the heart muscle stops functioning. This causes the circulatory system to fail. When the heart stops, other body systems will also start to fail. However, you can keep the person's respiratory system functioning artificially with rescue breathing.

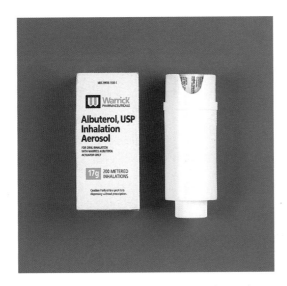

**Figure 6-3** An inhaler prescribed for asthma.

| Care for Respiratory Distress |
| --- |
| ◆ Complete a primary survey. |
| ◆ Contact more advanced personnel. |
| ◆ Help the casualty rest comfortably. |
| ◆ Do a secondary survey. |
| ◆ Reassure the casualty. |
| ◆ Assist with medication. |
| ◆ Maintain normal body temperature. |
| ◆ Monitor vital signs. |

# Rescue Breathing

***Rescue breathing*** is a technique of breathing air into a person to supply him or her with the oxygen needed to survive. Rescue breathing is given to casualties who are not breathing but still have a pulse.

Rescue breathing works because the air you breathe into the casualty contains more than enough oxygen to keep that person alive. The air you take in with every breath contains about 21 percent oxygen, but your body uses only a small part of that. The air you breathe out of your lungs and into the lungs of the casualty contains about 16 percent oxygen, enough to keep someone alive.

A first responder should always use a resuscitation mask when giving rescue breaths. You also should be able to perform rescue breathing in the event a resuscitation mask is not available. In this chapter, you will learn how to do rescue breathing. You will learn how to use a resuscitation mask in Chapter 8.

You will discover if you need to give rescue breathing during the first two steps of the ABCs in the primary survey, when you open the airway and check for breathing. If you cannot see, hear, or feel signs of breathing, give 2 slow breaths immediately to get air into the casualty's lungs. Then check for signs of circulation,

feel for the pulse, and look for severe bleeding. Call advanced medical personnel if you have not already done so.

If the casualty is not breathing but has a pulse, begin rescue breathing. To give breaths, keep the airway open with the head-tilt/chin-lift (Fig. 6-4, *A*). The ***head-tilt/chin-lift*** not only opens the airway by moving the tongue away from the back of the throat, but also moves the epiglottis from the opening of the trachea. Gently pinch the casualty's nose shut with the thumb and index finger of your hand that is on the casualty's forehead. Next, make a tight seal around the casualty's mouth with your mouth. Breathe slowly into the casualty until you see the casualty's chest gently rise (Fig. 6-4, *B*). Each breath should last a full 2 seconds, with a pause between breaths to let the air flow back out. Watch the casualty's chest rise each time you breathe to make sure that your breaths are actually going in.

If you do not see the casualty's chest rise and fall as you give a breath, you may not have the head tilted back far enough to open the airway adequately. Retilt the casualty's head and attempt to ventilate again. If air still does not go in, the casualty's airway is obstructed. You must give the care for the obstructed airway that is described later in this chapter.

A
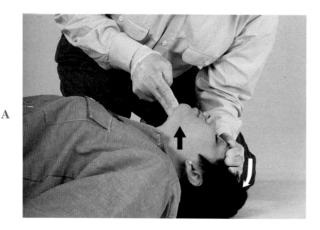
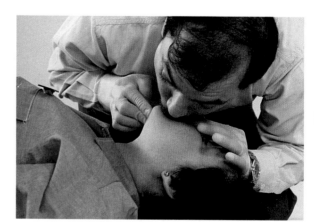
B

**Figure 6-4**  **A,** The head-tilt/chin-lift opens the casualty's airway. **B,** To breathe for a non-breathing casualty, seal your mouth around the casualty's mouth and breathe slowly into the casualty.

Once you are able to give 2 breaths, check for signs of circulation. If the casualty has signs of circulation but is not breathing, continue rescue breathing by giving 1 breath every 5 seconds. A good way to time the breaths is to count, "one one-thousand, two one-thousand, three one-thousand." Then take a breath on "four one-thousand," and breathe into the casualty on "five one-thousand." Counting this way ensures that you give 1 breath about every 5 seconds. Remember, breathe slowly into the casualty. Each breath should last a full 2 seconds.

After 1 minute of rescue breathing (about 12 breaths), recheck for signs of circulation to make sure the heart is still beating. If the casualty still has circulation but is not breathing, continue rescue breathing. Check for signs of circulation every minute. Do not stop rescue breathing unless one of the following occurs:

♦ The casualty begins to breathe on his or her own.
♦ The casualty has no signs of circulation. Begin CPR (described in Chapter 7).
♦ Another rescuer with training equal to or greater than yours takes over for you.
♦ You are too exhausted to continue.

# Special Considerations for Rescue Breathing

## Air in the Stomach

When you do rescue breathing, air normally enters the casualty's lungs. Sometimes, air may enter the casualty's stomach. There are several reasons why this may occur. First, breathing into the casualty longer than 2 seconds may cause extra air to fill the stomach. Do not overinflate the lungs. Stop the breath when the chest rises. Second, if the casualty's head is not tilted back far enough, the airway will not open completely. As a result, the chest may only rise slightly. This will cause you to breathe more forcefully, causing air to enter the stomach. Last, breaths given too quickly create more pressure in the airway, causing air to enter the stomach. Long, slow breaths minimize pressure in the air passages.

Air in the stomach is called **gastric distention.** Gastric distention can be a serious problem because it can make the casualty vomit. When an unconscious casualty vomits, stomach contents may get into the lungs, obstructing breathing. Taking such foreign material into the lungs is called *aspiration.* Because aspiration can hamper rescue breathing, it may eventually be fatal.

| **Table 6-2** How to Differentiate Among Breathing Emergencies | | |
|---|---|---|
| **Problem** | **Signs and symptoms** | **Care** |
| Respiratory distress | Gasping, wheezing<br>Fast and slow breathing<br>Deep or shallow breathing | Help casualty rest comfortably<br>Assist with prescribed medication, such as an inhalant or oxygen |
| Respiratory arrest | No apparent breathing | Begin rescue breathing |
| Choking—conscious casualty, partial obstruction | Coughing forcefully<br>Can speak and breathe<br>Wheezing | Encourage casualty to continue coughing |
| Choking—conscious casualty, complete obstruction | Coughing weakly<br>Cannot speak or breathe | Begin abdominal thrusts |
| Choking—unconscious casualty | No breathing<br>Breaths will not go in | Begin CPR sequence |
| Summon advanced medical personnel when necessary. | | |

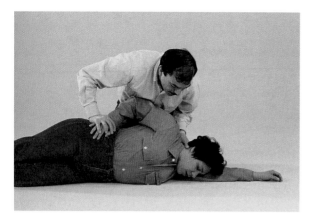

**Figure 6-5**   If vomiting occurs, turn the casualty on his or her side and clear the mouth of any matter.

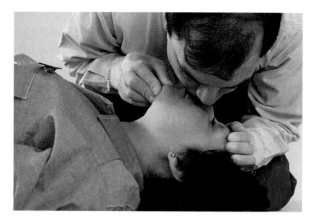

**Figure 6-6**   For mouth-to-nose breathing, close the casualty's mouth and seal your mouth around the casualty's nose. Breathe full breaths, watching the chest to see if the air goes in.

To avoid forcing air into the stomach, be sure to keep the casualty's head tilted back far enough. Breathe slowly into the casualty, just enough to make the chest rise. Pause between breaths long enough for the casualty's lungs to empty and for you to take another breath.

## Vomiting

When you give rescue breathing, the casualty may vomit. If this happens, turn the casualty's head and body together as a unit to the side (Fig. 6-5). This helps prevent vomit from entering the lungs. Quickly wipe the casualty's mouth clean, carefully reposition the casualty on his or her back, and continue with rescue breathing.

## Mouth-to-Nose Breathing

Sometimes you may not be able to make an adequate seal over a casualty's mouth to perform rescue breathing. For example, the person's jaw or mouth may be injured or shut too tightly to open, or your mouth may be too small to cover the casualty's. If so, provide mouth-to-nose rescue breathing as follows:

Maintain the head-tilt position with one hand on the forehead. Use your other hand to close the casualty's mouth, making sure to push on the chin, not on the throat.

Open your mouth wide, take a deep breath, seal your mouth tightly around the casualty's nose, and breathe full breaths into the casualty's

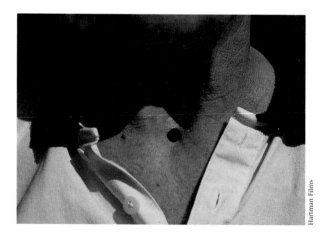

**Figure 6-7**   You may need to perform rescue breathing on a casualty with a stoma.

nose (Fig. 6-6). Open the casualty's mouth between breaths, if possible, to let air escape.

## Mouth-to-Stoma Breathing

Some people have had an operation that removed all or part of the **larynx,** the upper end of the windpipe. They breathe through an opening in the front of the neck called a **stoma** (Fig. 6-7). Air passes directly into the trachea through the stoma instead of through the mouth and nose.

Most people with a stoma wear a medical alert bracelet or necklace or carry a card identifying this condition. You may not see the stoma immediately. You will probably notice the opening in the neck as you tilt the head back to check for breathing.

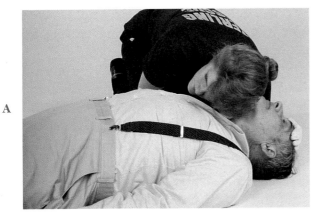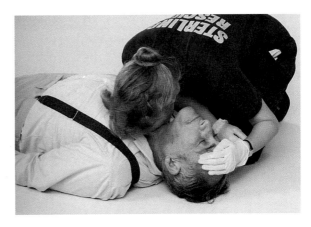

A                                                                                                                                    B

**Figure 6-8  A,** Look, listen, and feel for breathing with your ear over the stoma. **B,** Seal your mouth around the stoma and breathe into the casualty. You may need to tilt the head back to get the chin out of the way.

To give rescue breathing to someone with a stoma, you must give breaths through the stoma instead of the mouth or nose. Follow the same basic steps as in mouth-to-mouth breathing, except—

1. Look, listen, and feel for breathing with your ear over the stoma (Fig. 6-8, *A*).
2. Give breaths into the stoma, breathing at the same rate as for mouth-to-mouth breathing (Fig. 6-8, *B*).
3. Remove your mouth from the stoma between breaths to let air flow back out.

If the chest does not rise when you give rescue breaths, suspect that the casualty may have had only part of the larynx removed. That means that some air continues to flow through the larynx to the lungs during normal breathing. When giving mouth-to-stoma breathing, air may leak through the nose and mouth, diminishing the amount of oxygen that reaches the lungs. If this occurs, you need to seal the nose and mouth with your hand to prevent air from escaping during rescue breathing (Fig. 6-9).

## Casualties with Dentures

If you know or see the casualty is wearing **dentures,** do not automatically remove them. Dentures help rescue breathing by supporting the casualty's mouth and cheeks during mouth-to-mouth breathing. If the dentures are loose,

the head-tilt/chin-lift may help keep them in place. Remove the dentures *only* if they become so loose that they block the airway or make it difficult for you to give breaths.

## Suspected Head or Spinal Injuries

You should suspect head or spinal injuries in casualties who have suffered a violent force, such as that caused by a motor vehicle crash, a fall, or a diving or other sports-related incident. If you suspect the casualty may have an injury to the head, neck, or spine, you should try to minimize movement of the head and neck when opening the airway. This requires you to change the way you open the airway.

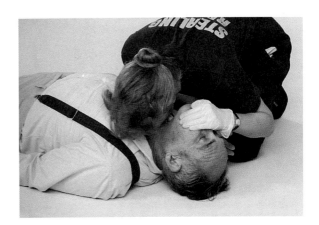

**Figure 6-9**  When performing rescue breathing on a casualty with a stoma, you may need to seal the casualty's nose and mouth to prevent air from escaping.

Open the airway by placing your fingers under the angles of the jaw and lifting (Fig. 6-10, *A*). Place your mouth over the casualty's, using your cheek to close the nose, and breathe (Fig. 6-10, *B*). This technique allows you to open the airway and provides rescue breathing without moving the head. Resuscitation masks may also be used when opening the airway in this manner.

## Infants and Children

Rescue breathing for infants and children follows the same general procedure as that for adults. The minor differences take into account the infant's or child's undeveloped physique and moderately faster heartbeat and breathing

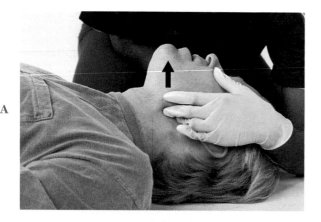

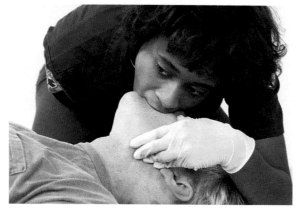

**Figure 6-10  A,** Use a two-handed jaw thrust when a chin-lift fails to open the airway of a casualty with a suspected head or spinal injury. **B,** Seal the nose with your cheek, and breathe into the casualty.

rate. Rescue breathing for infants and children uses less air in each breath, and breaths are delivered at a slightly faster rate.

You do not need to tilt a child's or infant's head as far back as an adult's to open the airway. Tilt the head back only far enough to allow your breaths to go in. Tipping the head back too far in a child or infant may cause injury that will obstruct the airway. Give 1 slow breath every 3 seconds for both a child and an infant. Figure 6-11 shows rescue breathing for an adult, a child, and an infant.

It is easier to cover both the mouth and nose of an infant with your mouth when giving breaths. Remember to breathe slowly into the casualty. Each breath should last about 1½ seconds. Be careful not to overinflate a child's or infant's lungs. Breathe only until you see the chest rise. After 1 minute of rescue breathing (about 20 breaths in a child or in an infant), recheck for signs of circulation.

## ◆ AIRWAY OBSTRUCTION

*Airway obstructions* are the most common cause of respiratory emergencies. The two types of airway obstruction are anatomical and mechanical.

An **anatomical obstruction** occurs when the airway is blocked by an anatomical structure, such as the tongue or swollen tissues of the mouth and throat. This type of obstruction may result from injury to the neck or a medical emergency, such as anaphylactic shock. The most common obstruction in an unconscious person is the tongue, which may drop to the back of the throat and block the airway. This occurs because muscles, including the tongue, relax when deprived of oxygen.

A **mechanical obstruction** occurs when the airway is blocked by a foreign object, such as a piece of food or a small toy, or fluids such as vomit, blood, mucus, or saliva. Someone with a mechanical obstruction may be choking.

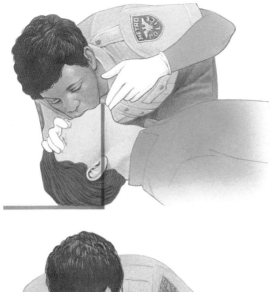

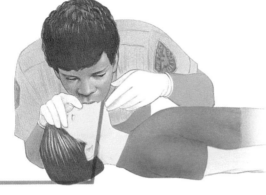

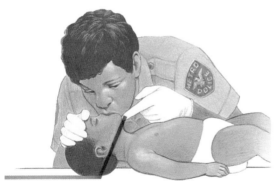

**Figure 6-11**   There are only minor differences in rescue breathing for adults, children, and infants. Often, the older the casualty, the greater the head tilt needed to help open the airway.

Common causes of choking include—

- Trying to swallow large pieces of poorly chewed food.
- Drinking alcohol before or during meals. Alcohol dulls the nerves that aid swallowing, making choking on food more likely.
- Wearing dentures. Dentures make it difficult for you to sense whether food is fully chewed before you swallow it.

- Eating while talking excitedly or laughing or eating too fast.
- Walking, playing, or running with food or objects in the mouth.

A casualty whose airway is blocked by a piece of food or another object can quickly stop breathing, lose consciousness, and die. You must be able to recognize that the airway is obstructed and give care immediately. This is why checking the airway comes first in the ABCs of the primary survey.

A casualty who is choking may have either a complete or partial airway obstruction. A casualty with a complete airway obstruction is not able to breathe at all. With a partial airway obstruction, the casualty's ability to breathe depends on how much air can get past the obstruction into the lungs.

## Partial Airway Obstruction

A casualty with a **partial airway obstruction** can still move air to and from the lungs. This air allows the person to cough in an attempt to dislodge the object. The casualty may also be able to move air past the vocal cords to speak. The narrowed airway causes a wheezing sound as air moves in and out of the lungs. As a natural reaction to choking, the casualty may clutch at the throat with one or both hands. This is universally recognized as a distress signal for choking (Fig. 6-12). If the casualty is coughing forcefully or wheezing, do not interfere with attempts to cough up the object. A casualty who has enough air to cough forcefully or speak also has enough air entering the lungs to breathe. Stay with the casualty and encourage him or her to continue coughing to clear the obstruction. If coughing persists, call for more advanced medical personnel.

## Complete Airway Obstruction

A partial airway obstruction can quickly become a complete airway obstruction. A casualty with a completely blocked airway is unable to speak,

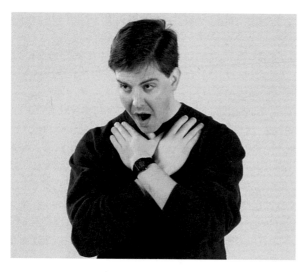

**Figure 6-12** Clutching the throat with one or both hands is universally recognized as a distress signal for choking.

cry, breathe, or cough effectively. Sometimes the casualty may cough weakly and ineffectively or make high-pitched noises. All of these signs tell you the casualty is not getting enough air to the lungs to sustain life. Act immediately. If you have not already done so, have a bystander call for more advanced medical personnel while you begin to give care.

## Care for Choking Casualties

When someone is choking, you must try to reopen the airway as quickly as possible. Give abdominal thrusts. This technique is also called the **Heimlich manoeuvre**. **Abdominal thrusts** compress the abdomen, increasing pressure in the lungs and airway. This simulates a cough, forcing trapped air in the lungs to push the object out of the airway like a cork from a bottle of champagne (Fig. 6-13).

The method you use depends on whether the casualty is conscious, unconscious and is an adult, child or infant. Variations are used for large adults or pregnant women who are conscious.

### Care for a Conscious Choking Adult

To give abdominal thrusts to a conscious choking adult, stand behind the casualty and wrap your arms around his or her waist (Fig. 6-14, *A*). The

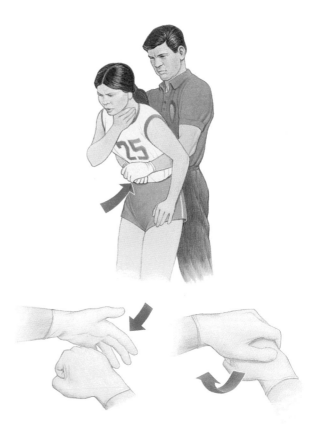

**Figure 6-13** Abdominal thrusts simulate a cough, forcing air trapped in the lungs to push the object out of the airway.

casualty may be seated or standing. Make a fist with one hand and place the thumb side against the middle of the casualty's abdomen just above the navel and well below the lower tip of the breastbone (Fig. 6-14, *B*). Grab your fist with your other hand, and give quick upward thrusts into the abdomen (Fig. 6-14, *C*). Repeat these thrusts until the object is dislodged or the casualty becomes unconscious.

### If You Are Alone and Choking

If you are choking and no one is around who can help, you can give yourself abdominal thrusts in two ways:

(1) Make a fist with one hand and place the thumb side on the middle of your abdomen slightly above your navel and well below the tip of your breastbone. Grasp your fist with your other hand and give a quick upward thrust.

(2) Lean forward and press your abdomen over any firm object, such as the back of a chair, a

railing, or a sink (Fig. 6-15). Be careful not to lean over anything with a sharp edge or a corner that might injure you.

## Care for a Conscious Choking Adult Who Becomes Unconscious

While giving abdominal thrusts to a conscious choking adult casualty, anticipate that the casualty will become unconscious if the obstruction is not removed. If this occurs, lower the casualty to the floor on his or her back. Have someone summon for advanced medical personnel immediately if this has not already been done.

Open the airway by grasping the lower jaw and lifting the jaw up. Look for an object at the back of the throat. If an object is seen, attempt to dislodge and remove the object by sweeping it out with your finger. This action is called a **finger sweep** (Fig. 6-16). Use a hooking action to remove the object. Be careful not to push the object deeper into the airway. A finger sweep should not be performed if the casualty is conscious or convulsing. Next, try to open the casualty's airway, using the head-tilt/chin-lift method and check for effective breathing. Attempt to ventilate. Often the throat muscles relax enough after the person becomes unconscious, allowing air past the obstruction and into the lungs. If the air does not go into the lungs, re-tilt and try again. If air still does not go in, assume that the airway is obstructed and begin the CPR sequence (15 chest compressions).

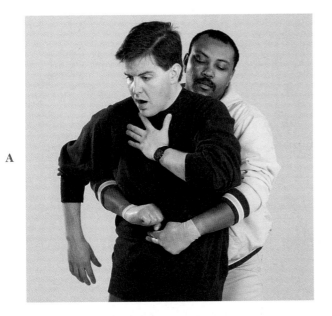
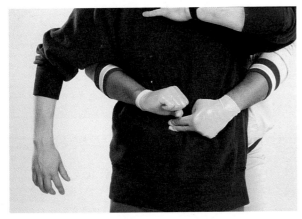
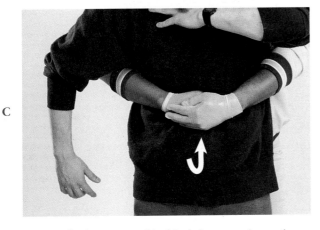

**Figure 6-14 A,** Stand behind the casualty and wrap your arms around his or her waist to give abdominal thrusts. **B,** Place the thumb side of your fist against the middle of the casualty's abdomen. **C,** Grasp your fist with your other hand and give quick upward thrusts into the abdomen.

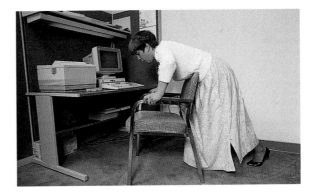

**Figure 6-15** To give yourself abdominal thrusts, press your abdomen onto a firm object, such as the back of a chair.

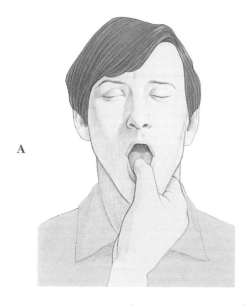

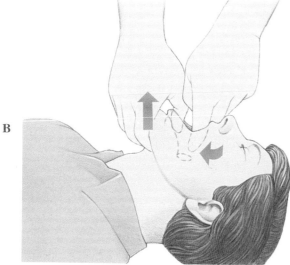

**Figure 6-16 A,** To do a finger sweep, first lift the lower jaw. **B,** Use a hooking action to sweep the object out of the airway.

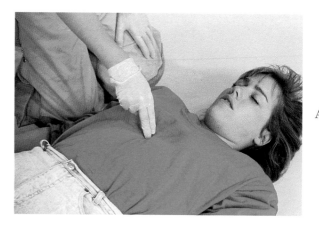

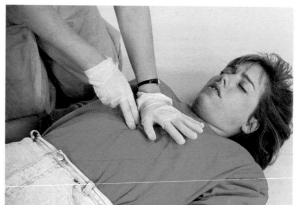

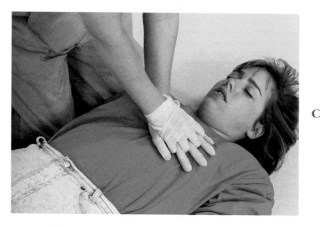

**Figure 6-17** To locate compression position, **A,** find the notch where the lower ribs meet the sternum. **B,** Place the heel of your hand on the sternum, next to your index finger. **C,** Place your other hand over the heel of the first hand. Use the heel of your bottom hand to apply pressure on the sternum.

Chest compressions are performed just as they are in CPR (Fig. 6-17) and are proven to be effective in dislodging an object in the throat. Many casualties who have an obstructed airway will also not have circulation, so chest compressions will not only be effective in dislodging the obstruction, but will also provide necessary care for absence of circulation.

After 15 chest compressions, open the airway and look in the mouth. If you see an object, remove it, then attempt to ventilate. Remember, if necessary, to reposition the head to adjust the airway. If you are still not able to get air into the casualty's lungs, continue the CPR sequence, always looking in the mouth prior to the ventilation attempt. Repeat the sequence until the object is expelled, you can breathe into the casualty, or other trained personnel arrive and take over. If you see any change in the person's condition, stop CPR and reassess the ABCs.

## Care for an Unconscious Adult with an Obstructed Airway

During your primary survey, you may discover that an unconscious adult casualty is not breathing and that the first breath you give will not go in. If this happens, re-tilt the head and attempt to ventilate again. You may not have tilted the casualty's head back correctly. If air still does not go in, assume the casualty's airway is obstructed and begin the CPR sequence (15 chest compressions).

After giving 15 chest compressions, look in the mouth. If you see an object, it should be carefully removed but not discarded. Use a finger sweep then attempt to ventilate. Remember, if necessary, to reposition the head to adjust the airway. If you are still not able to breathe air into the casualty's lungs, repeat the CPR sequence, always looking in the mouth prior to the ventilation attempt.

If your first attempts to clear the airway are unsuccessful, *do not stop.* The longer the casualty goes without oxygen, the more the muscles will relax, making it easier to clear the airway.

Once you are able to breathe air into the casualty's lungs, give 2 full breaths. Then complete the primary survey by checking the casualty for signs of circulation and checking and caring for any severe bleeding. If there are no signs of circulation, begin CPR (see Chapter 7). If the casualty has signs of circulation but is not breathing on his or her own, continue rescue breathing.

If the casualty starts breathing on his or her own, maintain an open airway and continue to monitor both breathing and circulation until more advanced medical personnel arrive and take over. Place the casualty in the recovery position, as described in Chapter 5.

### When to Stop Care

Stop giving chest thrusts or chest compressions immediately if the object is dislodged or if the person begins to breathe or cough. Make sure the object is cleared from the airway, and the person is breathing freely again. Even after the object is coughed up, the person may still have breathing problems that you do not immediately see. You should also realize that abdominal thrusts, chest compressions and chest thrusts (described in the next section) may cause internal injuries. *Therefore, anytime this type of care is used to dislodge an object, the casualty should be taken to the nearest hospital emergency department for follow-up care, even if he or she seems to be breathing without difficulty.*

## Special Considerations for Choking Casualties

In some instances, abdominal thrusts are not the best method of care for choking casualties. Some choking casualties need chest thrusts. For example, if you cannot reach far enough around the casualty to give effective abdominal thrusts, you should give chest thrusts. You should also give chest thrusts instead of abdominal thrusts to noticeably pregnant choking casualties.

### Chest Thrusts for a Conscious Casualty

To give **chest thrusts** to a conscious casualty, stand behind the casualty and place your arms

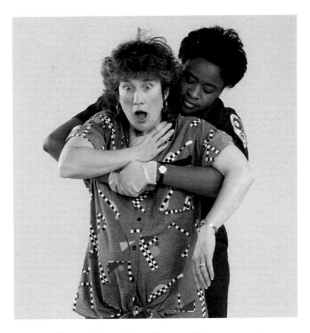

**Figure 6-18**   Give chest thrusts if you cannot reach around the casualty to give abdominal thrusts or if the casualty is noticeably pregnant.

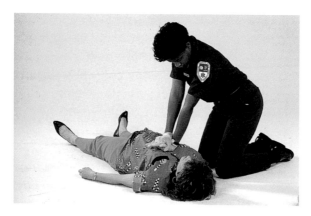

**Figure 6-19** Use the same technique for all types of unconscious adult casualties with an obstructed airway.

under the casualty's armpits and around the chest. As for abdominal thrusts, make a fist with one hand, placing the thumb side against the centre of the casualty's breastbone. Be sure that your thumb is centered on the breastbone, not on the ribs. Also, make sure that your fist is not near the lower tip of the breastbone. Grab your fist with your other hand and thrust inward

(Fig. 6-18). Repeat these thrusts until the object is dislodged or the casualty becomes unconscious.

If the casualty becomes unconscious, position the casualty on his or her back. Once positioned, use the same techniques as described earlier in this chapter (Fig 6-19).

# Children and Infants

Choking emergencies are common in children and infants. Emergency care for a choking child is similar to the care for a choking adult. The only significant difference involves considering the child's size. Obviously, you cannot use the same force when giving abdominal thrusts to a child to expel the object. Care for infants who are choking includes a combination of chest thrusts given with two fingers and back blows. Abdominal thrusts are not used for a choking infant because of their potential to cause injury.

## Care for a Conscious Choking Child

If you suspect that a child is choking, begin the primary survey by asking, "Are you choking?" If

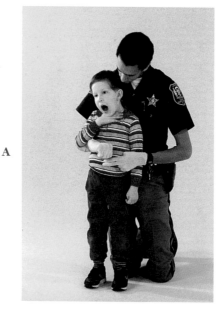
A

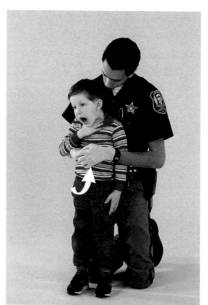
B

**Figure 6-20** To give abdominal thrusts to a child, **A,** stand or kneel behind the child. Wrap your arms around the child's waist. Make a fist with one hand. Place the thumb side of your fist against the middle of the child's abdomen, just above the navel and well below the tip of the breastbone. **B,** Grasp your fist with your other hand and give quick upward thrusts into the abdomen.

you have not already done so, call more advanced medical personnel for help. Continue care as you would for an adult.

Give abdominal thrusts. Stand or kneel behind the child. Wrap your arms around the child's waist. Make a fist with one hand. Place the thumb side of your fist against the middle of the child's abdomen, just above the navel and well below the lower tip of the breastbone. Grasp your fist with your other hand and give quick upward thrusts into the abdomen (Fig. 6-20). Repeat the thrusts until the obstruction is cleared or the child becomes unconscious.

If the child coughs up the object or starts to breathe or cough, continue to watch the child to ensure that he or she is breathing again. Even though the child may be breathing well, remember that he or she may have other problems that will require a doctor's attention. It is best that the child be examined by more advanced medical personnel.

## Care for Unconscious Child with an Obstructed Airway

If during the primary survey, you determine that an unconscious child has a complete airway obstruction, begin the CPR sequence (5 chest compressions), look in the mouth, do a finger sweep if you see the object, open the airway and attempt to ventilate (Fig. 6-21). If necessary, reposition the head to adjust the airway.

Repeat the CPR sequence until the obstruction is removed, the child starts to breathe or cough, or advanced medical personnel take over. Once you are able to breathe air into the casualty's lungs, give 2 full breaths. Check for signs of circulation and bleeding and care for any conditions you find.

## Care for a Conscious Choking Infant

If, during the primary survey, you determine that a conscious infant cannot breathe, cough, or cry, give care for a complete airway obstruc-

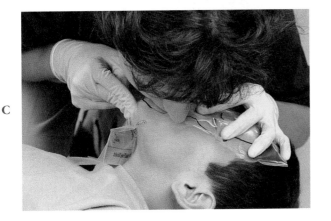

A

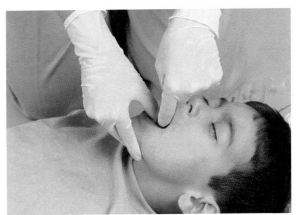

B

C

**Figure 6-21** To care for an unconscious child with a complete airway obstruction, **A,** give 5 chest compressions. **B,** Do a finger sweep if you see the object. **C,** Open the airway and attempt to ventilate.
*Courtesy of the American Red Cross.*
*All rights reserved in all countries.*

A

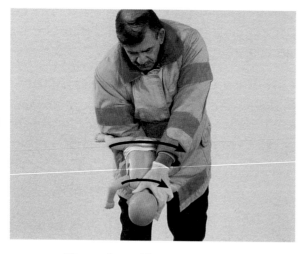

B

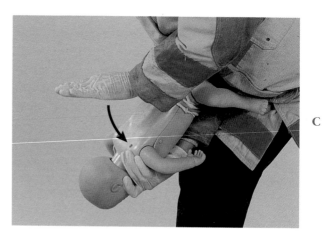

C

**Figure 6-22** To give back blows, **A,** sandwich the infant between your forearms. Support the infant's head and neck by holding the jaw between your thumb and forefinger. **B,** Turn the infant over so that he or she is face down on your forearm. **C,** Give 5 firm back blows with the heel of your hand while supporting your arm that is holding the infant on your thigh.

tion. Begin by giving 5 back blows followed by 5 chest thrusts.

Start by positioning the infant faceup on your forearm. Place your other arm on top of the infant, using your thumb and fingers to hold the infant's jaw while sandwiching the infant between your forearms (Fig. 6-22, *A*). Turn the infant over so that he or she is facedown on your forearm (Fig. 6-22, *B*). Lower your arm onto your thigh so that the infant's head is lower than his or her chest. Give 5 firm back blows with the heel of your hand between the infant's

shoulder blades (Fig. 6-22, *C*). Maintain support of the infant's head and neck by firmly holding the jaw between your thumb and forefinger.

To give chest thrusts, you will need to turn the infant back over. Start by placing your free hand and forearm along the infant's head and back so that the infant is sandwiched between your two hands and forearms. Continue to support the infant's head between your thumb and fingers from the front while you cradle the back of the head with your other hand (Fig. 6-23, *A*).

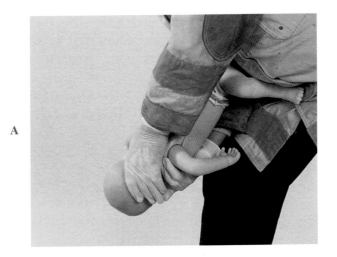

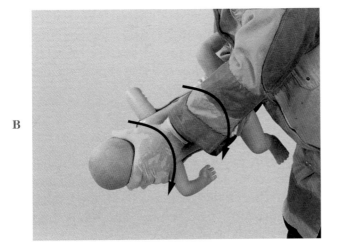

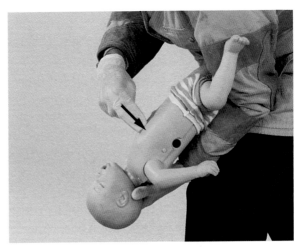

**Figure 6-23**  To give chest thrusts, **A,** sandwich the infant between your forearms. Continue to support the infant's head. **B,** Turn the infant onto his or her back and support your arm on your thigh. The infant's head should be lower than the chest. **C,** Give 5 chest thrusts.

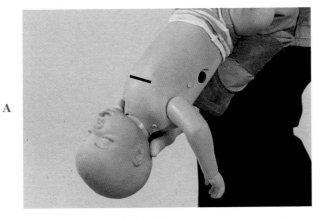

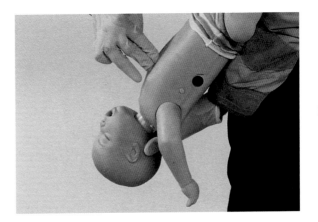

**Figure 6-24**  To locate the correct place to give chest thrusts, **A,** imagine a line running across the infant's chest between the nipples. **B,** Place the pad of your ring finger on the breastbone just under this imaginary line. Place the pads of the two fingers next to the ring finger just under the nipple line. Raise the ring finger.

Turn the infant onto his or her back. Lower your arm that is supporting the infant's back onto your thigh. The infant's head should be lower than his or her chest (Fig. 6-23, *B*). Give 5 chest thrusts (Fig. 6-23, *C*).

To locate the correct place to give chest thrusts, imagine a line running across the infant's chest between the nipples (Fig. 6-24, *A*). Place the pad of your ring finger on the breastbone just under this imaginary line. Then place the pads of the two fingers next to the ring finger just under the nipple line. Raise the ring finger (Fig. 6-24, *B*). If you feel the notch at the end of the infant's breastbone, move your fingers up a little bit.

Use the pads of the two fingers to compress the breastbone. Compress the breastbone 1.2 to 2.5 cm (1/2 to 1 inch), then let the breastbone return to its normal position. Keep your fingers in contact with the infant's breastbone. Compress 5 times. You can give back blows and chest thrusts effectively whether you stand up or sit. If the infant is large or your hands are too small to adequately support the infant, you may prefer to sit. Place the infant in your lap to give back blows and chest thrusts. The infant's head should be lower than the chest (Fig. 6-25).

Keep giving back blows and chest thrusts until the object is coughed up or the infant begins to breathe or cough. Summon more advanced medical personnel if you have not already done so. Even if the infant seems to be breathing well, he or she should be examined by more advanced medical personnel.

## Care for Unconscious Infant with an Obstructed Airway

Like the care for an adult and a child, the care for an unconscious infant with a complete airway obstruction begins with a primary survey. If, while doing the ABC steps, you determine that you cannot get air into the lungs, retilt the head and reattempt the ventilation. If you still cannot breathe air into the infant, start the CPR sequence. Give 5 chest compressions, then look in the mouth. Next, do a foreign body check, open the airway and attempt to ventilate. Remember, if necessary, to reposition the head to adjust the airway.

To do a foreign-body check—

♦ Stand or kneel beside the infant's head.
♦ Open the infant's mouth, using your hand that is nearer the infant's feet. Put your thumb into the infant's mouth and hold both the tongue and the lower jaw between the thumb and fingers. Lift the jaw upward (Fig. 6-26, *A*).
♦ Look for an object. If you can see it, try to remove it by doing a finger sweep with the little finger (Fig. 6-26, *B*).

If your first attempts to clear the airway are unsuccessful, *do not stop*. Repeat the CPR sequence until you are able to get air in the infant's lungs.

If you are able to breathe air into the infant's lungs, finish the primary survey. Give 2 slow puffs as you did for rescue breathing, and check the infant's signs of circulation and brachial pulse. Next, check and care for any severe bleeding. If the infant has no circulation, begin CPR, which you will learn in Chapter 7. If the infant has signs of circulation and is not breathing on his or her own, continue rescue breathing.

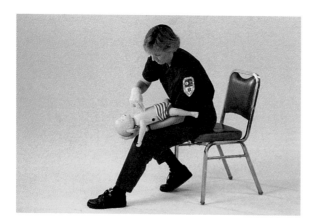

**Figure 6-25** If you cannot adequately support the infant, put him or her on your lap with the head lower than the chest.

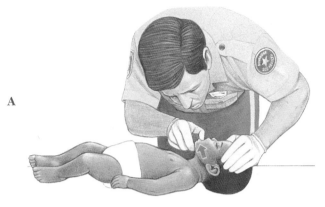

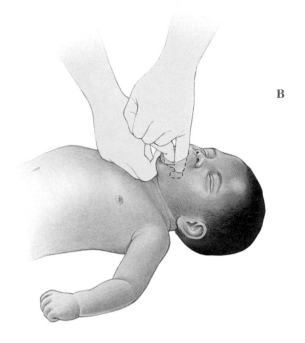

A

B

**Figure 6-26** To do a finger sweep on an infant, **A,** put your thumb into the infant's mouth and hold the tongue and lower jaw between the thumb and fingers. Lift the jaw upward. **B,** If you see an object, try to remove it by doing a finger sweep using the little finger.

If the infant starts breathing on his or her own, complete a secondary survey, continue to maintain an open airway, and monitor breathing and circulation until more advanced personnel arrive and take over.

## ◆ SUMMARY

In this chapter, you learned how to recognize and provide care for breathing emergencies. You now know to look for a breathing emergency in the primary survey because it can be life threatening. You learned the signs and symptoms of respiratory distress and respiratory arrest and the appropriate care for each condition. You also learned the basic techniques for rescue breathing and for special situations. Finally, you learned how to care for choking casualties, both conscious and unconscious. By knowing how to care for breathing emergencies, you are now better prepared to care for other emergencies. You will learn about cardiac emergencies in Chapter 7.

### YOU ARE THE RESPONDER

*You arrive at a scene to find a distraught mother who says, "I can't wake my baby up." You determine that the baby is unconscious, is not breathing, but has a pulse. What do you do?*

◆ **NOTES:**

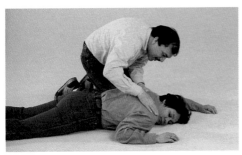

1. Check for responsiveness and call for help. If alone, "CALL FIRST.".

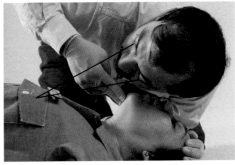

2. Open airway—check for breathing.

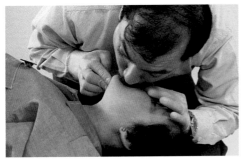

3. No breathing—give 2 slow breaths.

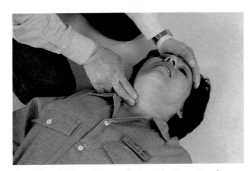

4. Check for signs of circulation (and carotid pulse).

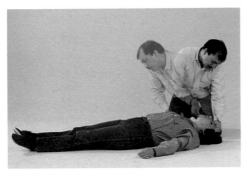

5. Check for severe bleeding.

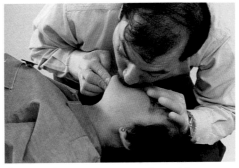

6. Circulation present, no breathing—begin rescue breathing. Give 1 slow breath every 5 seconds for an adult (1 slow breath every 3 seconds for a child).

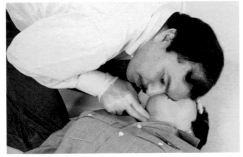

7. Recheck breathing and circulation after each minute.

# Rescue Breathing for an Infant

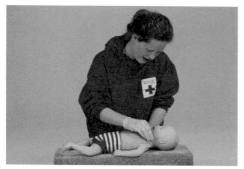

**1.** Check for responsiveness and call for help. If alone, "CALL FIRST."

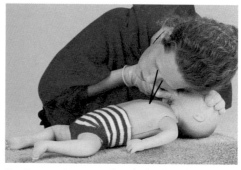

**2.** Open airway—check for breathing.

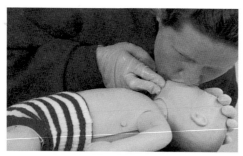

**3.** No breathing—give 2 slow puffs.

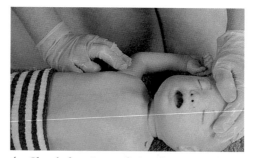

**4.** Check for signs of circulation (and brachial pulse).

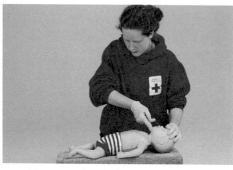

**5.** Check for severe bleeding.

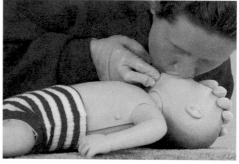

**6.** Circulation present, no breathing—begin rescue breathing. Give 1 slow puff every 3 seconds.

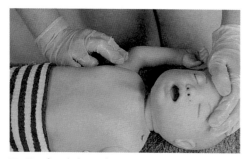

**7.** Recheck breathing and circulation after each minute.

120

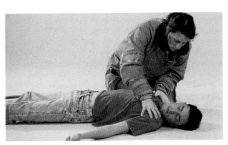

1. Check for responsiveness and call for help. If alone, "CALL FIRST."

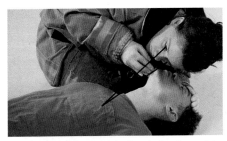

2. Open airway and check for breathing.

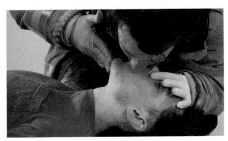

3. Attempt to ventilate.

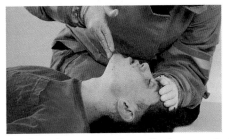

4. If air does not go in, retilt the casualty's head and try again.

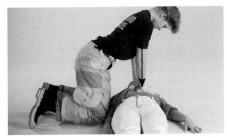

5. Begin CPR. For an adult, give 15 chest compressions.

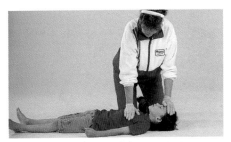

6. For a child, give 5 chest compressions.

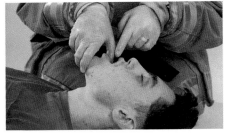

7. Look in the mouth. If you see an object, sweep it out.

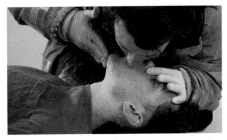

8. Open airway and attempt to ventilate. Remember, if necessary, to reposition the head to adjust the airway.

If air still does not go in, repeat the CPR sequence (Adult: 15 compressions, Child: 5 compressions) looking into the mouth prior to the ventilation attempt.

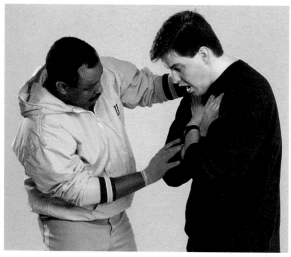

**1.** Determine if casualty is choking.

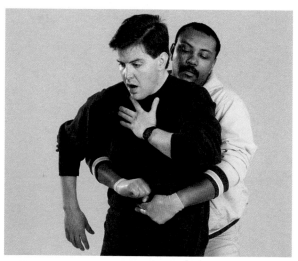

**2.** Position yourself to give abdominal thrusts.

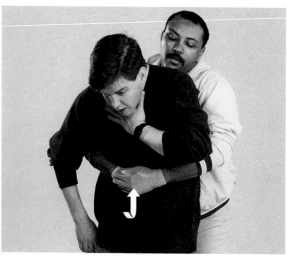

**3.** Give abdominal thrusts.

Repeat thrusts until object is expelled or casualty becomes unconscious.

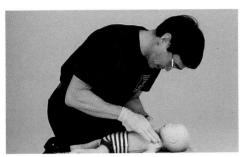

1. Check for responsiveness and call for help. If alone, "CALL FIRST."

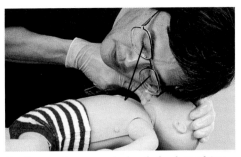

2. Open airway and check for breathing.

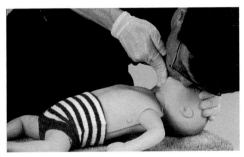

3. Attempt to ventilate.

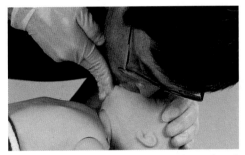

4. If air does not go in, retilt infant's head and try again.

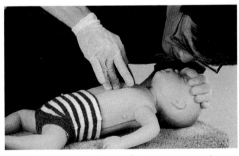

5. Begin CPR with 5 chest compressions.

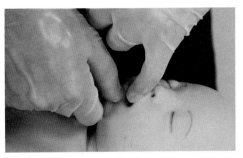

6. Look in the mouth. If you see an object, sweep it out.

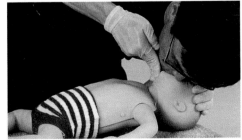

7. Open airway and attempt to ventilate. Remember, if necessary, to reposition the head to adjust the airway.

If air still does not go in, repeat the CPR sequence looking in the mouth prior to the ventilation attempt.

# Cardiac Emergencies

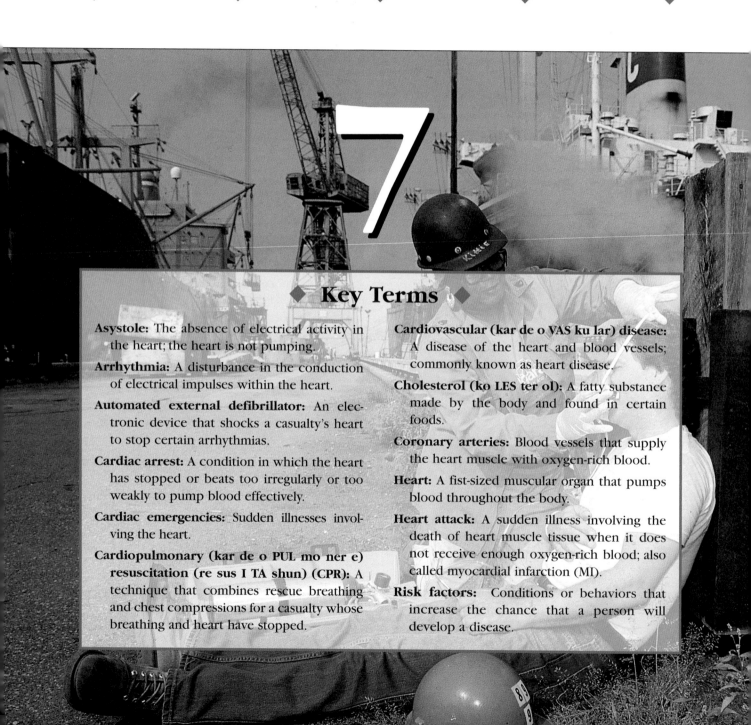

7

## Key Terms

**Asystole:** The absence of electrical activity in the heart; the heart is not pumping.

**Arrhythmia:** A disturbance in the conduction of electrical impulses within the heart.

**Automated external defibrillator:** An electronic device that shocks a casualty's heart to stop certain arrhythmias.

**Cardiac arrest:** A condition in which the heart has stopped or beats too irregularly or too weakly to pump blood effectively.

**Cardiac emergencies:** Sudden illnesses involving the heart.

**Cardiopulmonary (kar de o PUL mo ner e) resuscitation (re sus I TA shun) (CPR):** A technique that combines rescue breathing and chest compressions for a casualty whose breathing and heart have stopped.

**Cardiovascular (kar de o VAS ku lar) disease:** A disease of the heart and blood vessels; commonly known as heart disease.

**Cholesterol (ko LES ter ol):** A fatty substance made by the body and found in certain foods.

**Coronary arteries:** Blood vessels that supply the heart muscle with oxygen-rich blood.

**Heart:** A fist-sized muscular organ that pumps blood throughout the body.

**Heart attack:** A sudden illness involving the death of heart muscle tissue when it does not receive enough oxygen-rich blood; also called myocardial infarction (MI).

**Risk factors:** Conditions or behaviors that increase the chance that a person will develop a disease.

## ◆ Key Terms ◆

**Sternum:** The long, flat bone in the middle of the front of the rib cage; also called the breastbone.

**Ventricular fibrillation:** A life-threatening arrhythmia in which the heart muscle quivers rather than pumping blood.

**Ventricular tachycardia:** A life-threatening arrhythmia in which the heart muscle contracts too quickly for an adequate pumping of blood to the body.

## ◆ For Review ◆

Before reading this chapter, you should have a basic understanding of how the respiratory and circulatory systems function (Chapter 3) and be able to do a primary survey (Chapter 5) and rescue breathing (Chapter 6).

## ◆ INTRODUCTION

In the primary survey, you identify and care for immediate threats to a casualty's life. Your priorities are to care for the casualty's airway, breathing, and circulation (the ABCs). In Chapter 5, you learned how to open a casualty's airway and assess breathing. In Chapter 6, you learned how to provide rescue breathing for a casualty who has signs of circulation but is not breathing.

In this chapter, you will learn how to recognize and provide care for *cardiac emergencies,* sudden illnesses involving the heart. You will learn the care for a casualty with persistent chest pain and for a casualty whose heart stops beating. The condition in which the heart stops, known as *cardiac arrest,* sometimes results from a heart attack. To provide care for a cardiac arrest casualty, you need to learn how to perform cardiopulmonary resuscitation (CPR). Properly performed, CPR can keep a casualty's vital organs supplied with oxygen-rich blood until more highly trained personnel arrive to provide advanced care.

This chapter also identifies the important risk factors for cardiovascular disease. It is as important to prevent heart attack and cardiac arrest as it is to learn how to recognize them when they occur and provide appropriate care. Learn to modify your behavior to prevent cardiovascular disease.

## ◆ HEART ATTACK

The *heart* is a muscular organ about the size of your fist that functions like a pump. It lies between the lungs, in the middle of the chest, behind the lower half of the **sternum** (breastbone). The heart is protected by the ribs and sternum in front and by the spine in back (Fig. 7-1). It has four chambers and is separated into right and left halves. Oxygen-poor blood enters the right side of the heart and is pumped to the lungs, where it picks up oxygen. The now oxygen-rich blood returns to the left side of the heart, from where it is pumped to all parts of the body. One-way valves direct the flow of blood as it moves through each of the heart's four chambers (Fig. 7-2). For the circulatory system to be effective, the respiratory

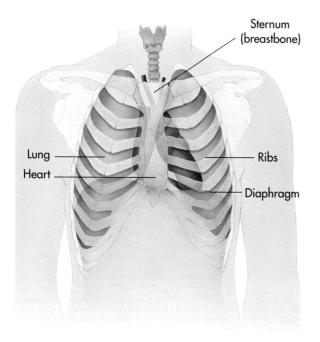

**Figure 7-1** The heart is located in the middle of the chest, behind the lower half of the sternum.

system must also be working so that the blood can pick up oxygen in the lungs.

Like all living tissue, the cells of the heart need a continuous supply of oxygen. The *coronary arteries* supply the heart muscle with oxygen-rich blood (Fig. 7-3, *A*). If heart muscle tissue is deprived of this blood, it dies and the casualty often develops certain signs and symptoms. If too much tissue dies, the heart will not be able to pump effectively. When heart tissue dies, it is called a *heart attack.*

A heart attack interrupts the heart's electrical system. This may result in an irregular heartbeat, which prevents blood from circulating effectively.

## Common Causes of Heart Attack

Heart attack usually results from cardiovascular disease. *Cardiovascular disease*—disease of the heart and blood vessels—is a leading cause of death for adults in Canada. About 80,000 deaths in Canada each year are attributed to cardiovascular disease. Of these, more than half are due to heart attack, and most of them are sudden deaths.

Cardiovascular disease develops slowly. Deposits of **cholesterol,** a fatty substance made by the body, and other material may gradually build up on the inner walls of the arteries. This condition, called **atherosclerosis,** is the progressive narrowing of these vessels. Narrowing of the coronary arteries is a common form of coronary artery disease. When coronary arteries narrow, a heart attack may occur (Fig. 7-3, *B*). Atherosclerosis can also involve arteries in other parts of the body, such as the brain. Diseased arteries in the brain can lead to **stroke,** a disruption of blood flow to a part of the brain.

Because atherosclerosis develops gradually, it can go undetected for many years. Even with significantly reduced blood flow to the heart muscle, there may be no signs and symptoms of heart trouble. Most people with atherosclerosis are unaware of it. As the narrowing progresses, some people experience symptoms, such as chest pain, an early warning sign that the heart is not receiving enough oxygen-rich blood. Others may suffer a heart attack or even cardiac arrest without any previous warning. Fortunately, this process can be slowed or stopped by lifestyle changes, such as forming healthy eating habits.

## ◆ PREVENTING CARDIOVASCULAR DISEASE

Although a heart attack seems to strike suddenly, the conditions that lead to it may develop over years. Many people's lifestyles may gradually be endangering their hearts, which can eventually result in cardiovascular disease. Potentially harmful behaviors frequently begin early in life. For example, many children develop tastes for "junk" foods that are high in cholesterol and have little or no nutritional value. Sometimes children are not encouraged to exercise.

Several studies have shown that coronary artery disease actually begins in the teenage

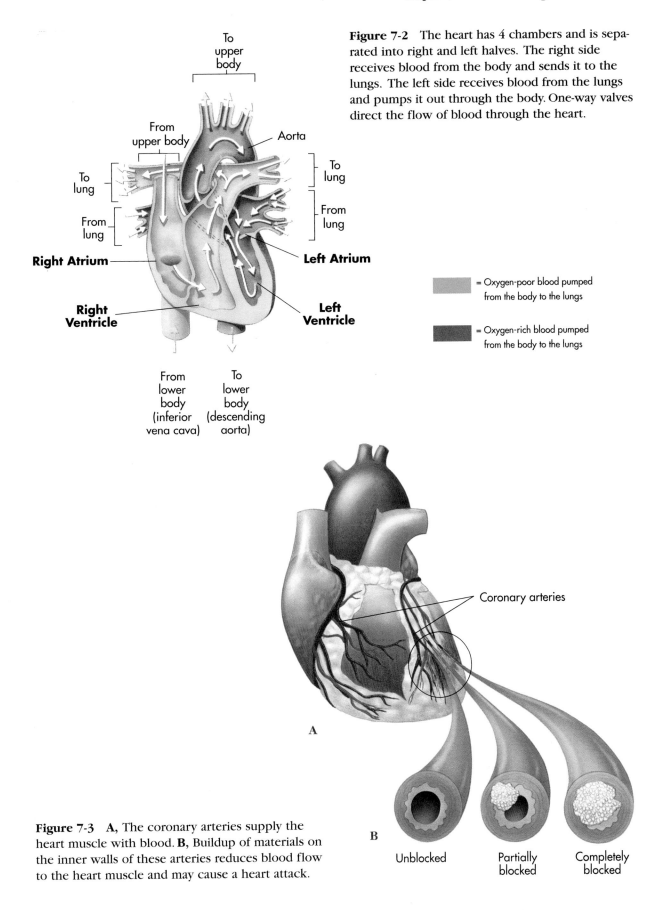

To
upper
body

From
upper body

Aorta

To
lung

From
lung

From
lung

**Right Atrium**

**Left Atrium**

**Right
Ventricle**

**Left
Ventricle**

From
lower
body
(inferior
vena cava)

To
lower
body
(descending
aorta)

= Oxygen-poor blood pumped
from the body to the lungs

= Oxygen-rich blood pumped
from the body to the lungs

**Figure 7-2**   The heart has 4 chambers and is separated into right and left halves. The right side receives blood from the body and sends it to the lungs. The left side receives blood from the lungs and pumps it out through the body. One-way valves direct the flow of blood through the heart.

Coronary arteries

A

B

Unblocked

Partially
blocked

Completely
blocked

**Figure 7-3**   **A,** The coronary arteries supply the heart muscle with blood. **B,** Buildup of materials on the inner walls of these arteries reduces blood flow to the heart muscle and may cause a heart attack.

years, when most smoking begins. Teenagers are more likely to begin smoking if their parents smoke. Smoking contributes to cardiovascular disease, as well as to other diseases.

# Risk Factors of Heart Disease

Scientists have identified many factors that increase a person's chances of developing heart disease. These are known as *risk factors.* Some risk factors for heart disease cannot be changed. For instance, men have a higher risk for heart disease than do women. Having a history of heart disease in your family also increases your risk.

But people can control many risk factors for heart disease. Smoking, diets high in fats, high blood pressure, obesity, and lack of routine exercise are all linked to increased risk of heart disease. When one risk factor, such as high blood pressure, is combined with other risk factors, such as obesity or cigarette smoking, the risk of heart attack or stroke is greatly increased.

## Controlling Risk Factors

Controlling your risk factors involves adjusting your lifestyle to minimize the chance of future cardiovascular disease. The three major risk factors you can control are cigarette smoking, high blood pressure, and high blood cholesterol levels.

Cigarette smokers are more than twice as likely to have a heart attack as nonsmokers and 2 to 4 times as likely to have cardiac arrest. The earlier a person starts using tobacco, the greater the risk to his or her future health. Giving up smoking will rapidly reduce the risk of heart disease. After a number of years, the risk becomes the same as if the person had never smoked. If you do not smoke, do not start. If you do smoke, quit.

Uncontrolled high blood pressure can damage blood vessels in the heart, kidneys, and other organs. You can often control high blood pressure by losing excess weight and by changing your diet. When these are not enough, medications can be prescribed. It is important to have regular checkups to guard against high blood pressure and its harmful effects.

Diets high in saturated fats and cholesterol increase the risk of heart disease. These diets raise the level of cholesterol in the blood and increase the chances that cholesterol and other fatty materials will be deposited on blood vessel walls and cause atherosclerosis.

Some cholesterol in the body is essential. The amount of cholesterol in the blood is determined by how much your body produces and by the food you eat. Foods high in cholesterol include egg yolks, shrimp, lobster, and organ meats, such as liver.

More important to an unhealthy blood cholesterol level is saturated fat. **Saturated fats** raise blood cholesterol level by interfering with the body's ability to remove cholesterol from the blood. Saturated fats are found in beef, lamb, veal, pork, ham, whole milk, and whole milk products.

Rather than eliminating saturated fats and cholesterol from your diet, limit your intake. This is easier than you think. Moderation is the key. Make changes whenever you can by substituting low-fat milk or skim milk for whole milk, margarine for butter, trimming visible fat from meats, and broiling or baking rather than frying. Read labels carefully. A "cholesterol-free" product may be high in saturated fat.

Two additional ways to help prevent heart disease are to control your weight and exercise regularly. You store excess calories in your diet as fat. In general, overweight people have a shorter life expectancy. Obese middle-aged men have nearly three times the risk of a fatal heart attack as do normal-weight middle-aged men.

Routine exercise has many benefits, including increased muscle tone and weight control. Exercise can also help you survive a heart attack because the increased circulation of blood through the heart develops additional channels for blood flow. If the primary channels that supply the heart are blocked in a heart attack, these additional channels can supply the heart tissue with oxygen-rich blood.

# How the Heart Functions

Too often we take our hearts for granted. The heart is extremely reliable. The heart beats about 70 times each minute, or more than 100,000 times a day. During the average lifetime, the heart will beat nearly 3 billion times. The heart moves about 4 litres of blood per minute through the body. This is about 160 million litres in an average lifetime. The heart moves blood through about 100,000 kilometers of blood vessels.

## Results of Managing Risk Factors

Managing your risk factors for cardiovascular disease really works. During the past 20 years, deaths from cardiovascular disease have decreased substantially.

Why did deaths from these causes decline? Probably they declined as a result of improved detection and treatment, as well as lifestyle changes. People are becoming more aware of their risk factors for heart disease and are taking action to control them. If you do this, you can improve your chances of living a long and healthy life. If you suffer a cardiac arrest, your chances of survival are poor. Begin today to reduce your risk of cardiovascular disease.

## Signs and Symptoms of a Heart Attack

The most prominent symptom of a heart attack is persistent chest pain or discomfort. However, it may not always be easy for you to distinguish between the pain of a heart attack and chest pain caused by indigestion, muscle spasms, or other conditions. Brief, stabbing chest pain or pain that feels more intense when the casualty bends or breathes deeply is usually not caused by a heart attack.

The pain of heart attack can range from mild discomfort to an unbearable crushing sensation in the chest. The casualty may describe it as an uncomfortable pressure, squeezing, tightness, aching, constricting, or heavy sensation in the chest. Often, the casualty feels pain in the centre of the chest behind the sternum. It may spread to the shoulder, arm, neck, or jaw (Fig. 7-4). The pain is constant and usually not relieved by resting, changing position, or taking oral medication. Any severe chest pain, chest pain that lasts longer than 10 minutes, or chest pain that is accompanied by other heart attack signs and symptoms should receive immediate emergency medical care.

Although a heart attack is often dramatic, heart attack casualties can have relatively mild symptoms. The casualty often mistakes the symptoms for indigestion. Some heart attack casualties feel little or no chest pain or discomfort.

Some people with coronary artery disease may experience chest pain or pressure that comes and goes and is not generally caused by a heart attack. This type of pain is called angina pectoris, a medical term for pain in the chest.

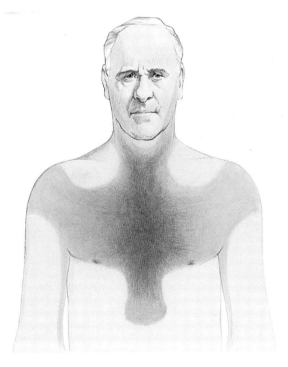

**Figure 7-4** Heart attack pain is most often felt in the centre of the chest, behind the sternum. It may spread to the shoulder, arm, neck, or jaw.

Angina pectoris develops when the heart needs more oxygen-rich blood than it gets, such as during physical activity or emotional stress. This lack of oxygen can cause a constricting chest pain that may spread to the neck, jaw, and arms.

Pain associated with angina usually lasts less than 10 minutes. A casualty who knows he or she has angina will often have a prescribed medication to help relieve the pain. Reducing the heart's demand for oxygen, such as by stopping physical activity and by taking prescribed medication, often relieves angina. Administering oxygen to casualties experiencing angina helps relieve chest pain.

Another sign of a heart attack is difficulty breathing. The casualty may be breathing faster than normal because the body tries to get much-needed oxygen to the heart. Depending on the casualty's general condition, the casualty's pulse may be faster or slower than normal or irregular. The casualty's skin may be pale or bluish, particularly around the face. The face may also be moist from perspiration. Some heart attack casualties sweat profusely. These signs result from the stress the body experiences when the heart does not work effectively.

Since any heart attack may lead to cardiac arrest, it is important to recognize and act on these signs and symptoms. Prompt action may prevent cardiac arrest. A heart attack casualty whose heart is still beating has a far better chance of living than a casualty whose heart has stopped. Most casualties who die from a heart attack die within 1 to 2 hours after the first signs and symptoms appear. Many could have been saved if bystanders or the casualty had been aware of the signs and symptoms of a heart attack and acted promptly. Since most heart attacks result from blood clotting within arteries, early treatment of an attack with medication that dissolves clots has been helpful in minimizing damage to the heart.

Many heart attack casualties delay seeking care. Nearly half of them wait 2 or more hours before going to the hospital. Casualties often do not realize they are having a heart attack. They may dismiss the symptoms as indigestion or muscle soreness.

Remember, the key symptom of a heart attack is persistent chest pain. If the casualty states that chest pain is severe or chest discomfort has been present for more than 10 minutes, summon more advanced medical personnel immediately and begin to care for the casualty.

## Care for a Heart Attack

The most important step in providing care is to recognize that any of the signs and symptoms listed in Table 7-1 may be those of a heart attack. You must take immediate action if any of these appear. A heart attack casualty will probably deny the seriousness of the symptoms he or she is experiencing. Do not let this

| **Table 7-1** Signs and Symptoms of a Heart Attack | |
|---|---|
| **Signs and Symptoms** | **Characteristics** |
| Persistent chest pain or discomfort | Persistent pain or pressure in the chest that is not relieved by resting, changing position, or oral medication<br>Pain may range from discomfort to an unbearable crushing sensation<br>Pain may radiate to the shoulders, arms, neck, or jaw |
| Breathing difficulty | Casualty's breathing is noisy<br>Casualty feels short of breath<br>Casualty breathes faster than normal |
| Changes in pulse rate | Pulse may be faster or slower than normal or may be irregular |
| Skin appearance | Casualty's skin may be pale or bluish in color<br>Casualty's face may be moist, or casualty may sweat profusely |

NOTE: Compared to men, women may feel less chest discomfort. They may experience more neck, shoulder, abdominal or back pain, nausea and/or shortness of breath.

influence you. If you think there is a possibility that a casualty is having a heart attack, you must act. First, have the casualty stop what he or she is doing and rest comfortably. Many heart attack casualties find it easier to breathe while sitting (Fig. 7-5). Second, summon more advanced medical personnel.

Continue with your secondary survey. Talk to bystanders and the casualty, if possible, to get more information. If the casualty is experiencing persistent chest pain, ask him or her the following:

Ask the casualty if he or she has a history of heart disease. Some casualties who have heart disease have prescribed medications for chest pain. Although you should not administer the medication, you can help by getting any medication for the casualty. A medication often prescribed for angina is nitroglycerin, a small tablet that is dissolved under the tongue. Sometimes nitroglycerin patches are placed on the chest. The most common form of the medication is a spray delivered under the tongue. Once absorbed into the body, nitroglycerin enlarges the blood vessels to make it easier for blood to reach heart muscle tissue. The pain is relieved because the heart does not have to work so hard and oxygen delivery to the heart is increased.

Administer oxygen if it is available and you are trained to do so. Ensure that advanced medical personnel have been summoned. Surviving a heart attack often depends on how soon the casualty receives **advanced cardiac life support (ACLS),** the use of special equipment and medications to maintain breathing and circulation for the casualty of a cardiac emergency.

Be calm and reassuring when caring for a heart attack casualty. Comforting the casualty helps reduce anxiety and eases some of the discomfort. Continue to monitor the vital signs until advanced medical personnel arrive. Watch for any changes

## Questions About Pain: PQRST

| Acronym | Question to ask |
| --- | --- |
| Provoke | What provokes the pain or causes it to get worse? |
| Quality | What does the pain feel like? (sharp, dull, stabbing, moving, etc.) |
| Region (or Radiate) | Where exactly is the pain located? Does it radiate to other areas? |
| Severity | How bad is the pain? |
| Time | When did the pain begin? |

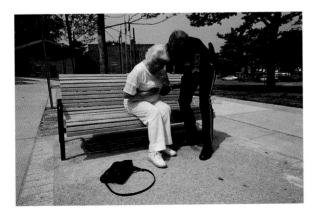

**Figure 7-5** The heart attack casualty should rest in a position that helps breathing.

## Care for a Heart Attack

- ◆ Recognize the signals of a heart attack.
- ◆ Convince the casualty to stop activity and rest.
- ◆ Help the casualty to rest comfortably.
- ◆ Try to obtain information about the casualty's condition.
- ◆ Comfort the casualty.
- ◆ Administer oxygen if available and you are trained to do so.
- ◆ Call for advanced medical personnel.
- ◆ Assist with medication, if prescribed.
- ◆ Monitor vital signs.
- ◆ Be prepared to give CPR if the casualty's heart stops beating.

in appearance or behavior. Since the heart attack may cause cardiac arrest, be prepared to give CPR.

## ◆ CARDIAC ARREST

### What Is Cardiac Arrest?

Cardiac arrest occurs when the heart stops beating or beats too irregularly or too weakly to circulate blood effectively. Without a heartbeat, breathing soon ceases. The condition when the heart stops beating and breathing stops is referred to as **clinical death.** Cardiac arrest is a life-threatening emergency because the body's vital organs are no longer receiving oxygen-rich blood. Every year, tens of thousands of Canadians die of cardiac arrest before reaching a hospital.

### Common Causes of Cardiac Arrest

Cardiovascular disease is the most common cause of cardiac arrest. Other causes include drowning, suffocation, certain drugs, severe injuries to the chest, severe blood loss, and electrocution. Stroke and other types of brain damage can also stop the heart.

### Signs of Cardiac Arrest

A casualty in cardiac arrest is not breathing and does not have a pulse. The casualty's heart has either stopped beating or is beating so weakly or irregularly that it cannot produce a pulse. The absence of a pulse is the primary sign of cardiac arrest. No matter how hard you try, you will not be able to feel a pulse. If you cannot feel a carotid pulse, no blood is reaching the brain. The casualty will be unconscious and breathing will stop.

Although cardiac arrest can result from a heart attack, cardiac arrest can also occur suddenly, independent of a heart attack. Therefore, the casualty may not have shown the signs and symptoms of a heart attack before the cardiac arrest. This is called **sudden death.**

### Care for Cardiac Arrest

A casualty who is not breathing and has no pulse is clinically dead. However, the cells of the brain and other vital organs will continue to live for a few minutes until the oxygen in the bloodstream is depleted. This casualty needs ***cardiopulmonary resuscitation (CPR)***. The term *cardio* refers to the heart, and *pulmonary* refers to the lungs. CPR is a combination of rescue breathing and chest compressions. Chest compressions are a method of making the blood circulate when the heart is not beating. Given together, rescue breathing and chest compressions artificially take over the functions of the lungs and heart.

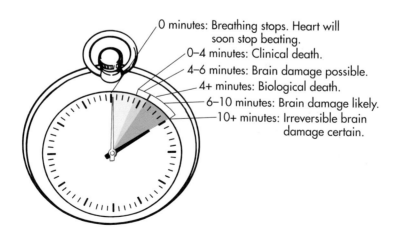

0 minutes: Breathing stops. Heart will soon stop beating.
0–4 minutes: Clinical death.
4–6 minutes: Brain damage possible.
4+ minutes: Biological death.
6–10 minutes: Brain damage likely.
10+ minutes: Irreversible brain damage certain.

**Figure 7-6**   In clinical death the heart and breathing stop. Clinical death can lead to biological death, which is the irreversible death of brain cells.

CPR increases a cardiac arrest casualty's chances of survival by keeping the brain supplied with oxygen until the casualty receives advanced medical care. Without CPR, the brain will begin to die within 4 to 6 minutes. The irreversible damage caused by brain cell death is known as **biological death** (Fig. 7-6). Be aware, that at best, CPR only generates about one third of the normal blood flow to the brain.

CPR alone is not enough to help someone survive cardiac arrest. Advanced medical care is needed immediately. Trained emergency personnel can provide ACLS. Acting as an extension of a hospital emergency department, EMTs and paramedics can administer medications or use a defibrillator as part of their emergency care (Fig. 7-7).

A **defibrillator** is a device that sends an electric shock through the chest to the heart to start the heart beating effectively again. Defibrillation given as soon as possible is the key to helping some casualties survive cardiac arrest. Immediate CPR must be combined with early defibrillation and other forms of ACLS to give the casualty of cardiac arrest the best chance for survival.

First responders in some communities are trained to use new defibrillators called **automated external defibrillators (AEDs)**. Today, AEDs are available for use by trained individuals in places such as factories, stadiums, and other places where large numbers of people gather. The use of defibrillators is described in a later section.

In all cases of cardiac arrest, it is very important to start CPR promptly and continue it until a defibrillator is available. When a defibrillator is not available, CPR should be continued. Effective rescue breathing and chest compressions can help keep the brain, heart, and other vital organs supplied with oxygen-rich blood. Any delay in starting CPR, or unnecessary delays in continuing it, reduces the casualty's chance for survival.

Even in the best of situations, when CPR is started promptly and advanced medical personnel arrive quickly, casualties of cardiac arrest do not often survive. Controlling your emotions and accepting death are not easy. Remember that any attempt to resuscitate is worthwhile. Since performing CPR and summoning more advanced medical personnel are not the only factors that determine whether a cardiac arrest casualty survives, you should feel assured that you did everything you could to help.

## ◆ CPR FOR ADULTS

### Chest Compressions

It is not entirely understood why giving CPR circulates blood. The theory that is most widely held today is that chest compressions create pressure within the chest cavity that moves blood through the circulatory system. For compressions to be most effective, the casualty should be flat on his or her back on a firm surface. The casualty's head should be on the same level as the heart, or lower. CPR is much less effective if the casualty is on a soft surface, such as a sofa or mattress, or is sitting up in a chair.

### Finding the Correct Hand Position

Using the correct hand position allows you to give the most effective compressions without causing injury. The correct position for your hands is over the lower half of the sternum (breastbone). At the lowest point of the sternum

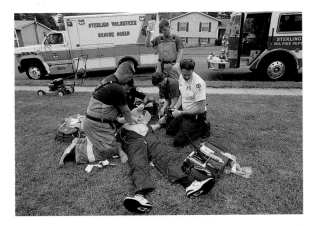

**Figure 7-7** Use of a defibrillator and other advanced measures may restore a heartbeat in a casualty of cardiac arrest.

is an arrow-shaped piece of hard tissue called the **xiphoid.** You should avoid pressing directly on the xiphoid, which can break and injure underlying tissues.

To locate the correct hand position for chest compressions—

◆ Find the lower edge of the casualty's rib cage. Slide your middle and index fingers up the edge of the rib cage to the notch where the ribs meet the sternum (Fig. 7-8, *A*). Place your middle finger on this notch. Place your index finger next to your middle finger.

◆ Place the heel of your other hand on the sternum next to your index finger (Fig. 7-8, *B*). The heel of your hand should rest along the length of the sternum.

◆ Once the heel of your hand is in position on the sternum, place your other hand directly on top of it (Fig. 7-8, *C*).

◆ Use the heel of your hand to apply pressure on the sternum. Try to keep your fingers off the chest by interlacing them or holding them upward. Applying pressure with your fingers can cause inefficient chest compressions or unnecessary damage to the chest.

Positioning the hands correctly provides the most effective compressions. It also decreases the chance of pushing the xiphoid into the delicate organs beneath it, although this rarely occurs.

If you have arthritis or a similar condition in your hands or wrists, you may use an alternative hand position. Find the correct hand position, as above, then grasp the wrist of the hand on the chest with the other hand (Fig. 7-9).

The casualty's clothing will not necessarily interfere with your ability to position your hands correctly. If you can find the correct position without removing thin clothing, such as a T-shirt, do so. Sometimes a layer of thin clothing will help keep your hands from slipping, since the casualty's chest may be moist with sweat. However, if you are not sure that you can find the correct hand position, bare the casualty's chest. You should not be overly concerned about being able to find the correct position if the casualty is obese, since fat does not accumulate over the sternum.

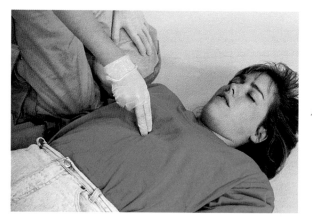

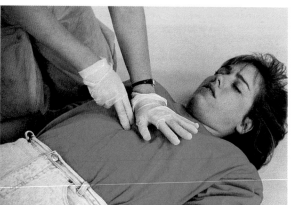

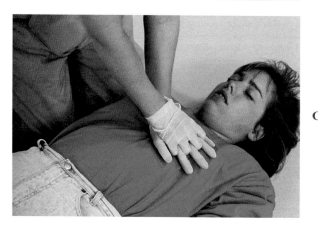

**Figure 7-8** To locate compression position, **A,** find the notch where the lower ribs meet the sternum. **B,** Place the heel of your hand on the sternum, next to your index finger. **C,** Place your other hand over the heel of the first hand. Use the heel of your bottom hand to apply pressure on the sternum.

## Position of the Rescuer

Your body position is important when giving chest compressions. Compressing the chest straight down provides the best blood flow. The correct body position is also less tiring for you.

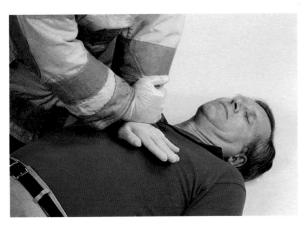

**Figure 7-9**   Grasping the wrist of the hand positioned on the chest is an alternate hand position for giving chest compressions.

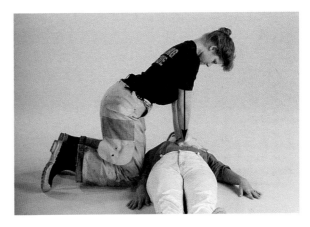

**Figure 7-10**   With your hands in place, position yourself so that your shoulders are directly over your hands, arms straight and elbows locked.

Kneel at the casualty's chest with your hands in the correct position. Straighten your arms and lock your elbows so that your shoulders are directly over your hands (Fig. 7-10). When you press down in this position, you are pushing straight down onto the casualty's sternum. Locking your elbows keeps your arms straight and prevents you from tiring quickly.

Compressing the chest requires little effort in this position. When you press down, the weight of your upper body creates the force needed to compress the chest. Push with the weight of your upper body, not with the muscles of your arms. Push straight down. Do not rock back and forth. Rocking results in less effective compressions and uses unnecessary energy. If your arms and shoulders tire quickly, you are not using the correct body position. After each compression, release the pressure on the chest without losing contact with it and allow the chest to return to its normal position before you start the next compression (Fig. 7-11).

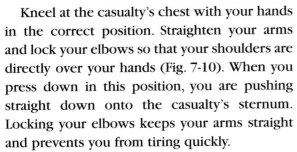

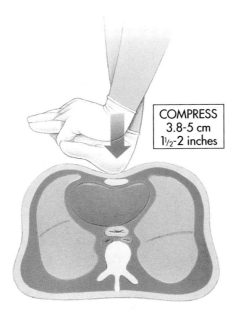

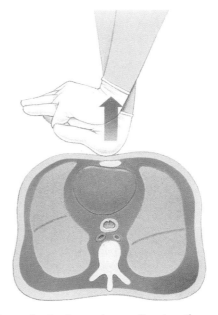

**Figure 7-11**   Push straight down with the weight of your body, then release, allowing the chest to return to the normal position.

# Recommendation on ASA and Nitroglycerin for Chest Pain

In 2001, Health Canada approved the use of **acetylsalicylic acid (ASA)** to treat acute heart attacks. Current research has shown that early administration of ASA (e.g., Aspirin®) during a heart attack can reduce the risk of death by as much as 25%. It is then recommended that all individuals who are experiencing acute onset of chest pain that is cardiac in origin be encouraged to chew 160–325 mg of ASA regardless of whether they take ASA or not. Therefore, an individual who is experiencing chest pain should be assisted with his/her prescribed medications and ASA (whether prescribed or not) in the following way:

- As soon as chest pain is detected, summon for advanced medical personnel.
- While waiting for medical help, assist the person to the most comfortable position, usually semi-sitting with the head and shoulders raised and supported. Loosen tight clothing at the neck, chest, and waist. Reassure the person. Assist the fully conscious person to take appropriate medications as described below. *If your profession is governed by regulations that preclude this action, you should not proceed.*
- Ask the **fully conscious person** if he/she carries **nitroglycerin**. If yes, determine if the person has taken Viagra® within the last 24 hours. If yes, explain to the person that they must not take their nitroglycerin because they may develop low blood pressure. Ensure that you have the correct medication before assisting the person. If the person has not taken Viagra®, help them administer nitroglycerin by either tablets or spray. Nitroglycerin tablets are placed under the tongue where they quickly dissolve. Nitroglycerin spray is sprayed under the tongue and is rapidly absorbed. Nitroglycerin starts working within 1 to 2 minutes and works for about 5 to 6 minutes. The nitroglycerin dose may be repeated every 5 minutes until the pain is relieved or until a maximum of three doses have been administered.

- Ask the **fully conscious person** if he/she carries ASA. Ask if he/she is allergic to ASA and/or has asthma. ASA can trigger an asthmatic attack in some people. If the **fully conscious person** does not carry nitroglycerin or if the pain is not relieved by the first dose of nitroglycerin, suggest the person chew two children's ASA tablets (80 mg each) or one ASA tablet (regular strength adult dose = 325 mg). You may offer Aspirin® but you are cautioned to only recommend that the person take Aspirin® and explain why. The individual must make the decision whether or not to take the medication. NOTE: Acetaminophen (e.g., Tylenol®) or ibuprofen (e.g., Advil®) do not have the same effect as ASA in reducing damage due to heart attacks: do not substitute!
- When advanced medical personnel arrive, advise them of any actions or medications that have been taken.
- Monitor respiration and circulation (pulse) and be ready to provide rescue breathing or CPR.

**REFERENCE**

Adapted from ECC Coalition, *"Recommendation on ASA and Nitroglycerin for Chest Pain,"* November 22, 1999.

## Compression Technique

Each compression should push the sternum down from 3.8 to 5 centimetres (1½ to 2 inches). The downward and upward movement should be smooth, not jerky. Maintain a steady down-and-up rhythm, and do not pause between compressions. When you press down, the chambers of the heart empty. When you come up, release all pressure on the chest, which lets the chambers of the heart fill with blood between compressions.

Keep your hands in their correct position on the sternum. If your hands slip, find the notch as you did before and reposition your hands.

Give compressions at the rate of about 100 per minute. As you do compressions, count aloud, "One and two and three and four and five and six and. . ." up to 15. Counting aloud will help you pace yourself. Push down as you say the number and come up as you say "and." You should be able to do the 15 compressions in about 9 seconds. Even though you are compressing the chest at a rate of about 100 times per minute, you will actually perform only 70 compressions in a minute. This is because you must take the time to do rescue breathing, giving 2 slow breaths between each group of 15 compressions.

## Compression/Breathing Cycles

When you give CPR, do cycles of 15 compressions and 2 breaths. You should be positioned midway between the chest and the head to move easily between compressions and breaths (Fig. 7-12). For each cycle, give 15 chest compressions; then open the airway with a head-tilt/chin-lift, and give 2 slow breaths. This cycle should take about 15 seconds. When you are alone and using a resuscitation mask, the cycle may take a little longer. For each new cycle of compressions and breaths, use the correct hand position by first finding the notch at the lower end of the sternum.

After doing 4 signs of continuous CPR, check to see if the casualty has signs of circulation (pulse). These 4 cycles (of 15 compressions and 2 breaths) should take about 1 minute. Tilt the casualty's head to open the airway, and take no more than 10 seconds to check for signs of circulation. If there are no signs of circulation, continue CPR, beginning with compressions. Check circulation and breathing again every few minutes. If the casualty has signs of circulation but is not breathing, give rescue breathing. If the casualty is breathing, keep his or her airway open, and continue to monitor breathing and circulation closely. The Skills Summaries at the end of this chapter provide a guide for step-by-step practice of CPR.

## When to Stop CPR

Once you begin CPR, try not to interrupt the blood flow you are creating artificially. However, you can stop CPR—

- ◆ If another trained person takes over CPR for you. (Continue to assist by calling advanced medical personnel for help if this has not already been done.)
- ◆ If advanced medical personnel arrive and take over care of the casualty.
- ◆ If an automated external defibrillator (AED) is available and someone there is trained and authorized to use it.
- ◆ If you are exhausted and unable to continue.
- ◆ If the scene suddenly becomes unsafe.
- ◆ If the casualty's heart starts beating.

## ◆ AUTOMATED EXTERNAL DEFIBRILLATION

Studies show that ***early defibrillation*** is the most likely step to improve the survival of adult casualties in cardiac arrest. Each minute that defibrillation is delayed the chance of survival is reduced by about 7 to 10 percent.

Until recently, only health care professionals performed defibrillation. Contemporary technology has produced automated external defibrillators (AEDs), devices suitable for first responders and other rescuers in the community to provide early defibrillation while waiting for more advanced medical personnel to arrive (Fig. 7-13).

During defibrillation, an electrical shock is delivered to the heart. The shock is not intended to start a dead heart; one without any electrical activity. Instead, it is intended to briefly stop the abnormal electrical activity (e.g., ventricular fibrillation or pulseless ven-

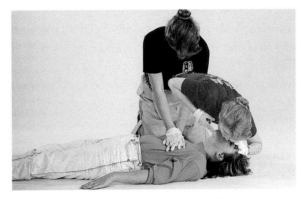

**Figure 7-12**  Give 15 compressions, then give 2 breaths.

tricular tachycardia) long enough to allow the heart to spontaneously develop an effective rhythm on its own.

# The Heart's Electrical System

To better understand both the limitations of CPR and how defibrillators work, it is helpful to understand how the heart's electrical system functions. The electrical system determines the pumping action of the heart. Under normal conditions, specialized cells of the heart initiate and carry on electrical activity. The normal point of origin of the electrical impulse is the sinoatrial (SA) node, which is situated in the upper part of the right atrium.

The current is conducted to the atrioventricular (AV) node, which is situated between the atria and ventricles, through conduction pathways within the heart muscle. From the AV node the electrical signal is sent to the ventricles through other pathways. These electrical impulses are the stimulus that cause the heart muscle to contract and pump the blood out of its chambers and throughout the body (Fig. 7-14).

Cardiac monitors are used to read the electrical impulses in the heart to produce an *electrocardiogram* (ECG), which is a picture of the conduction of the electrical current through the pathways of the heart. The normal conduction of electrical impulses without any disturbances is called *normal sinus rhythm* (NSR) (Fig. 7-15).

In NSR the impulse is initiated in the SA node and transmitted to the atria. The stimulus from the electrical impulse causes the atria to contract and expel the blood to the ventricles. Meanwhile, the electrical current continues to travel through the atria and the AV node to the ventricles. When the ventricles receive the impulse, they contract to expel the blood throughout the body's blood vessels. This process normally takes place 60 to 100 times per minute.

## Alarming Disturbances in Heart Rhythm

The healthy adult heart usually displays NSR on the ECG. Disturbances or variations in the con-

duction of electrical impulses within the heart are called arrhythmias. Although arrhythmias can be either benign or have serious consequences, there are three major conduction disturbances that are immediately life threatening: asystole, ventricular tachycardia, and ventricular fibrillation.

### Asystole

*Asystole* is the absence of electrical activity in the heart. It is not corrected by defibrillation and indicates a dead heart (Fig. 7-16).

### Ventricular tachycardia without pulse

*Ventricular tachycardia (VT)* is a rhythm of fast-paced contractions of the heart's ventricles. The contractions are too rapid to allow for the ventricles to fill with blood to pump an adequate supply of blood to the body (Fig. 7-17). This type of arrhythmia can occur in a casualty who is pulseless and may soon deteriorate to ventricular fibrillation.

### Ventricular fibrillation

*Ventricular fibrillation (VF)* is a chaotic discharge of electrical activity that causes the heart muscle to quiver (Fig. 7-18). Casualties with this arrhythmia have no pulse. Ventricular fibrillation will deteriorate to asystole within a few minutes if not treated promptly.

## Correcting the Problem

Although defibrillators can be used only with certain arrhythmias, such as ventricular fibrilla-

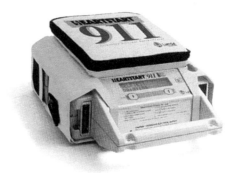

**Figure 7-13** Automated external defibrillator (AED).

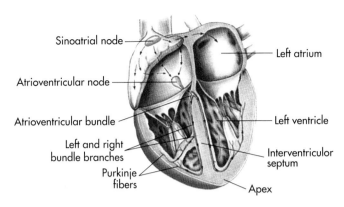

**Figure 7-14** Conduction system of heart.

tion and ventricular tachycardia, these rhythms occur commonly enough to warrant the use of defibrillators in prehospital settings. In over 80 percent of all sudden cardiac deaths, the initial rhythm is ventricular tachycardia or ventricular fibrillation. Because the treatment of choice for both of these rhythms in cases of cardiac arrest is defibrillation along with CPR, early response with an AED is important. Unfortunately, defibrillation does not correct asystole, and CPR must be initiated until more advanced help arrives or ambulance transportation is available. The successful resuscitation of casualties of cardiac arrest with a shockable arrhythmia (e.g., ventricular fibrillation or ventricular tachycardia) depends greatly on how much time has passed from the start of the arrhythmia until defibrillation is initiated. The availability of AEDs to a wider range of responders can greatly reduce the response time from collapse to defibrillation.

## Using an Automated External Defibrillator (AED)

In a situation involving cardiac arrest, an AED should be put to use as soon as it is available. To defibrillate a casualty of cardiac arrest by using an AED, take the following steps.

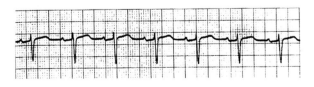

**Figure 7-15** Normal sinus rhythm.

. **Confirm cardiac arrest.** Check for responsiveness, airway, breathing, and circulation (including pulse).
. **Turn on the AED.**
. **Attach the AED to large defibrillator electrode pads and apply the pads to the casualty's bare, dry chest.**
   - ◆ Wipe the casualty's chest dry.
   - ◆ Attach the electrode pads to the chest.
   - ◆ Place one pad on the upper-right side of the chest, and the other pad on the lower-left side of the chest. (Fig. 7-19)
   - ◆ Plug the electrode cable to the AED.
4. **Let the AED analyze the heart rhythm** (or push the "analyze" button).
   - ◆ Make sure no one is touching the casualty.
   - ◆ Say "Everyone stand clear".
5. **Clear the casualty and deliver a shock if indicated.** If the AED advises a shock is needed...
   - ◆ Make sure no one (rescuers and bystanders) is touching the casualty.
   - ◆ Say "Everyone stand clear".

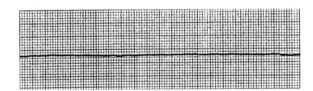

**Figure 7-16** Asystole.

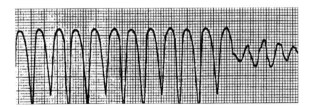

**Figure 7-17** Ventricular tachycardia.

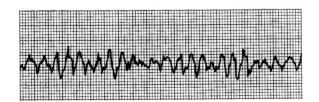

**Figure 7-18** Ventricular fibrillation.

- Deliver a shock by pushing the "shock" button when prompted by the AED.
- Repeat up to three times if advised.
- Check for signs of circulation.
- If no signs, do CPR for 1 minute.
- Clear the casualty, analyze.

If the AED advises no shock is needed...
- Check for signs of circulation.
- If no signs, do CPR for 1 minute.
- Clear the casualty, analyze.

First Responders using AEDs are encouraged to have medical supervision provided on a local, regional or province-wide basis. Defibrillation is currently an act that is under a degree of medical supervision. You must follow local protocols that establish how many shocks are delivered, the energy setting of each shock, and how CPR and other lifesaving measures are used.

## Special Resuscitation Situations

Some situations require rescuers to pay special attention when using an AED. It is important that rescuers be familiar with these situations and be able to respond appropriately.

### Hypothermia

Casualties of severe hypothermia should receive only three shocks if defibrillation is indicated. Following the three shocks continue with the CPR sequence. The remaining shocks will be delivered by advanced medical personnel according to local protocol.

### Children

Children under 8 years of age or weighing less than 25 kg (55 lbs) should not be defibrillated. Follow local protocol.

### Transdermal medications

AED electrodes should not be placed over a transdermal medication patch (e.g., nitroglycerin, nicotine), as the patch may block delivery of energy or cause burns to the skin. With a gloved hand, remove any patches from the chest before attaching the device.

### Implanted pacemakers and ICDs

The casualty may have a pacemaker or implanted cardioverter-defibrillator (ICD) implanted in the area where one of the electrodes is intended to go. If you observe a small scar and a matchbox-size lump on the chest, reposition the electrode at least 2.5 cm (1 in) away. If an ICD is in shock sequence, allow 30 to 60 seconds for the ICD to complete the treatment cycle.

### Single rescuer

In some situations, one rescuer with immediate access to an AED may respond to a cardiac arrest. The rescuer should quickly summon more advanced medical personnel. A single rescuer responding with an AED should confirm the cardiac arrest, attach the AED, and follow the standard defibrillation protocol.

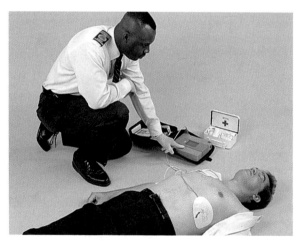

**Figure 7-19** Place one AED electrode pad on the upper-right side of the chest (above the nipple, below the collarbone). Place the other on the lower-left side of the chest, below the nipple at the level of the xiphoid.
*Courtesy of the American Red Cross.*
*All rights reserved in all countries.*

## Trauma casualties

The standard defibrillation protocol along with spinal precautions can be initiated in traumatized casualties in cardiac arrest. Your local medical director, however, may not include these casualties in the standing orders due to the low incidence of a shocking rhythm being present and to other treatment needed in this setting.

## Maintenance

For defibrillators to perform optimally, they must be maintained like any other machine. The AEDs that are available today require minimal maintenance. These devices have various self-testing features. However, it is important that operators are familiar with any visual or audible warning prompts that the AED may have to warn of malfunction or a low battery. It is important to read the operator's manual thoroughly and check with the manufacturer to obtain all necessary information regarding maintenance.

## Other Precautions

The following precautions must be taken when using an AED:

- Do not defibrillate a casualty lying on a conductive surface. Casualties lying on conductive surfaces such as puddles of water or sheet metal should either be moved to a nonconductive surface, or the lead rescuer must ensure that no one is in contact with the surface. Remember, if the casualty's chest is wet, dry it before using the AED.
- Do not use alcohol pads to clean the chest before attaching the pads. The alcohol is flammable.
- Stand clear of the casualty while analyzing and defibrillating.
- Do not analyze the heart rhythm or defibrillate in a moving vehicle.
- Do not defibrillate a casualty in the presence of flammable materials (such as gasoline).

- Avoid radio transmissions while defibrillating, including cell phones, within 2 m (6 feet) of the victim.
- Keep breathing devices with free flowing oxygen away from the victim during defibrillation.
- Avoid the use of supplemental, free flowing oxygen and use of an AED in a confined space.

## ♦ CARDIAC EMERGENCIES IN INFANTS AND CHILDREN

A child's heart is usually healthy. Unlike adults, children do not often initially suffer a cardiac emergency. Instead, the child suffers a respiratory emergency. Then a cardiac emergency develops.

The most common cause of cardiac emergencies in children is injury from motor vehicle crashes. Other common causes of cardiac emergencies for both infants and children include injuries from near-drowning, smoke inhalation, burns, poisoning, airway obstruction, firearms, and falls. Rarely, a cardiac emergency results from a medical condition or illness, such as severe **croup** (a respiratory infection that occurs mainly in children and infants), severe asthma, or certain respiratory infections.

Most cardiac emergencies in infants and children are preventable. One way to prevent them in this age group is to prevent injuries. Another is to make sure that infants and children receive proper medical care. A third is to recognize the early signs of a respiratory emergency. These signs include—

- Agitation.
- Drowsiness.
- Change in skin colour (to pale, blue, or grey).
- Increased difficulty breathing.
- Increased heart and breathing rates.

If you recognize that an infant or child is in respiratory distress or respiratory arrest, provide the care you learned in Chapter 6 for those

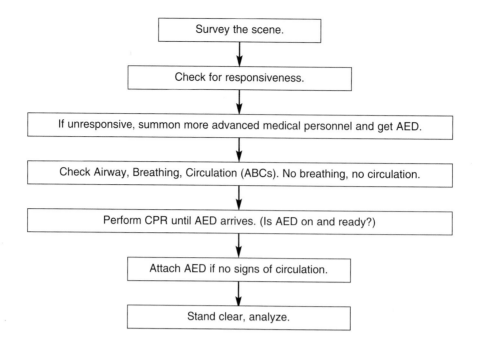

Survey the scene.

Check for responsiveness.

If unresponsive, summon more advanced medical personnel and get AED.

Check Airway, Breathing, Circulation (ABCs). No breathing, no circulation.

Perform CPR until AED arrives. (Is AED on and ready?)

Attach AED if no signs of circulation.

Stand clear, analyze.

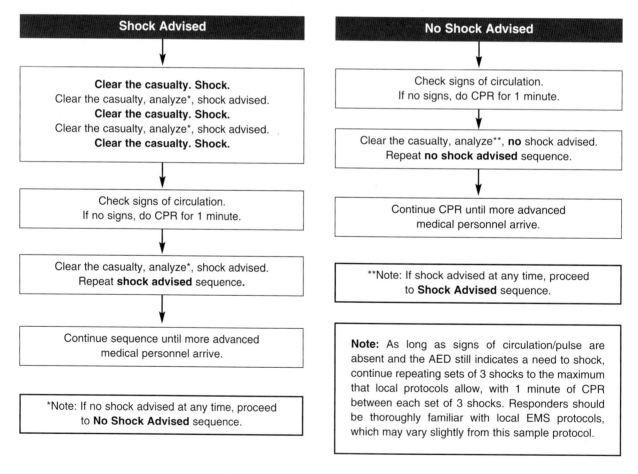

**Shock Advised**

**Clear the casualty. Shock.**
Clear the casualty, analyze*, shock advised.
**Clear the casualty. Shock.**
Clear the casualty, analyze*, shock advised.
**Clear the casualty. Shock.**

Check signs of circulation.
If no signs, do CPR for 1 minute.

Clear the casualty, analyze*, shock advised.
Repeat **shock advised** sequence.

Continue sequence until more advanced
medical personnel arrive.

*Note: If no shock advised at any time, proceed
to **No Shock Advised** sequence.

**No Shock Advised**

Check signs of circulation.
If no signs, do CPR for 1 minute.

Clear the casualty, analyze**, **no** shock advised.
Repeat **no shock advised** sequence.

Continue CPR until more advanced
medical personnel arrive.

**Note: If shock advised at any time, proceed
to **Shock Advised** sequence.

**Note:** As long as signs of circulation/pulse are
absent and the AED still indicates a need to shock,
continue repeating sets of 3 shocks to the maximum
that local protocols allow, with 1 minute of CPR
between each set of 3 shocks. Responders should
be thoroughly familiar with local EMS protocols,
which may vary slightly from this sample protocol.

**Figure 7-20** Sample AED protocol.

emergencies. If the infant or child is in cardiac arrest, start CPR immediately. In either event, summon more advanced medical personnel.

## ◆ CPR FOR INFANTS AND CHILDREN

The CPR technique for infants and children is similar to the technique for adults. As in rescue breathing, you need to modify the techniques to accommodate the smaller body size and faster breathing and heart rates. Figure 7-21 compares the adult, child, and infant CPR techniques.

## CPR for Children

To find out if a child needs CPR, begin with a primary survey. If you determine that there are no signs of circulation, begin CPR.

To give compressions, kneel beside the child's chest with your knees against the child's side. Maintain an open airway with one hand and find the correct hand position with the other (Fig. 7-22). To locate hand position on a child, slide your middle finger up the lower edge of the ribs until you locate the notch where the ribs meet the sternum (breastbone). Place the index finger next to it. The two fingers should be resting on the lower end of the sternum (Fig. 7-23, *A*).

Visually mark the place where you put your index finger. Lift your fingers off the sternum and put the heel of the same hand on the sternum immediately above where you had your index finger (Fig. 7-23, *B*). Keep your fingers off the child's chest. Only the heel of your hand should rest on the sternum.

When you compress the chest, use only the hand that is on the child's sternum. You do *not* use both hands to give chest compressions to a child. Push straight down, making sure your shoulder is directly over your hand (Fig. 7-24). Each compression should push the sternum down from 2.5 to 3.8 centimetres (1 to 1½

inches). The down-and-up movement should be smooth, not jerky. Release the pressure on the chest completely, but do not lift your hand off the child's chest (Fig. 7-25).

When you give CPR to a child, do cycles of 5 compressions and 1 breath at a rate of about 100 compressions per minute. While giving compressions with one hand, keep your other hand on the child's forehead to help maintain an open airway. After giving 5 compressions, remove your compression hand from the chest, lift the chin, and give 1 slow breath. The breath should last 1–1½ seconds. Always use a chin-lift with a head-tilt to ensure that the child's airway is open. After giving the breath, place your hand in the same position as before and continue compressions. You do not have to measure your hand position each time by sliding your fingers up the rib cage, unless you lose your place.

Keep repeating the cycle of 5 compressions and 1 breath (Fig. 7-26). Each cycle of 5 compressions and 1 breath should take about 5 seconds. After you do about 1 minute of continuous CPR (about 20 cycles), recheck the child's signs of circulation (pulse) for no more than 10 seconds. If there are no signs of circulation, continue CPR, beginning with compressions. Recheck circulation and breathing every few minutes.

If the child has signs of circulation, keep the airway open and monitor breathing and circulation closely. Cover the child, and keep the child warm and as quiet as possible.

## CPR for Infants

To find out if an infant needs CPR, begin with a primary survey to check the ABCs. To check the pulse in an infant, locate the brachial pulse in the arm. If the infant has no signs of circulation (brachial pulse), begin CPR.

Position the infant face up on a firm, flat surface. The infant's head must be on the same level as the heart or lower. Stand or kneel facing

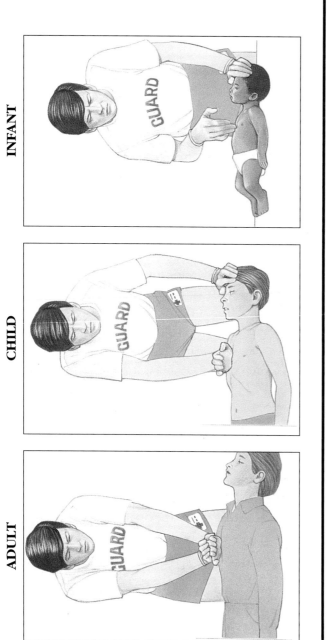

| | **ADULT** | **CHILD** | **INFANT** |
|---|---|---|---|
| **HAND POSITION:** | Two hands on lower half of sternum | One hand on lower half of sternum | Two fingers on lower half of sternum (one finger width below nipple line) |
| **COMPRESS:** | 3.8 - 5 cm (1½ – 2 in) | 2.5 - 3.8 cm (1–1½ in) | 1.2 - 2.5 cm (½ –1 in) |
| **BREATHE:** | Slowly until chest gently rises (about 2 seconds per breath) | Slowly until chest gently rises (about 1–1.5 seconds per breath) | Slowly until chest gently rises (about 1–1.5 seconds per breath) |
| **CYCLE:** | 15 compressions 2 breaths | 5 compressions 1 breath | 5 compressions 1 puff |
| **RATE:** | 15 compressions in about 9 seconds | 5 compressions in about 3 seconds | 5 compressions in about 3 seconds |

**Figure 7-21** The technique for chest compressions differs for adults, children, and infants.

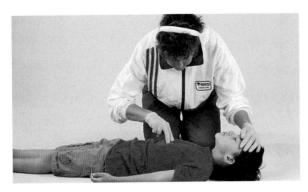

**Figure 7-22** While kneeling beside the child, maintain an open airway with one hand and find the correct hand position with the other.

the infant from the side. Keep one hand on the infant's head to maintain an open airway. Use your other hand to give compressions.

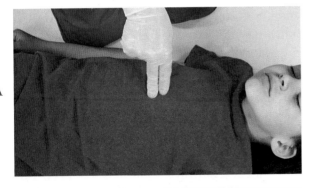

A

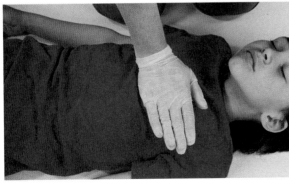

B

**Figure 7-23** To locate compression position, **A,** find the notch where the lower rib meets the sternum with your middle finger. Place the index finger next to it, so that both fingers rest on the lower end of the breastbone. **B,** Place the heel of the same hand on the breastbone immediately above where you had your index finger.

To find the correct place to give compressions, imagine a line running across the chest between the infant's nipples (Fig. 7-27, *A*). Place your index finger on the sternum in line with this imaginary line. Then place the pads of the middle and ring fingers one finger width below the imaginary line on the sternum. Use your index finger as a guide. Raise the index finger (Fig. 7-27, *B*). If you feel the notch at the end of the infant's sternum, move your fingers up a little bit.

Use the pads of two fingers to compress the chest (Fig. 7-27, *C*). Compress the chest 1.2 to 2.5 centimetres (½ to 1 inch), then let the sternum return to its normal position. When you compress, push straight down. The down-and-up movement of your compressions should be smooth, not jerky. Keep a steady rhythm. Do not pause between compressions. When you are coming up, release pressure on the infant's chest completely, but do not let your fingers lose contact with the chest (Fig. 7-28). Keep your fingers in the compression position. Use your other hand to keep the airway open using a head-tilt.

When you give CPR, do cycles of 5 compressions and 1 puff (Fig. 7-29). Compress at a rate of at least 100 compressions per minute. When you complete 5 compressions, give 1 slow puff, covering the infant's nose and mouth with your

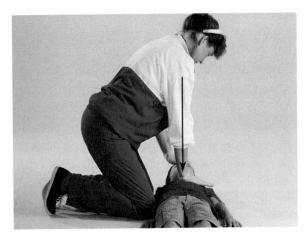

**Figure 7-24** When you compress the chest, use the heel of your hand. Push straight down, making sure your shoulder is directly over your hand.

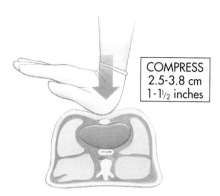
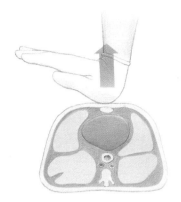

COMPRESS
2.5-3.8 cm
1-1½ inches

**Figure 7-25** Push straight down with the weight of your body and then release, allowing the chest to return to its normal position.

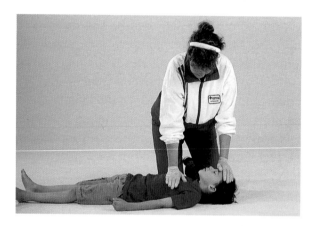

**Figure 7-26** Give 5 compressions and then 1 breath.

mouth. The puff should take 1–1½ seconds. Keep repeating cycles of 5 compressions and 1 puff. A complete cycle of 5 compressions and 1 puff should take about 5 seconds.

Recheck for signs of circulation (brachial pulse) and breathing after about 1 minute of continuous CPR (about 20 cycles). Check for signs of circulation (brachial pulse) for no more than 10 seconds with the hand that was giving compressions. If there are no signs of circulation, continue CPR, starting with compressions. Recheck circulation and breathing every few minutes.

If the infant has signs of circulation but is not breathing, give rescue breaths. If the infant is breathing, keep the airway open and monitor breathing and circulation closely. Maintain normal body temperature.

## ◆ TWO-RESCUER CPR

When two professional rescuers are available, they give two-rescuer CPR. They share the responsibility for performing rescue breathing and chest compressions (Fig. 7-30). You should be able to perform two-rescuer CPR in each of the following situations:

1. CPR is *not* being given, and two or more rescuers arrive on the scene at the same time and begin CPR together.
2. One rescuer is giving CPR, and a second rescuer is available to begin two-rescuer CPR.
3. Either rescuer tires and the rescuers change position.

### Two-Rescuer Techniques

In two-rescuer CPR for an adult, the cycle involves 15 compressions and 2 breaths (a ratio of 15 to 2). Compressions are stopped at the upstroke of the 15th compression, and the rescuer giving breaths immediately gives 2 slow breaths. The compressor then continues giving compressions.

Chest compressions are given at a rate of about 100 per minute and at a depth of 3.8 to 5 centimetres (1½ to 2 inches), the same as in one-rescuer CPR. The compressor uses the same counting rhythm as for one-rescuer CPR.

During two-rescuer CPR, the person giving breaths (the ventilator) checks the effectiveness

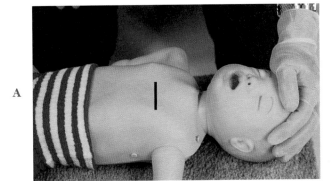

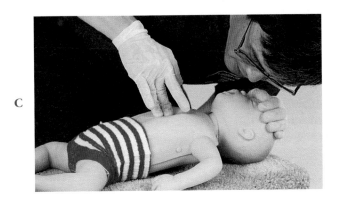

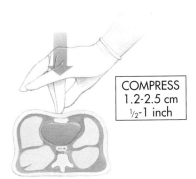

**Figure 7-27** To locate compression position, **A,** imagine a line running across the chest between the infant's nipples. Place your index finger on the sternum in line with the line. **B,** Place the pads of the middle and ring fingers next to your index finger on the breastbone. Raise the index finger. **C,** Use the pads of the remaining two fingers to compress the chest.

of the compressions by feeling for the carotid pulse while the compressor is giving chest compressions (Fig. 7-31). He or she advises the compressor whether the compressions are effective. If the casualty has lost a significant amount of blood, a carotid pulse may not be felt even though compressions are effective.

The ventilator also check for signs of circulation (pulse) after the first minute of compressions and repeats the check every few minutes after that to determine if circulation has returned. This is done by communicating that he or she is performing a circulation check, then the compressor stops compressing after the 15th compression. The ventilator checks for signs of circulation (pulse) for no more than 10 seconds. If there is no circulation, they continue CPR, starting with compressions.

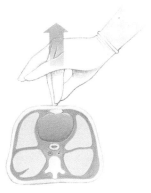

COMPRESS
1.2-2.5 cm
½-1 inch

**Figure 7-28** Push straight down with your fingers and then release the pressure on the chest completely.

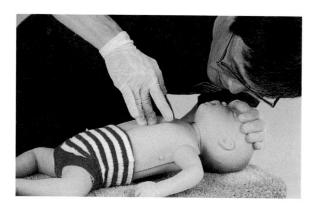

**Figure 7-29** Give 5 compressions and then 1 breath.

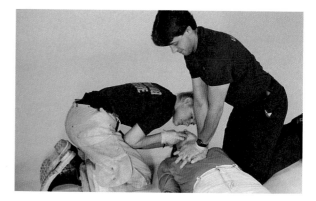

**Figure 7-30** During two-rescuer CPR, the rescuers share the responsibility for performing rescue breathing and chest compressions.

## When Two Rescuers Arrive on the Scene at the Same Time

If CPR is not being performed when you arrive, one rescuer should do a primary survey and, if appropriate, begin CPR. The other rescuer should manage other responsibilities at the scene, such as scene safety, communications, and setting up equipment and supplies. Then the second rescuer can assist with CPR.

## Two Rescuers Beginning CPR Together

When both rescuers are available to begin CPR at the same time, the first rescuer does a primary survey. While the first rescuer is doing the primary survey, the second rescuer gets into position to give chest compressions and locates the correct hand position. He or she should begin chest compressions when the first rescuer communicates that there are no signs of circulation (pulse). Both rescuers continue CPR together.

## When CPR Is in Progress by One Rescuer

When a rescuer is giving CPR and a second rescuer arrives, that rescuer should ask whether advanced medical personnel have been summoned. If not, he or she should summon them or send someone else to call. Then the second rescuer should either *replace* the first rescuer or *assist* him or her in giving two-rescuer CPR.

If the second rescuer is going to assist with two-rescuer CPR, he or she enters immediately after the first rescuer has completed a cycle of 15 compressions and 2 breaths.

The second rescuer gets into position at the casualty's chest and finds the correct hand position. The first rescuer remains at the casualty's head and checks for signs of circulation (pulse). If there are still no signs of circulation, the first rescuer signals to begin CPR. The second rescuer, at the chest, begins chest compressions. Both rescuers continue giving two-rescuer CPR.

## Changing Positions

If a rescuer becomes tired, he or she can change position with the other rescuer. When the rescuers change, the rescuer at the casualty's head completes 2 breaths and then moves immediately to the chest. The rescuer at the chest moves immediately to the head. Both rescuers move quickly into position without changing sides. The sequence for changing positions is the following:

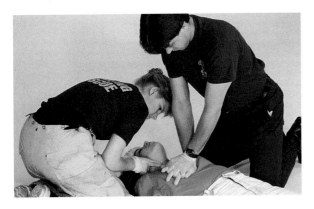

**Figure 7-31** The ventilator periodically checks the effectiveness of compressions by feeling for the carotid pulse while the compressor gives chest compressions.

1. Compressor says to change positions. He or she begins the cycle of compressions by saying, *"Change and, two and, three and, four and, five and, six...."*
2. Change positions. The ventilator completes one breath at the end of the *"change"* cycle and moves to the chest. He or she locates the correct hand position and waits for the other rescuer to signal before beginning compressions. The compressor moves to the casualty's head to become the ventilator. He or she checks for signs of circulation (pulse) for no more than 10 seconds. If there is no circulation, he or she communicates that there are no signs of circulation (pulse) and prompts the second resuer to continue CPR.
3. They continue two-rescuer CPR. The new compressor begins compressions. The new ventilator gives 2 breaths after each set of 15 compressions. The new ventilator continues to check the effectiveness of the compressions.

Two-rescuer CPR can also be performed on a child as on an adult. Use the child CPR technique (one hand) at a ratio of 5 chest compressions to 1 breath.

Skill Summaries for all two-rescuer skills are at the end of this chapter.

## ◆ SUMMARY

It is important to recognize signs and symptoms that may indicate a heart attack. If you think someone is suffering from a heart attack or if you are unsure, summon more advanced medical personnel without delay. Provide care by helping the casualty rest in the most comfortable position until help arrives.

When heartbeat and breathing stop, it is called cardiac arrest. A casualty who suffers a cardiac arrest is clinically dead, since no oxygen is reaching the cells of vital organs. Irreversible brain damage will occur from lack of oxygen. By starting CPR immediately, you can help keep the brain supplied with oxygen. By summoning more advanced medical personnel, you can increase the cardiac arrest casualty's chances for survival.

If the casualty does not have signs of circulation, start CPR.

If two rescuers are available, begin two-rescuer CPR as soon as possible. If either of you tires, quickly change positions and continue.

Once you start CPR, do not stop unnecessarily. Continue CPR until you are relieved by another trained rescuer, you are exhausted, the casualty's heart starts beating, more advanced medical personnel arrive and take over, or an AED is available.

### YOU ARE THE RESPONDER

1. You arrive on the scene to find a bystander giving CPR. You confirm that the casualty is in cardiac arrest and take over CPR. Advanced medical personnel have not yet arrived. You are tiring and do not think you can continue. What do you do?
2. You initiate CPR on an older casualty of cardiac arrest. You estimate him to be in his seventies. As you do compressions, you hear the chest crack and pop. What do you do?

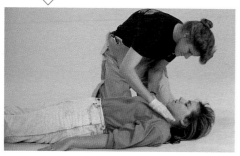

1. Check for responsiveness and call for help. If alone, "CALL FIRST."

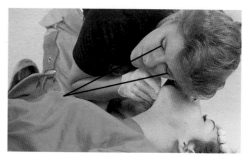

2. Open airway and check for breathing.

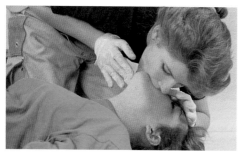

3. Give 2 slow breaths.

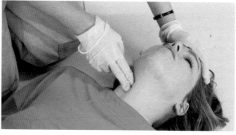

4. Check for signs of circulation (carotid pulse) and severe bleeding.

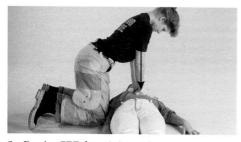

5. Begin CPR by giving 15 compressions.

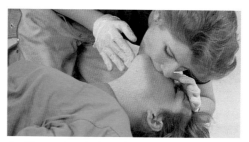

6. Then give 2 slow breaths.

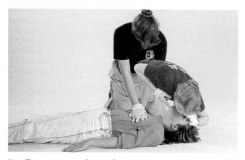

7. Repeat cycles of 15 compressions and 2 breaths.

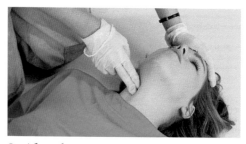

8. After about 1 minute, recheck for signs of circulation for no more than 10 seconds.

If there are still no signs of circulation (pulse),
continue CPR, beginning with chest compressions.

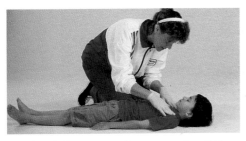

1. Check for responsiveness and call for help. If alone, "CALL FIRST."

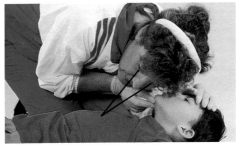

2. Open airway and check for breathing.

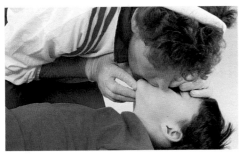

3. Give 2 slow breaths.

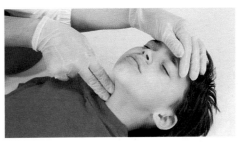

4. Check for signs of circulation (carotid pulse) and severe bleeding.

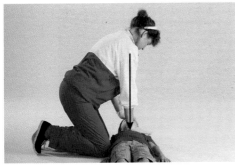

5. Begin CPR by giving 5 compressions

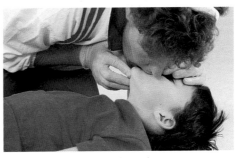

6. Then give 1 slow breath.

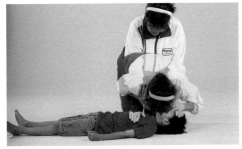

7. Repeat cycles of 5 compressions and 1 breath.

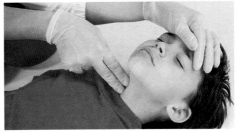

8. After about 1 minute, recheck for signs of circulation (pulse) for no more than 10 seconds.

If there are still no signs of circulation (pulse), continue CPR, beginning with chest compressions.

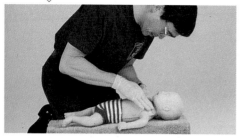

1. Check for responsiveness and call for help. If alone, "CALL FIRST."

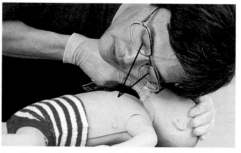

2. Open airway and check for breathing.

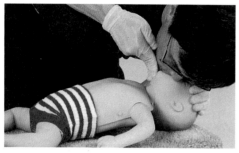

3. Give 2 slow puffs.

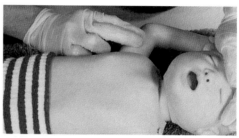

4. Check for signs of circulation (brachial pulse) and severe bleeding.

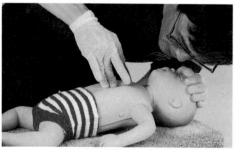

5. Begin CPR by giving 5 compressions.

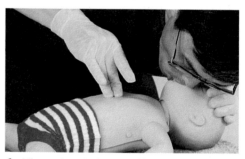

6. Then give 1 slow puff.

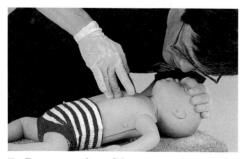

7. Repeat cycles of 5 compressions and 1 puff.

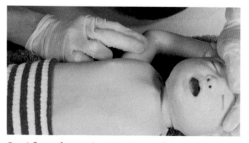

8. After about 1 minute, recheck signs of circulation (pulse) for no more than 10 seconds.

If there are still no signs of circulation (pulse),
continue CPR, beginning with chest compressions.

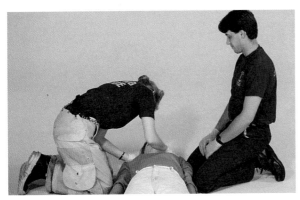

1. First rescuer checks for responsiveness.

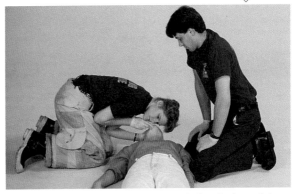

2. First rescuer opens airway and checks breathing.

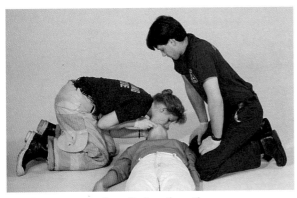

3. First rescuer gives 2 slow breaths.

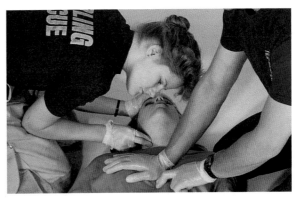

4. First rescuer checks for signs of circulation (carotid pulse). Second rescuer locates proper hand placement.

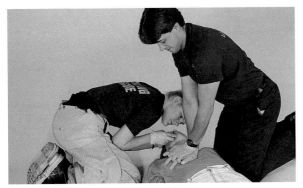

5. Second rescuer does 15 chest compressions for an adult casualty.

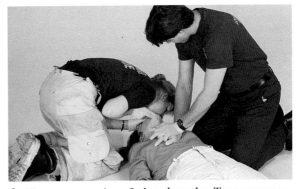

6. First rescuer gives 2 slow breaths. Two rescuers repeat cycles of CPR.

After about 1 minute of CPR, the rescuer at the head checks for signs of circulation (pulse). If there are still no signs of circulation (pulse), both rescuers continue CPR, beginning with chest compressions. Two-rescuer CPR can also be performed on a child as on an adult. Use the child CPR technique (one hand) at a ratio of 5 chest compressions to 1 breath.

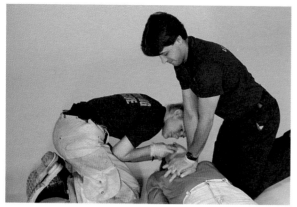

1. Rescuer at chest calls, "Change," and finishes compressions.

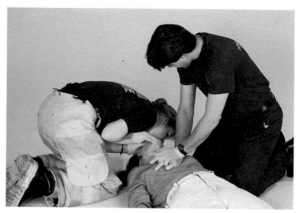

2. Rescuer at head gives breaths.

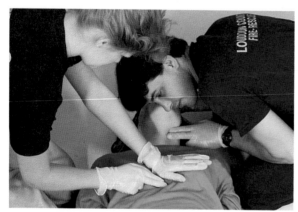

3. Rescuers change positions. New ventilator rechecks for signs of circulation (pulse).

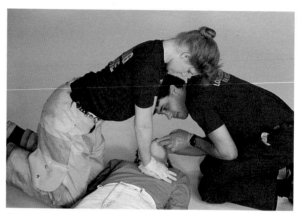

4. Compressor continues with chest compressions.

Repeat cycles of CPR. After about 1 minute of CPR, the rescuer at the head rechecks for signs of circulation (pulse). If there are still no signs of circulation, both rescuers continue CPR, beginning with chest compressions.

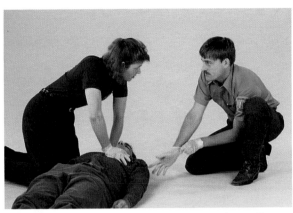

**1.** Second rescuer identifies himself or herself.

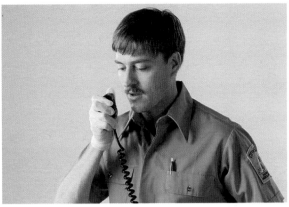

**2.** Second rescuer summons advanced medical personnel (if necessary).

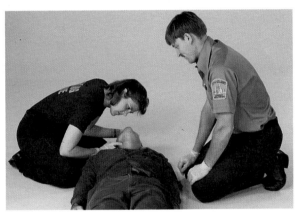

**3.** First rescuer completes CPR cycle and checks for signs of circulation (pulse). Second rescuer gets into position.

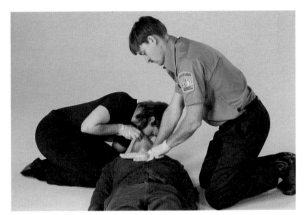

**4.** Second rescuer locates proper hand placement and does 15 chest compressions for an adult (5 chest compressions for a child).

Repeat cycles of CPR. After about 1 minute of CPR, the first rescuer rechecks for signs of circulation (pulse). If there are still no signs of circulation (pulse), both rescuers continue CPR, beginning with chest compressions.

# Breathing Devices

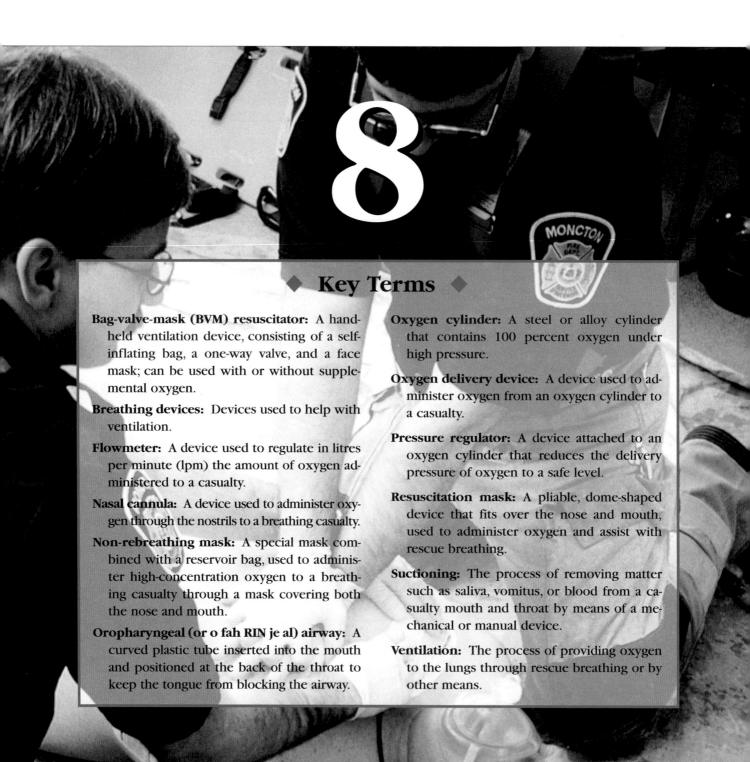

## ◆ Key Terms ◆

**Bag-valve-mask (BVM) resuscitator:** A hand-held ventilation device, consisting of a self-inflating bag, a one-way valve, and a face mask; can be used with or without supplemental oxygen.

**Breathing devices:** Devices used to help with ventilation.

**Flowmeter:** A device used to regulate in litres per minute (lpm) the amount of oxygen administered to a casualty.

**Nasal cannula:** A device used to administer oxygen through the nostrils to a breathing casualty.

**Non-rebreathing mask:** A special mask combined with a reservoir bag, used to administer high-concentration oxygen to a breathing casualty through a mask covering both the nose and mouth.

**Oropharyngeal (or o fah RIN je al) airway:** A curved plastic tube inserted into the mouth and positioned at the back of the throat to keep the tongue from blocking the airway.

**Oxygen cylinder:** A steel or alloy cylinder that contains 100 percent oxygen under high pressure.

**Oxygen delivery device:** A device used to administer oxygen from an oxygen cylinder to a casualty.

**Pressure regulator:** A device attached to an oxygen cylinder that reduces the delivery pressure of oxygen to a safe level.

**Resuscitation mask:** A pliable, dome-shaped device that fits over the nose and mouth, used to administer oxygen and assist with rescue breathing.

**Suctioning:** The process of removing matter such as saliva, vomitus, or blood from a casualty mouth and throat by means of a mechanical or manual device.

**Ventilation:** The process of providing oxygen to the lungs through rescue breathing or by other means.

## ◆ For Review ◆

Before reading this chapter, you should have a basic understanding of the respiratory system and the interrelationship of the body systems (Chapter 3). You should also know how to care for a casualty in respiratory distress or arrest (Chapter 6).

## ◆ INTRODUCTION

*A 45-year-old man is experiencing chest pain. He states that it started about 30 minutes ago as a mild, squeezing sensation. Now the pain is severe and he is gasping for breath. You recognize that these signs and symptoms suggest a serious condition. While waiting for an ambulance to arrive, you do what you can for the casualty. You help him get into the most comfortable position and ask him to remain still. You open a nearby window to circulate fresh air into the stuffy room.*

*You are called to assist a co-worker with an unknown medical emergency. You find a 60-year-old unconscious woman who has vomited and is not breathing. You know what must be done, but the sight of vomit causes you to hesitate. You overcome your reluctance, sweep out her mouth, and begin rescue breathing.*

What do both of these situations have in common? Both are examples of situations in which **breathing devices,** used to help with ventilation, would have been desirable and could have enhanced the care you were providing. Although most of the care that you give will not require the use of breathing devices, there are situations in which they can be used effectively as part of your care. Breathing devices include resuscitation masks and supplemental oxygen. Such devices can contribute significantly to the survival and recovery of a seriously ill or injured casualty.

As you learned in previous chapters, airway management is critical in life-threatening situations. In this chapter, you learn when and how to use various breathing devices to increase the effectiveness of the airway management you give a casualty who is injured or has suddenly become ill.

## ◆ BREATHING DEVICES

Many different breathing devices are commonly used in the prehospital setting. Which breathing devices are routinely available to you will depend on your local standards and protocols. This chapter focuses on those breathing devices that you are likely to have immediately available or be asked to assist with in providing care. *You should not delay care because a specific breathing device is not available.* Instead, you should start basic care, adding any breathing devices when they become available.

Breathing devices include resuscitation masks, bag-valve-mask resuscitators, oropharyngeal airways, suctioning devices, and oxygen. In general, they provide several advantages. They can help you—

- Maintain an open airway.
- Perform rescue breathing.
- Limit the potential for disease transmission.
- Increase the oxygen concentration in a person's bloodstream.

With all breathing devices, give the same number of ventilations as you would for rescue breathing.

### Resuscitation Masks

One of the most readily available, simple breathing devices for first responders is the *resuscitation mask.* Resuscitation masks are pliable, dome-shaped devices that fit over a person's mouth and nose, aiding *ventilation* (providing oxygen to the lungs). Several types of resuscitation masks are available, varying in size, shape, and features (Fig. 8-1).

Resuscitation masks offer you several advantages. These include—

• Increasing the flow of air to the lungs by permitting air to travel through a person's mouth and nose at the same time.

• Providing an adequate seal for ventilation, even when a person has facial injuries.

• Providing an effective and easily accessible alternative to other methods of ventilation, such as mouth-to-mouth or mouth-to-nose breathing or bag-valve-mask resuscitation.

• Permitting easy delivery of supplemental oxygen to either a breathing or a nonbreathing casualty.

• Reducing the possibility of disease transmission by providing a barrier between the rescuer and the casualty.

### Selecting a Resuscitation Mask

For a resuscitation mask to be most effective, it should meet the following criteria:

• Be made of a transparent, pliable material that allows you to make a tight seal on the casualty's face when you perform rescue breathing or supply supplemental oxygen.

• Have a one-way valve for releasing a casualty's exhaled air.

• Have a standard 15-mm or 22-mm coupling assembly (the diameter of the opening that receives the one-way valve).

• Have an inlet for the delivery of supplemental oxygen.

• Work well under a variety of environmental conditions, such as extreme heat or cold.

• Be easy to assemble and use.

Figure 8-2 shows the features of an effective resuscitation mask.

### Using a Resuscitation Mask

When using a resuscitation mask, begin by attaching the one-way valve to the mask. Next, place the mask so that it covers the casualty's mouth and nose. Position one rim of the mask between the lower lip and chin. The opposite end of the mask should cover the nose. Figure 8-3 shows how to assemble and position the resuscitation mask.

When you use a resuscitation mask to give rescue breathing, you must maintain a good seal to prevent air from leaking at the edges of the mask. Use both hands to hold the mask in place and to maintain an open airway. You do this by following three steps. They involve—

• Tilting the casualty's head back.
• Lifting the jaw upward.
• Keeping the casualty's mouth open.

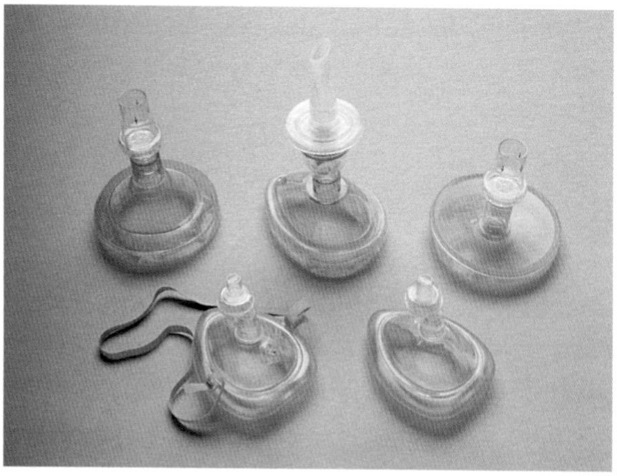

**Figure 8-1** Resuscitation masks vary in size, shape, and features.

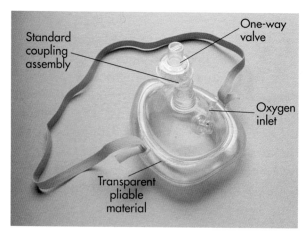

**Figure 8-2** A resuscitation mask should meet specific criteria.

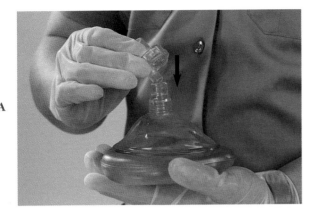

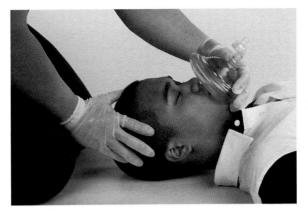

**Figure 8-3**  To use a resuscitation mask, **A,** begin by attaching the one-way valve to the mask. **B,** Position the mask to cover the mouth and nose.

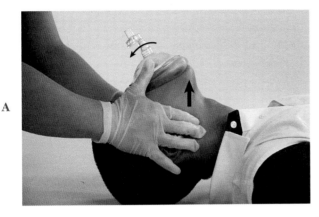

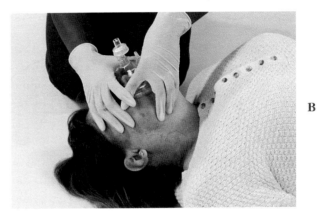

**Figure 8-4**  **A,** Tilt the head back, and lift the jaw to open the airway. **B,** Holding the mask from the side is an alternative method for using a resuscitation mask, for example, during one-rescuer CPR.

Figure 8-4 shows two methods for using a resuscitation mask.

If you suspect the casualty has a head or spinal injury, use the two-handed jaw thrust technique without head-tilt, described in Chapter 6. This technique can also be used with a resuscitation mask (Fig. 8-5). However, because the success of this technique depends on one's hand size and strength, some people will find it difficult to perform a two-handed jaw thrust using a resuscitation mask.

## Bag-Valve-Mask Resuscitators

There may be times when you will have a bag-valve-mask resuscitator available or be asked to assist with one. A ***bag-valve-mask (BVM) resuscitator*** is a hand-held device, like the resuscitation mask, primarily used to ventilate a nonbreathing casualty. It is also used to assist ventilation of a casualty who is in respiratory distress.

The device has three main components: a bag, valve, and mask. The bag is self-inflating. Once compressed, it reinflates automatically. The one-way valve allows air to move from the bag to the casualty but prevents the casualty's exhaled air from entering the bag. The mask is similar to the resuscitation masks described earlier in this chapter. An oxygen reservoir bag should be attached to the BVM when supplemental oxygen is administered (Fig. 8-6).

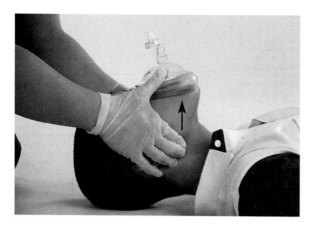

**Figure 8-5** If you suspect a head or spine injury, lift the jaw but do not tilt the head back.

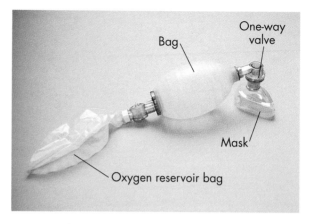

**Figure 8-6** A bag-valve-mask (BVM) resuscitator consists of a bag, valve, and mask. An oxygen reservoir bag should be attached at the end of the bag when delivering supplemental oxygen.

The principle of the BVM is simple. By placing the mask on the casualty's face and squeezing the bag, you open the one-way valve, forcing air into the casualty's lungs. When you release the bag, the valve closes and air from the atmosphere refills the bag. At approximately the same time, the casualty exhales. This exhaled air is diverted into the atmosphere through the closed one-way valve.

### Using a Bag-Valve-Mask Resuscitator

In the hands of a well-practised rescuer, the BVM resuscitator is effective. But studies have shown that without consistent practice, single rescuers have a difficult time maintaining a tight enough seal and also maintaining an open airway for effective ventilation. For this reason, it is best if a BVM is used by two rescuers when possible.

When two rescuers are using a BVM, one rescuer positions the mask and opens the casualty's airway. This is done in the same way as previously described for resuscitation masks. While the first rescuer maintains a tight seal with the mask on the casualty's face (Fig. 8-7, *A*), the second rescuer provides ventilations by squeezing the bag until the casualty's chest rises (Fig. 8-7, *B*). The bag should always be squeezed smoothly, not forcefully. This two-person technique is preferred because one rescuer can maintain an open

airway and a tight mask seal, while a second rescuer can provide ventilations.

If you must use a bag-valve-mask resuscitator alone, begin by assembling the bag, valve, and mask. Next, position the mask so that it covers the casualty's mouth and nose in the same way previously described for resuscitation masks. Open the airway. With one hand, hold the mask in place by making a "C-clamp" with your index finger and thumb around the mask. Maintain an open airway using your other fingers to lift the jaw. You can use your knees to help hold the casualty's head in this tilted position.

With one hand, press down on the mask to maintain a tight seal and help open the casualty's mouth. With your other hand, squeeze the bag slowly until the casualty's chest rises. People with small hands or poor grip strength may need to compress the bag against their thigh to adequately ventilate the casualty.

### Advantages and Disadvantages

Using the bag-valve-mask resuscitator has distinct advantages and disadvantages.

*Advantages:*

◆ It delivers a higher concentration of oxygen than that delivered during mouth-to-mouth or mouth-to-mask rescue breathing.

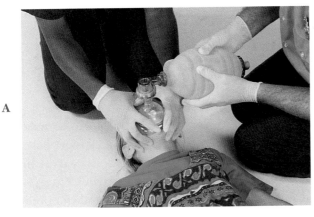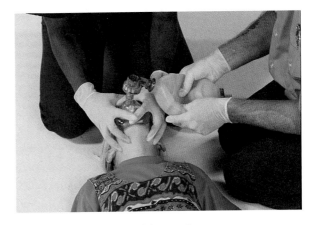

**Figure 8-7**  **A,** Position the mask over the casualty's mouth and nose. Hold it in place as you would a resuscitation mask. **B,** Second rescuer squeezes the bag slowly until the chest rises.

- It limits the potential for disease transmission.
- It is very effective when used by two rescuers.

*Disadvantages:*

- It is not an easy one-person skill to master.
- Without regular practice, you cannot stay proficient.
- It may take longer to assemble than other breathing devices.
- It is not a device readily available to you.

## Supplemental Oxygen

As you may recall, the normal concentration of oxygen in the air is approximately 21 percent. Under normal conditions, this is more than enough oxygen to sustain life. However, when serious injury or sudden illness occurs, the body does not function properly and can benefit from supplemental, or additional, oxygen. Without adequate oxygen, hypoxia will result. **Hypoxia** is a condition in which insufficient oxygen reaches the cells. Hypoxia causes increased breathing and heart rates, cyanosis, changes in consciousness, restlessness, and chest pain.

For example, delivery of a higher concentration of oxygen to a person experiencing difficulty breathing and chest pain because of a heart attack or angina may reduce this pain and breathing discomfort. Any patient with shortness of breath or chest pain should always receive supplemental oxygen. **Supplemental oxygen** delivered to the casualty's lungs may help meet the increased demand for oxygen for all body tissues.

If a heart attack casualty suddenly suffers cardiac arrest, then you must use rescue breathing to force air into the casualty's lungs. Whether you perform rescue breathing using the mouth-to-mouth or mouth-to-mask method, the oxygen concentration you deliver to the casualty is only 16 percent. This is adequate to sustain life in a healthy person. But, since chest compressions only circulate one third of normal blood flow under the best of conditions, body tissues are receiving only the bare minimum of oxygen required for short-term survival.

Using a bag-valve-mask resuscitator alone only improves this situation slightly, since it delivers atmospheric air (21 percent oxygen). A higher oxygen concentration helps to counter the effects of severe illness or injury to the body. Administering supplemental oxygen allows a substantially higher oxygen concentration, in some cases nearly 100 percent, to be delivered to the casualty (Fig. 8-8).

To deliver supplemental oxygen, you must have—

- An oxygen cylinder.
- A pressure regulator with flowmeter.
- A delivery device.

Figure 8-9 shows an oxygen cylinder, pressure regulator, flowmeter, and O-ring.

## Oxygen Cylinder

It is easy to recognize an *oxygen cylinder* because of its distinctive green or white colour and yellow diamond marking that says *oxidizer.* These cylinders are made of steel or an alloy. Depending on their size, those used in the prehospital setting can hold between 350 and 625 litres of oxygen. These cylinders have internal pressures of approximately 2000 pounds per square inch (psi).

## Pressure Regulator

The pressure inside the oxygen cylinder is far too great for a person to simply open the cylinder and administer the oxygen. Instead, a device must be attached to the cylinder to reduce the delivery pressure of the oxygen to a safe level. This regulating device is called a *pressure regulator.* The pressure regulator reduces the pressure from approximately 2000 psi inside the cylinder to less than 70 psi.

A pressure regulator has a gauge that indicates how much pressure is in the cylinder. By checking the gauge, you can determine if a cylinder is full (2000 psi), nearly empty (200 psi), or somewhere in between.

A pressure regulator has three metal prongs that fit into the valve at the top of the oxygen cylinder. The largest of these prongs must have a doughnut-shaped gasket, commonly called an "O-ring," attached. This gasket provides a tight seal between the oxygen cylinder and the pressure regulator.

## Flowmeter

A *flowmeter* controls the amount of oxygen administered in litres per minute (1pm). Flowmeters normally deliver from 1 to 15 1pm, but some of the newer flowmeters can deliver as much as 25 1pm.

## Oxygen Delivery Devices

Some *oxygen delivery devices* can deliver oxygen to either breathing or nonbreathing casualties. Two devices, the resuscitation mask

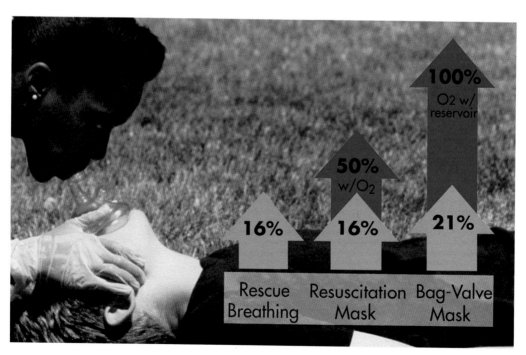

**Figure 8-8** Breathing devices and supplemental oxygen can greatly increase the concentration of oxygen that a casualty receives.

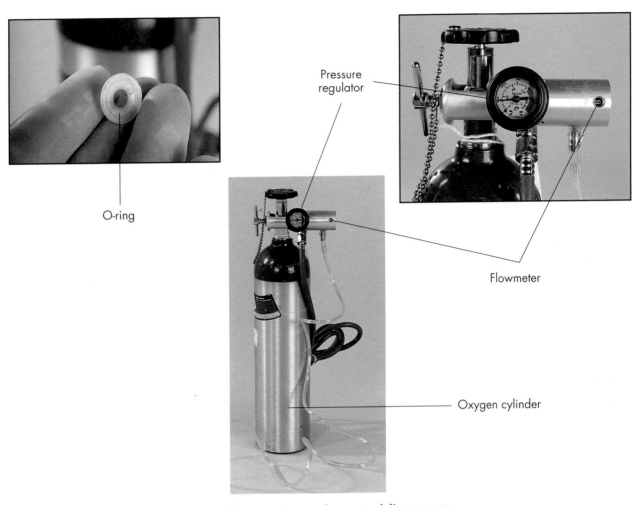

**Figure 8-9** Supplemental oxygen delivery system.

and the BVM, can deliver oxygen to both. For this reason, these devices are the most appropriate for you to use. Regardless of the device being used, a section of tubing is attached to the device at one end and to the flowmeter at the other end to create an oxygen-enriched environment for the casualty.

A resuscitation mask is capable of delivering approximately 50 percent oxygen to a breathing casualty, when delivered at 6 or more litres per minute. This is substantially higher than the normal 21 percent that the casualty is getting from the atmosphere. Some resuscitation masks have elastic straps attached to the mask. The elastic strap can be placed over the casualty's head and tightened to help keep the mask securely in place (Fig. 8-10, *A*). If the mask does not have a strap, either you or the casualty can hold it in place. When a resuscitation mask is used on a nonbreathing casualty, it will deliver an oxygen concentration of approximately 35 percent. The oxygen concentration is reduced because oxygen mixes with your exhaled air as you perform mouth-to-mouth rescue breathing.

The bag-valve-mask resuscitator with an oxygen reservoir bag is capable of supplying a minimum oxygen concentration of 90 percent when used at 10 or more litres per minute. The BVM can be held against the casualty's face, allowing a breathing casualty to inhale the supplemental oxygen (Fig. 8-10, *B*). A casualty breathing at a rate of less than 10 breaths per

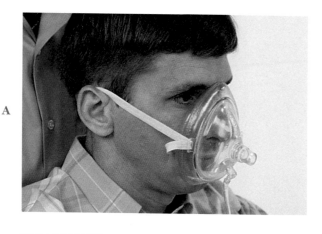

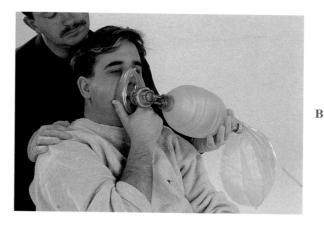

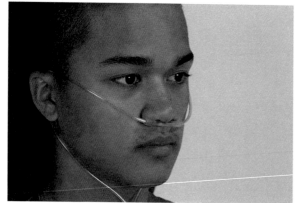

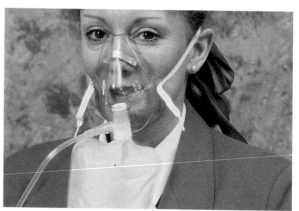

**Figure 8-10**  Common oxygen delivery devices include **A,** a resuscitation mask; **B,** a BVM; **C,** a nasal cannula; and **D,** a nonrebreather mask.

minute, or more than 30 per minute, should have his or her breathing assisted. This is done by squeezing the bag as the casualty breathes.

The high-concentration nonrebreather mask needs to have a flow rate of 10 or more litres a minute to ensure the proper reservoir bag inflation.

Some devices, such as the nasal cannula, can only be used to administer oxygen to breathing casualties. A ***nasal cannula*** is a device that delivers oxygen through the casualty's nostrils (Fig. 8-10, *C*). It is a plastic tube with two small prongs that are inserted into the nose. The use of a nasal cannula is limited, since it is normally used at a flow rate of 1 to 4 1pm. Under these conditions, it only delivers a peak oxygen concentration of approximately 36 percent. Flow rates above 4 1pm are not commonly used because of the tendency to quickly dry out mucous membranes. This can cause nosebleeds and headaches.

Because of its limitations, the nasal cannula is commonly used for casualties having only minor breathing difficulty. This device is not appropriate for casualties experiencing serious respiratory distress, since they are generally breathing through their mouths and need a device that can supply a greater concentration of oxygen. In addition, the nasal cannula can be ineffective if the casualty has a nasal airway obstruction, nasal injury, or bad cold causing blocked sinus passages. It should, however, be used if the casualty cannot tolerate a mask over his or her face.

It is sometimes difficult to remember how many litres of oxygen to deliver. To eliminate confusion over how many litres of oxygen to deliver per minute, remember this general rule:

**Table 8-1** Oxygen Delivery Devices

| Device | Common flow rate | Oxygen concentration | Function |
|--------|------------------|----------------------|----------|
| Nasal cannula | 1-4 lpm | 24-36 percent | Breathing casualties only |
| Resuscitation mask | 6+ lpm | 35-55 percent | Breathing and nonbreathing casualties |
| Bag-valve-mask resuscitator | 10+ lpm | 90+ percent | Breathing and nonbreathing casualties |
| Non-rebreathing mask | 10+ lpm | 90+ percent | Breathing casualties only |

*one to four and six or more.* For a nasal cannula, administering 1 to 4 1pm is appropriate. When using a mask that covers the casualty's face, you can safely administer 6 or more litres per minute. Table 8-1 provides an overview of each of the delivery devices presented.

## Administering Oxygen

Whether you are administering oxygen to a breathing or a nonbreathing casualty, the steps for preparing the equipment remain the same. Begin by examining the cylinder to be certain that it is labelled *oxygen* (Fig. 8-11, *A*). Next, check to see that the cylinder is full. Full cylinders come with a protective covering holding the plastic gasket (O-ring) in place. Remove this covering and save the gasket. Open the cylinder for 1 second (Fig. 8-11, *B*). This will remove any dirt or debris from the cylinder valve. Insert the gasket into the large opening of the cylinder (Fig. 8-12, *A*).

Next, examine the pressure regulator. Check to see that it is labelled *oxygen* pressure regulator (Fig. 8-12, *B*). Attach the pressure regulator to the cylinder, seating the three prongs inside the cylinder (Fig. 8-12, *C*). Hand tighten the screw until the regulator is snug (Fig. 8-12, *D*). Open the cylinder one full turn.

Check the pressure gauge to determine how much pressure is in the cylinder. A full cylinder should have approximately 2000 psi. Attach the chosen delivery device to the oxygen port near the flowmeter. Some devices, such as the resuscitation mask and the BVM, require that you attach a section of the tubing between the flowmeter and the device. Other devices, such as the nasal cannula, have this section of tubing already attached.

Turn on the flowmeter to the desired flow rate (Fig. 8-13). Listen and feel to make sure that oxygen is flowing into your delivery device. Finally, place the delivery device on the casualty.

A 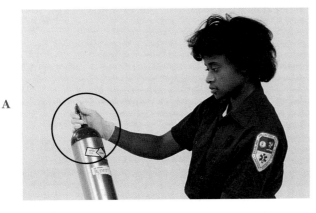 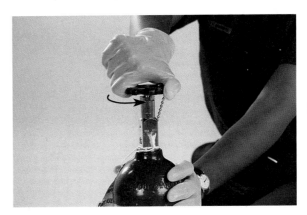 B

**Figure 8-11** **A,** An oxygen cylinder is usually green or white, with a yellow diamond indicating oxygen. **B,** When preparing oxygen equipment, clear the cylinder valve by turning it counterclockwise.

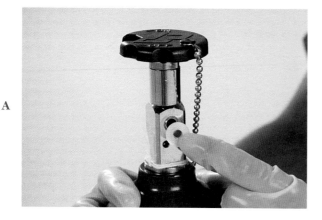

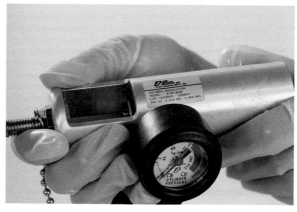

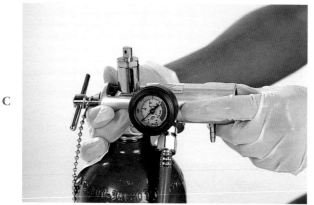

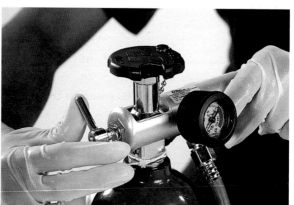

**Figure 8-12** To attach the pressure regulator to the oxygen cylinder, **A,** insert the gasket into the opening of the cylinder. **B,** Check to see that the pressure regulator is for use with oxygen. **C,** Seat the three prongs of the regulator inside the cylinder. **D,** Hand tighten the screw until the regulator is snug.

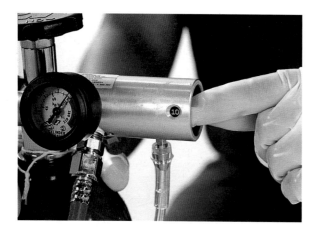

**Figure 8-13** Turn the flowmeter clockwise to the desired flow rate.

## Precautions

When administering oxygen, safety is a primary concern. Remember the following precautions:

- *Do not* operate oxygen equipment around an open flame or sparks. Oxygen causes fire to burn more rapidly.
- *Do not* stand oxygen cylinders upright unless they can be well secured. If the cylinder falls, it could damage the regulator or possibly loosen the cylinder valve.
- *Do not* use grease, oil, or petroleum products to lubricate any pressure regulator parts. Oxygen does not mix with these products, and a severe chemical reaction could cause an explosion.

# Oxygen-Powered Resuscitators: The Controversy Continues

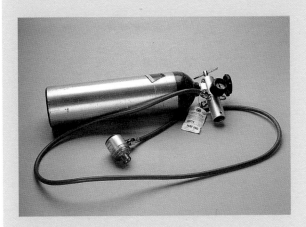

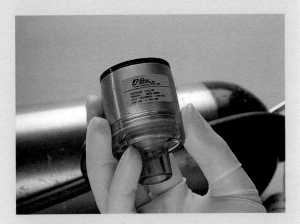

Oxygen-powered resuscitators, commonly called demand valves, have been the subject of controversy for several years. The points of controversy are whether these devices are as easy to use and safe as other oxygen delivery devices. As the name *demand valve* implies, the casualty can get oxygen on demand automatically.

A demand valve works in much the same way as a bag-valve-mask (BVM) resuscitator. However, instead of using a self-inflating bag as the ventilation source, it uses pressurized oxygen. The demand valve consists of a mask, a one-way valve, and an oxygen source. The mask is basically the same as that of the BVM unit. The one-way valve is designed to open and allow oxygen to flow to the breathing casualty upon inhalation. The rescuer must depress a button to force oxygen into the lungs of a nonbreathing casualty. The use of the demand valve to ventilate a nonbreathing casualty is commonly called positive pressure resuscitation.

There are both advantages and disadvantages to using a demand valve. Advantages include delivery of a high concentration of oxygen (approaching 100 percent), ease of use, and protection from disease transmission. Also, like the resuscitation mask and BVM, the demand valve can deliver oxygen to either breathing or non-breathing casualties.

The disadvantages include higher cost compared with other devices, requirement of a constant source of oxygen, and rapid depletion of a cylinder. In addition, because the oxygen is delivered under higher pressure, complications from overventilation have been reported. This resulted in manufacturers designing demand valves that restricted oxygen flow and installing relief valves to eliminate overinflation when ventilating nonbreathing casualties. However, this created another problem. This new restricted-flow demand valve did not always meet the needs of a casualty in severe respiratory distress. In addition, even with these restrictions, the device should not be used to ventilate nonbreathing children or infants because of the possibility that the device will overinflate the casualty.

Some EMS systems have stopped using demand valves. Others use both the newer restricted demand valve for nonbreathing casualties and the traditional demand valve for breathing casualties. Manufacturers are working to produce one demand valve more appropriate for both breathing and nonbreathing casualties.

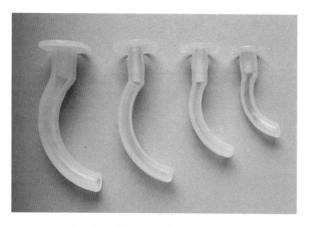

**Figure 8-14** Oropharyngeal airways come in a variety of sizes.

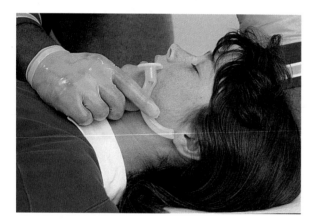

**Figure 8-15** Measure the oropharyngeal airway to see that it extends from the casualty's earlobe to the corner of the mouth.

◆ *Always check* to see that oxygen is flowing from the delivery device before placing the device over the casualty's face.

## Oropharyngeal Airways

As you may remember from Chapter 6, the tongue is the most common cause of airway obstruction in an unconscious casualty. An ***oropharyngeal airway*** is a device that is inserted into the mouth of an unconscious casualty and positioned to keep the tongue out of the back of the throat, keeping the airway open. An improperly placed airway device can compress the tongue into the back of the throat, further blocking the airway.

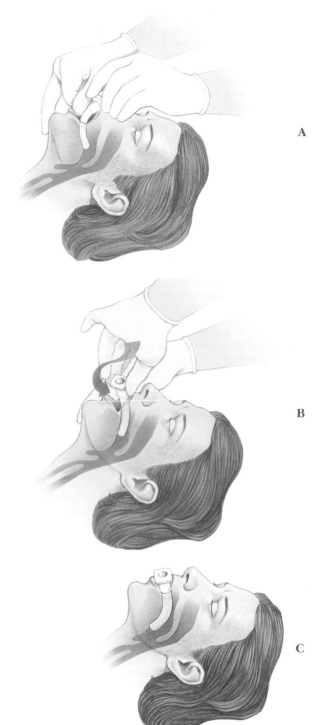

**Figure 8-16** **A,** Open the casualty's airway using the head-tilt/chin-lift. Insert the oropharyngeal airway with the curved end along the roof of the mouth. **B,** As the device approaches the back of the throat, rotate it a half turn. **C,** The device should drop into the throat without resistance. The flange end rests on the casualty's lower lip.

Oropharyngeal airways come in a variety of sizes (Fig. 8-14). The curved design fits the natural contour of the mouth and throat. Once you have positioned the device, you can use a resuscitation mask or bag-valve-mask resuscitator to ventilate a nonbreathing casualty.

When preparing to insert an oropharyngeal airway, first be sure the casualty is unconscious. Next, select the proper size of airway. Measure the device on the casualty to see that it extends from the casualty's earlobe to the corner of the mouth (Fig. 8-15). Grasp the casualty's lower jaw and tongue and lift upward. With the casualty's jaw raised, insert the oropharyngeal airway with the curved end along the roof of the mouth (Fig. 8-16, *A*). As the tip of the device approaches the back of the throat, rotate it a half turn (Fig. 8-16, *B*). If the casualty begins gagging as the device is positioned in the back of the throat, remove the device. The airway should drop into the throat without resistance. The flange end should rest on the casualty's lips (Fig. 8-16, *C*).

## Clearing the Airway

Sometimes injury or sudden illness results in foreign matter, such as mucus, vomitus, water, or blood, collecting in a casualty's airway. The most appropriate initial method of clearing the airway is to roll the casualty onto his or her side and sweep the secretions from the mouth. A more effective method is to suction the airway clear. ***Suctioning*** is the process of removing foreign matter by means of a mechanical or manual device. A variety of manual and mechanical devices are used to suction the airway.

Manual suction devices are lightweight, compact, and relatively inexpensive (Fig. 8-17, *A*). Mechanical suction devices use either battery-powered pumps or oxygen-powered aspirators (Fig. 8-17, *B*). These devices are normally found on ambulances. Attached to the end of any suction device is a suction tip. These come in various sizes and shapes. Some are rigid and others flexible.

Whether using a manual or mechanical suction device, perform these six steps:

1. Turn the casualty's head to one side. (If you suspect spinal injury, roll the casualty's body onto one side.)
2. Open the casualty's mouth.
3. Sweep large debris out of the mouth with your finger before suctioning.
4. Measure the distance of insertion from the casualty's ear lobe to the corner of the mouth.
5. Insert the suction tip into the back of the mouth.
6. Suction for no more than 10 seconds at a time.

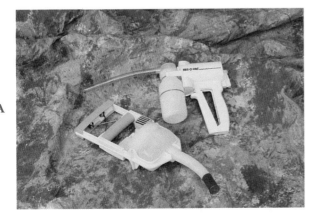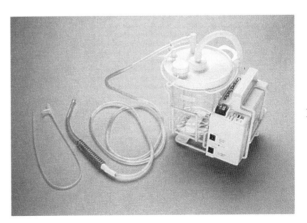

A

B

**Figure 8-17** **A,** Manual suction devices are lightweight and compact. **B,** Mechanical suction devices use either a battery-powered pump or an oxygen-powered aspirator.

## ◆ SUMMARY

Although they are not required, breathing devices can make the emergency care you provide safer, easier, and more effective. Airways help maintain an open airway by elevating the tongue away from the back of the throat. Suction equipment helps clear the airway of substances such as water, blood, saliva, or vomitus. The use of supplemental oxygen can relieve pain and breathing discomfort. The resuscitation mask and BVM are the most appropriate devices for first responders. They can significantly increase the oxygen concentration that an ill or injured casualty needs, help ventilate a nonbreathing casualty, and reduce the likelihood of disease transmission.

Breathing devices are appropriate for almost all types of injury or illness in which breathing may be impaired. Knowing how to use these devices will enable you to provide more effective care until advanced medical personnel arrive.

### YOU ARE THE RESPONDER

1. A 40-year-old man is experiencing chest pain and difficulty breathing. He is cyanotic (skin has a bluish colour), gasping for air, and breathing 28 times per minute. What breathing devices would you use to help this casualty?
2. The same casualty collapses, vomits, and stops breathing. How would you change your care for this casualty?

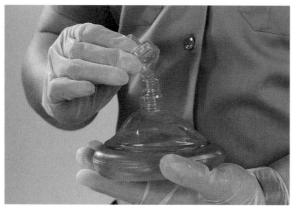

**1.** Assemble mask.

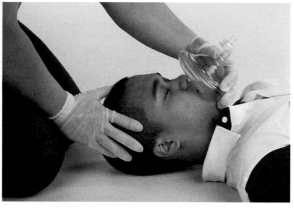

**2.** Kneel behind casualty's head. Position mask.

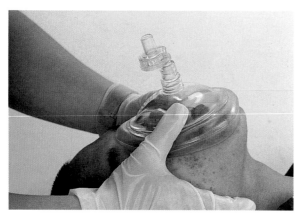

**3.** Seal mask. Tilt head back and lift jaw to open airway.

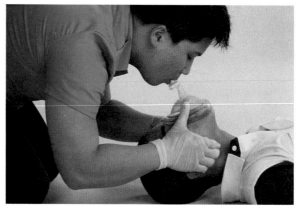

**4.** Begin rescue breathing.

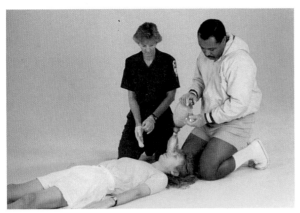

**1.** First rescuer assembles BVM.

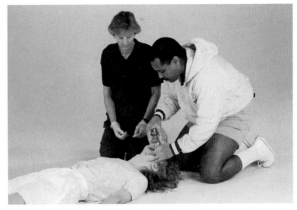

**2.** First rescuer positions mask.

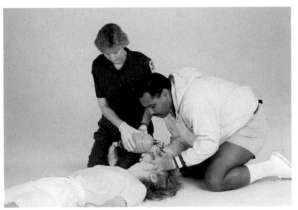

**3.** First rescuer tilts head, lifts jaw, and applies pressure to mask.

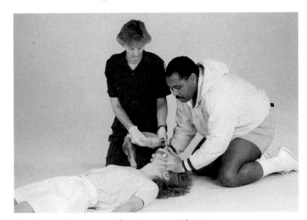

**4.** Second rescuer begins ventilations.

Give the same number of ventilations as you would for rescue breathing.

# Oxygen Delivery

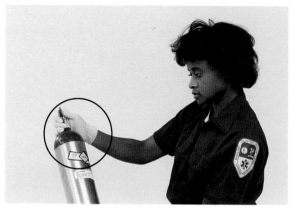

**1.** Check cylinder.

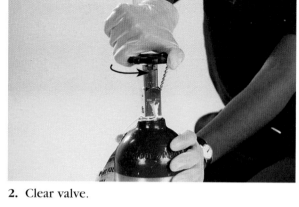

**2.** Clear valve.

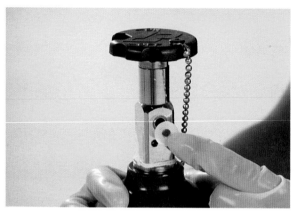

**3.** Insert gasket into cylinder.

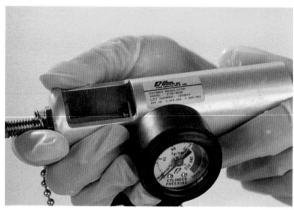

**4.** Check pressure regulator.

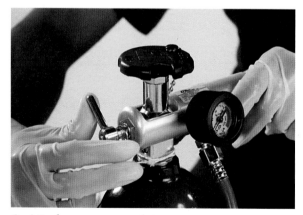

**5.** Attach pressure regulator.

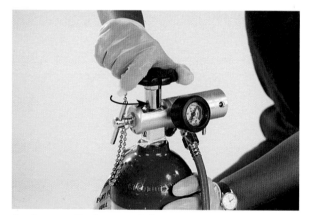

**6.** Open cylinder one full turn.

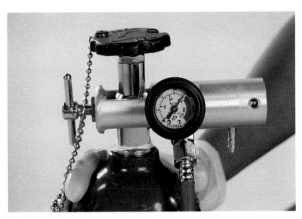

**7.** Check pressure gauge.

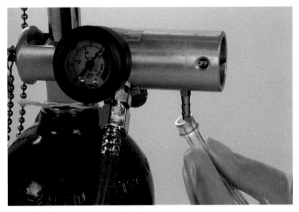

**8.** Attach delivery device to flowmeter.

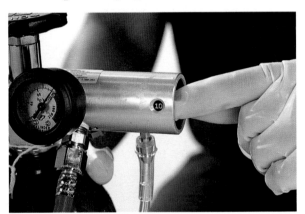

**9.** Adjust flowmeter.

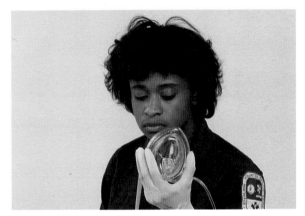

**10.** Verify oxygen flow.

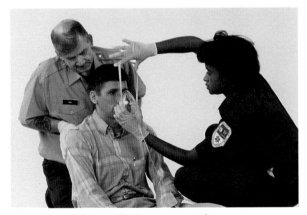

**11.** Place delivery device on casualty.

CAUTION: When breaking down the equipment, remove the delivery device from the casualty's face, turn off the flowmeter, close the cylinder, and then turn on the flowmeter to bleed the line. Finally, remove the regulator from the cylinder so that other participants may practice the complete skill.

# Bleeding

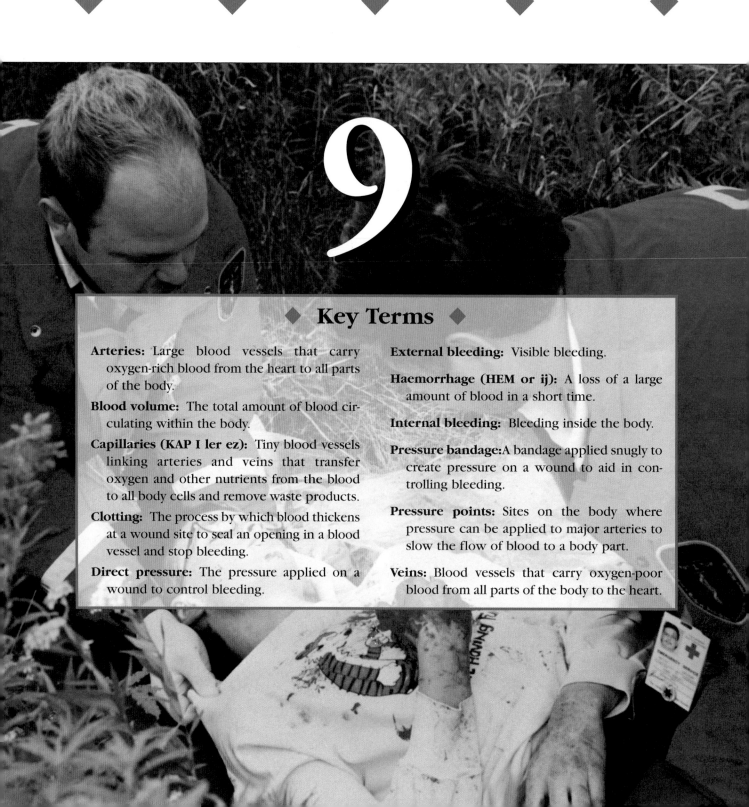

# 9

## ◆ Key Terms ◆

**Arteries:** Large blood vessels that carry oxygen-rich blood from the heart to all parts of the body.

**Blood volume:** The total amount of blood circulating within the body.

**Capillaries (KAP I ler ez):** Tiny blood vessels linking arteries and veins that transfer oxygen and other nutrients from the blood to all body cells and remove waste products.

**Clotting:** The process by which blood thickens at a wound site to seal an opening in a blood vessel and stop bleeding.

**Direct pressure:** The pressure applied on a wound to control bleeding.

**External bleeding:** Visible bleeding.

**Haemorrhage (HEM or ij):** A loss of a large amount of blood in a short time.

**Internal bleeding:** Bleeding inside the body.

**Pressure bandage:** A bandage applied snugly to create pressure on a wound to aid in controlling bleeding.

**Pressure points:** Sites on the body where pressure can be applied to major arteries to slow the flow of blood to a body part.

**Veins:** Blood vessels that carry oxygen-poor blood from all parts of the body to the heart.

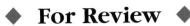

## ◆ For Review ◆

Before reading this chapter, you should have a basic understanding of how the circulatory system functions and how it interacts with other body systems (Chapter 3). You will also need to recall the emergency action principles (Chapter 5).

## ◆ INTRODUCTION

Bleeding is the loss of blood from arteries, veins, or capillaries. A large amount of bleeding occurring in a short time is called a ***haemorrhage.*** Bleeding is either internal or external. Internal bleeding is often difficult to recognize. External bleeding is usually obvious because it is typically visible. Uncontrolled bleeding, whether internal or external, is a life-threatening emergency.

As you learned in previous chapters, severe bleeding can result in death. Check for and control severe bleeding during the primary survey once you have checked for a pulse. You may not identify internal bleeding, however, until you perform a more detailed check during the secondary survey. In this chapter, you will learn how to recognize and care for both internal and external bleeding.

## ◆ BLOOD AND BLOOD VESSELS

### Blood Components

Blood consists of liquid and solid components and comprises approximately eight percent of the body's total weight. The liquid part of the blood is called plasma. The solid components are the red and white blood cells and cell fragments called platelets.

Plasma makes up about half of the ***blood volume,*** the total amount of blood circulating within the body. Composed mostly of water, plasma maintains the blood volume that the circulatory system needs to function normally. Plasma also contains nutrients essential for energy production, growth, and cell maintenance and carries waste products for elimination.

White blood cells are a key disease-fighting component of the immune system. They defend the body against invading microorganisms. They also aid in producing antibodies that help the body resist infection.

Red blood cells account for most of the solid components of the blood. They are produced in the marrow in the hollow centre of large bones such as the large bone of the arm (humerus) and of the thigh (femur). Red blood cells number nearly 260 million in each drop of blood. The red blood cells transport oxygen from the lungs to the body cells and carbon dioxide from the cells to the lungs. Red blood cells outnumber white blood cells about 1000 to 1.

Platelets are disk-shaped cells in the blood. Platelets are an essential part of the blood's clotting mechanism because they tend to bind together. ***Clotting*** is the process by which whole blood thickens at a wound site. Platelets help stop bleeding by forming blood clots at wound sites. Blood clots form the framework for healing. Until blood clots form, bleeding must be controlled artificially.

### Blood Functions

The blood has three major functions:

- Transporting oxygen, nutrients, and wastes.
- Protecting against disease by producing antibodies and defending against germs.
- Helping to maintain constant body temperature by circulating throughout the body.

### Blood Vessels

Blood is channeled through blood vessels. There are three major types of blood vessels: arteries, capillaries, and veins (Fig. 9-1). ***Arteries*** carry

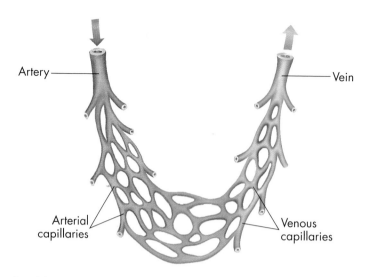

**Figure 9-1** Blood flows through the three major types of blood vessels: arteries, veins, and capillaries.

oxygen-rich blood away from the heart. Arteries become narrower the farther they extend from the heart until they connect to the capillaries. *Capillaries* are microscopic blood vessels linking arteries and veins that transfer oxygen and other nutrients from the blood to the cells. Capillaries pick up waste products, such as carbon dioxide, from the cells and transfer them to the veins. The *veins* carry waste products from the cells to the organs that eliminate waste from the body, such as the kidneys and lungs.

Blood in the arteries travels faster and under greater pressure than blood in the capillaries or veins. Blood flow in the arteries pulses with the heartbeat; blood in the veins flows more slowly and evenly.

## ♦ WHEN BLEEDING OCCURS

When bleeding occurs, the body begins a complex chain of events. The brain, heart, and lungs immediately attempt to compensate for blood loss to maintain the flow of oxygen-rich blood to the body, particularly to the vital organs.

Other important reactions also occur. Platelets collect at the wound site in an effort to stop blood loss through clotting. White blood cells try to prevent infection by attacking microorganisms that commonly enter through breaks in the skin. The body manufactures extra red blood cells to help transport more oxygen to the cells.

Blood volume is also affected by bleeding. Normally, excess fluid is absorbed from the bloodstream by the kidneys, lungs, intestines, and skin. However, when bleeding occurs, this excess fluid is reabsorbed into the bloodstream as plasma. This helps maintain the critical balance of fluids needed by the body to keep blood volume constant.

Bleeding severe enough to critically reduce the blood volume is life threatening. Severe bleeding can be either internal or external (Fig. 9-2).

## External Bleeding

External bleeding occurs when a blood vessel is opened externally, such as through a tear in the skin. You can usually see this type of bleeding. Most external bleeding you will encounter will be minor. Minor bleeding, such as occurs with small cuts, usually stops by itself within 10 minutes when the blood clots. Sometimes, the damaged blood vessel is too large or the blood is under too much pressure for effective clotting to occur. In these cases, you will need to recognize

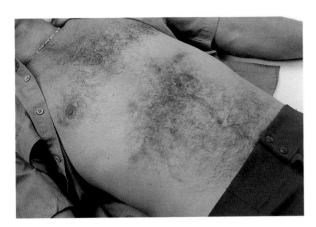 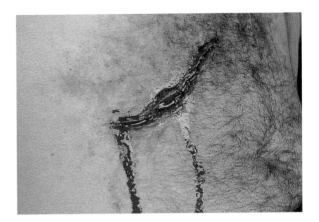

**Figure 9-2** Severe bleeding can be internal or external.

and control bleeding promptly. Look for severe bleeding during the check for circulation that is part of the primary survey.

### Recognizing External Bleeding

The signs of severe external bleeding include—

◆ Blood spurting from a wound.
◆ Blood that fails to clot after you have taken all measures to control bleeding.

Each type of blood vessel bleeds differently. Bleeding from arteries is often rapid and profuse. It is life threatening. Because arterial blood is under direct pressure from the heart, it usually spurts from the wound, making it difficult for clots to form. Because clots do not form rapidly, bleeding from arteries is harder to control than bleeding from veins and capillaries. Its high concentration of oxygen gives arterial blood a bright red colour.

Veins are damaged more often than arteries because they are closer to the skin's surface. Venous bleeding (bleeding from the veins) is easier to control than arterial bleeding. Venous blood is under less pressure than arterial blood and flows from the wound at a steady rate without spurting. Only damage to veins deep in the body, such as those in the trunk or thigh, produces profuse bleeding that is hard to control. Because it is oxygen-poor, venous blood is dark red or maroon.

Capillary bleeding is usually slow because the vessels are small and the blood is under low pressure. It is often described as "oozing" from the wound. Clotting occurs easily with capillary bleeding. The blood is usually dark red in colour.

### Controlling External Bleeding

External bleeding is usually easy to control. Generally, you can control it by applying pressure with your hand on the wound. This is called applying ***direct pressure.*** Pressure on the wound restricts the blood flow through the wound and allows normal clotting to occur. Elevating the injured area also slows the flow of blood and encourages clotting. You can maintain pressure on a wound by snugly applying a bandage to the injured area. A bandage applied to control bleeding is called a ***pressure bandage.*** This combination of pressure and elevation will control most bleeding.

In a few cases, direct pressure and elevation may not control severe bleeding. In these cases, you will have to take other measures. To further slow bleeding, you may compress the artery supplying the area against an underlying bone at specific sites on the body. These sites are called ***pressure points*** (Fig. 9-3, *A*).

The main pressure points used to control bleeding in the arms and legs are the brachial and femoral arteries (Fig. 9-3, *B*). Pressure points in other areas of the body may also be used to

# Blood: The Beat Goes On

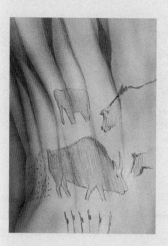

**The Ice Age—Prehistoric Man**
Primitive man draws a giant mammoth on a cave, with a red ochre marking resembling a heart in its chest.

**500 B.C.—Greek Civilization**
Ancient Greek physicians propound the theory of the humours, associating man's personality and health with four substances in the body—blood, black bile, yellow bile, and phlegm. An imbalance can cause diseases or emotional problems. A curious practice called bloodletting develops in which physicians open a patient's vein and let him or her bleed to fix an imbalance in the humours.

**900 to 1400—The Middle Ages**
Bloodletting flourishes during the Middle Ages. Astrology's influence grows, leading doctors to use astrological charts to determine when and where to open a vein. Medical schools sprout up in England. France, Belgium, and Italy.

**Circa 200 A.D.—Late Roman Civilization**
Galen, doctor of Roman Emperor Marcus Aurelius, theorizes that blood is continuously formed in the liver and then moves in two systems—one that combines with the air and a second that forms from food to nourish the body.

**1628—The Renaissance Period**
Dr. William Harvey cuts into live frogs and snakes to observe the heart. Through his studies. Harvey determines that blood circulates through the heart, the lungs, and rest of the body.

**3000 B.C.—The Fifth Dynasty**
Egyptians believe that blood is created in the stomach and that vessels running from the heart are filled with blood, air, feces, and tears.

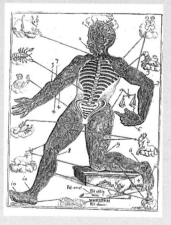

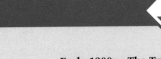

**Early 1900s—The Twentieth Century**

Dr. Karl Landsteiner discovers that all human blood is not compatible and names the blood types. His work helps make blood transfusions commonplace.

**1982**

Dr. William DeVries implants the first artificial heart in Barney Clark. The Seattle dentist survives 112 days, and the Jarvik-7 beats 12,912,499 times before Clark dies. In the 1980s, five artificial hearts are implanted. The longest survival period lasts 620 days. The body continues to treat the artificial heart as a "foreign body" and rejects it.

**1953**

Dr. John H. Gibbon invents a heart-lung machine to recirculate blood and provide oxygen during open-heart surgery, enabling more complex surgical techniques to develop.

**1661**

The invention of the microscope allows Italian-born physician Malpighi to see the tiny capillaries that link veins and arteries.

**1665**

The first blood transfusion mixes the blood of one dog with another. Transfusions range from successful to disastrous. One scientist proposes a transfusion between unhappily married people to try to reconcile the couple. After a man who receives sheep's blood dies, transfusion is outlawed in France.

**1967**

The first heart transplant is attempted by Dr. Christiaan Barnard in Cape Town, South Africa. Louis Washansky, a 54-year-old grocer, receives the heart of a woman hit by a speeding car. Washansky survives 18 days.

**The Future**

Through the ages, medical science has made extensive progress in saving lives. Many millions of people throughout the world receive blood transfusions each year. Several thousand people are living with another person's heart inside their chest. Several hundred thousand people are kept alive with an artificial kidney or a kidney transplant. The early medical experiments of yesterday have become commonplace lifesaving procedures today.

**1944**

When kidneys fail, poisons are released into the bloodstream that can cause vomiting, coma, and eventually death. Dr. Willem Kolff, a Dutch physician, develops one of the first artificial kidneys by sending the blood through a cellophane tubing that filters out the poisons.

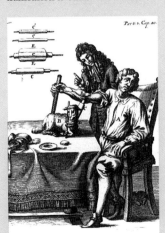

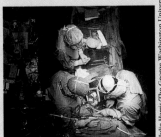

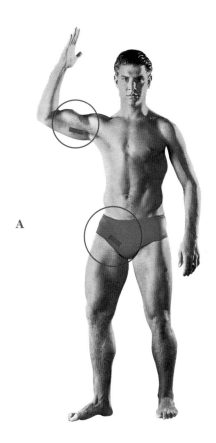

A

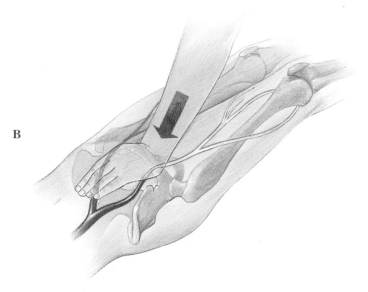

B

**Figure 9-3  A,** Pressure points are specific sites on the body where arteries lie close to the bone and the body's surface. **B,** Blood flow to an area can be controlled by applying pressure at one of these sites, compressing the artery against the bone.

control blood flow, but you are unlikely to need to use them. A **tourniquet,** a tight band placed around an arm or leg to constrict blood vessels to stop blood flow to a wound, is rarely used as part of emergency care because it too often does more harm than good.

To control external bleeding, follow these general steps:

1. Have the casualty sit or lie down and rest.
2. Place direct pressure on the wound with a sterile gauze pad or any clean cloth, such as a washcloth, towel, or handkerchief. Using gauze or a clean cloth keeps the wound free from germs. Place a hand over the gauze pad and apply firm pressure (Fig. 9-4, *A*). If you do not have gauze or cloth available, apply pressure with your gloved hand or have the injured casualty apply pressure with his or her hand. Use your bare hand only as a last resort.

3. Elevate the injured area above the level of the heart if you do not suspect a broken bone (Fig. 9-4, *B*).
4. Apply a pressure bandage. This bandage will hold the gauze pads or cloth in place while maintaining direct pressure (Fig. 9-4, *C*). If blood soaks through, add additional dressings and bandages with additional direct pressure. Do not remove any blood-soaked dressings or bandages.
5. If bleeding continues, apply pressure at a pressure point to slow the flow of blood (Fig. 9-4, *D*).

A good way to remember the basics of first aid for external bleeding is the acronym RED:

R - rest
E - elevate the injured area above the heart
D - direct pressure on the bleeding site

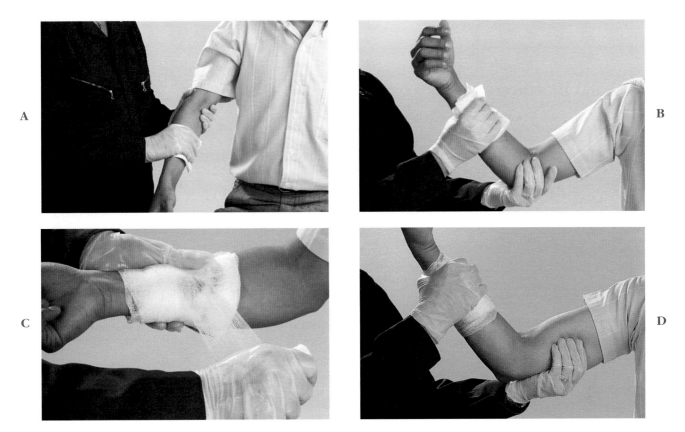

**Figure 9-4**  **A,** Apply direct pressure to the wound using a sterile gauze pad or clean cloth. **B,** Elevate the injured area above the level of the heart if you do not suspect a fracture. **C,** Apply a pressure bandage. **D,** If necessary, slow the flow of blood by applying pressure to the artery with your hand at the appropriate pressure point.

Continue to monitor the casualty's airway and breathing. Observe the casualty closely for signs that indicate a worsening condition. If bleeding is severe, administer supplemental oxygen to the casualty if available. Summon more advanced medical personnel if this has not already been done. If bleeding is not severe, provide additional care as needed.

### Preventing Disease Transmission

To reduce the risk of disease transmission when controlling bleeding, you should always follow the precautions you learned in Chapter 4. These include—

- Avoiding contacting the casualty's blood, directly or indirectly, by using barriers, such as gloves or goggles.
- Avoiding eating, drinking, and touching your mouth, nose, or eyes while providing care or before washing your hands.
- Always washing your hands thoroughly after providing care, even if you wore gloves or used other barriers.

Refer to Chapter 4 for a more detailed discussion of preventing disease transmission.

## Internal Bleeding

*Internal bleeding* is the escape of blood from arteries, veins, or capillaries into spaces in the body. Capillary bleeding, indicated by mild bruising, is just beneath the skin and is not serious. Deeper bleeding, however, involves arteries and veins and may result in severe blood loss.

Severe internal bleeding usually occurs in injuries caused by a violent blunt force, such as when the driver is thrown against the steering wheel in a car crash or when someone falls from a height. Internal bleeding may also occur when a sharp object, such as a knife, penetrates the skin and damages internal structures.

### Recognizing Internal Bleeding

Because internal bleeding is more difficult to recognize than external bleeding, you should always suspect internal bleeding in any serious injury. For example, if you find a motorcycle rider thrown from a bike, you may not see any serious external bleeding, but you should consider that the violent forces involved indicate the likelihood of internal injuries. Internal bleeding can occur from a fractured bone that ruptures an organ or blood vessels.

The body's inability to adjust to severe internal bleeding will eventually produce signs and symptoms that indicate shock. These signs and symptoms are less obvious and may take time to appear. These signs and symptoms include—

- Discolouration of the skin (bruising) in the injured area.
- Soft tissues, such as those in the abdomen, that are tender, swollen, or firm.
- Anxiety or restlessness.
- Rapid, weak pulse.
- Rapid breathing.

- Skin that feels cool or moist or looks pale or bluish.
- Nausea and vomiting.
- Excessive thirst.
- Declining level of consciousness.
- Drop in blood pressure.

Shock is discussed in detail in Chapter 10.

### Controlling Internal Bleeding

How you control internal bleeding depends on the severity and the site of the bleeding. For minor internal bleeding, such as a bruise on an arm, apply ice or a chemical cold pack to the injured area to help reduce pain and swelling. When applying ice, always remember to place something, such as a gauze pad or a towel, between the source of cold and the skin to prevent skin damage.

If you suspect internal bleeding caused by serious injury, summon more advanced medical personnel immediately. There is little you can do to control bleeding effectively. The casualty must be transported rapidly to the hospital. The casualty will often need immediate surgery to correct the problem. While waiting for more advanced medical personnel to arrive, follow the general guidelines for caring for any emergency. These are—

- Do no further harm.
- Monitor the ABCs and vital signs.
- Help the casualty rest in the most comfortable position.
- Maintain normal body temperature.
- Reassure the casualty.
- Provide care for other conditions.

In addition, administer oxygen if it is available and you are trained to do so.

## ◆ SUMMARY

One of the most important things you can do in any emergency is to recognize and control severe bleeding. External bleeding is easily recognized and should be cared for immediately. Check and care for severe bleeding during the primary survey. Severe external bleeding is life threatening. Although internal bleeding is less obvious, it also can be life threatening. Recognize when a serious injury has occurred and suspect internal bleeding. You may not identify internal bleeding until you perform the secondary survey. When you identify or suspect severe bleeding, request an ambulance so that the casualty can be transported quickly to a hospital. Continue to provide care until more advanced medical personnel arrive and take over.

## YOU ARE THE RESPONDER

1. *You are summoned to assist a worker who has been injured. She is bleeding severely from a large wound in her thigh. What care would you provide first?*
2. *The wound continues to bleed even after you have applied a pressure bandage and additional dressings. What further care would you provide?*

# Shock

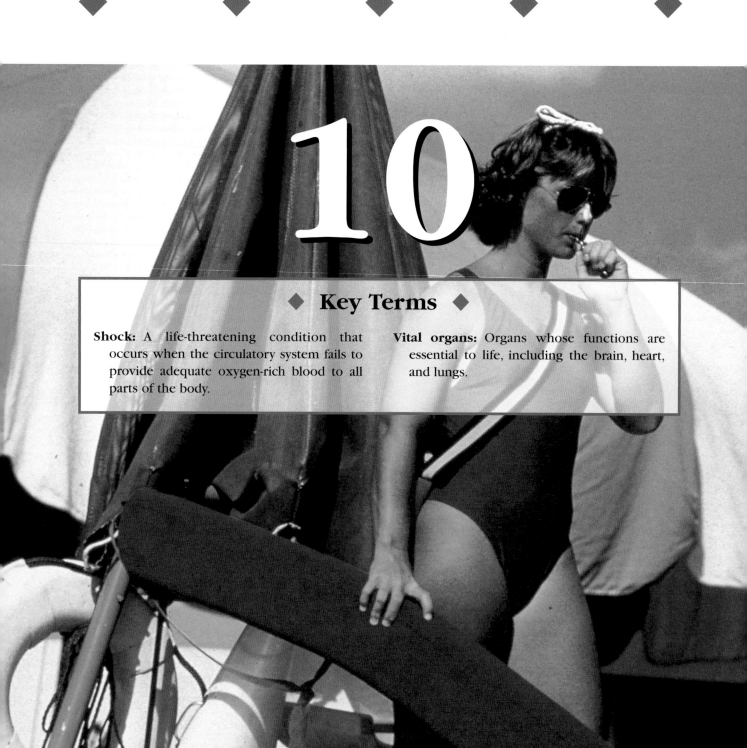

## ◆ Key Terms ◆

**Shock:** A life-threatening condition that occurs when the circulatory system fails to provide adequate oxygen-rich blood to all parts of the body.

**Vital organs:** Organs whose functions are essential to life, including the brain, heart, and lungs.

## ◆ **For Review** ◆

Before reading this chapter, you should have a basic understanding of how the respiratory and circulatory systems function and the interrelationship of body systems (Chapter 3).

## ◆ INTRODUCTION

***10:55 PM.*** *On an isolated road, a large deer leaps into the path of an oncoming car travelling 80 km per hour. The driver, a 21-year-old college student and track star, cannot avoid the collision. In the crash, both of her legs are broken and pinned in the wreckage.*

***11:15 PM.*** *Another car finally approaches. Seeing the wreck, the driver stops and comes forward to help. He finds the woman conscious but restless and in obvious pain. He says he will go to call an ambulance at the nearest house a kilometre or two down the road.*

***11:25 PM.*** *When the driver returns, he sees that the woman's condition has changed. She looks ill. He is unsure about what to do for her.*

***11:30 PM.*** *Having been dispatched, you arrive at the scene minutes before the ambulance. The man who found the wreck explains that the woman became drowsy and is no longer conscious. You check her and notice she is breathing fast, looks pale, and appears drowsy. Her skin is cold and moist. Her pulse is fast but so weak you can hardly feel it.*

***11:45 PM.*** *Finally, you and the other rescuers free her legs and remove her from the car. You notice that she looks worse. Her breathing has become very irregular. You know the hospital is still 15 minutes away.*

***12:30 AM.*** *Despite the best efforts of everyone involved, you hear the woman was pronounced dead. Her heart stopped beating enroute to the hospital. Although CPR and advanced life support measures were started,* *the ambulance personnel were unable to save her. She was a casualty of a progressively deteriorating condition called shock.*

I n preceding chapters, you learned that both medical emergencies and injuries can cause life-threatening conditions, such as cardiac and respiratory arrest and severe bleeding. Medical emergencies and injuries also can become life threatening in another way—as a result of shock. When the body experiences injury or sudden illness, it responds in a number of ways. Survival depends on the body's ability to adapt to the physical stresses of illness or injury. When the body's measures to adapt fail, the casualty can progress into a life-threatening condition called shock. Shock complicates the effects of injury or sudden illness. In this chapter, you will learn to recognize the signs and symptoms of shock and to provide care to minimize it.

## ◆ SHOCK

### What Is Shock?

Shock is a condition in which the circulatory system fails to adequately circulate oxygen-rich blood to all parts of the body. When ***vital organs,*** such as the heart, lungs, brain, and kidneys, do not receive oxygen-rich blood, they fail to function properly. This triggers a series of responses that produces specific signs and symptoms known as shock. These responses are the body's attempt to maintain adequate blood flow to the vital organs, preventing their failure.

When the body is healthy, three conditions are necessary to maintain adequate blood flow:

- The heart must be working well.
- An adequate amount of blood must be circulating in the body.
- The blood vessels must be intact and able to adjust blood flow.

Injury or sudden illness can interrupt normal body functions. In cases of minor injury or ill-

**Table 10-1** Types of Shock

| Type | Cause |
| --- | --- |
| Anaphylactic | Life-threatening allergic reaction to a substance; can occur from insect stings or from foods and drugs |
| Cardiogenic | Failure of the heart to effectively pump blood to all parts of the body; occurs with heart attack or cardiac arrest |
| Hypovolemic | Severe bleeding |
| Neurogenic | Failure of nervous system to control size of blood vessels, causing them to dilate; occurs with brain or nerve injuries |
| Psychogenic | Factor, such as emotional stress, causes blood to pool in the body in areas away from the brain, resulting in fainting |
| Respiratory | Failure of the lungs to transfer sufficient oxygen into the bloodstream; occurs with respiratory distress or respiratory arrest |
| Septic | Poisons caused by severe infections that cause blood vessels to dilate |

ness, this interruption is brief because the body is able to compensate quickly. With more severe injuries or illnesses, however, the body is unable to adjust. When the body is unable to meet its demands for oxygen because the blood fails to circulate adequately, shock occurs.

## Why Shock Occurs

There are different types of shock, as shown in Table 10-1. Although the first responder does not have to be able to identify each of these different types of shock, it may be helpful to know that there are different ways in which casualties can develop shock. Each causes a decrease in the amount of blood that effectively circulates in the body. For instance, shock caused by severe bleeding is called **hypovolemic shock.** If shock is caused by the heart failing to pump blood properly, it is called **cardiogenic shock.** When the nervous system fails to control the diameter of blood vessels, it is called **neurogenic shock.** Regardless of the cause, when the body cells receive inadequate oxygen, it triggers shock.

How does shock develop? You learned in Chapter 3 that the heart pumps blood by con-

tracting and relaxing in a consistent, rhythmic pattern. The heart adjusts its speed and the force of its contractions to meet the body's changing demands for oxygen. For instance, when a person exercises, the heart beats faster and more forcefully because the working muscles demand more oxygen (Fig. 10-1).

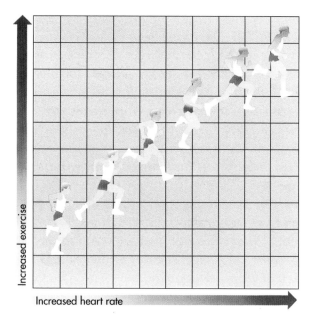

**Figure 10-1** The heartbeat changes to meet the body's demands for oxygen.

Similarly, when someone suffers a severe injury or sudden illness that affects the flow of blood, the heart beats faster and stronger at first to adjust to the increased demand for more oxygen (Fig. 10-2). Because the heart is beating faster, breathing must also speed up to meet the body's increased demands for oxygen. You can detect these changes by feeling the pulse and listening to breathing when you check vital signs during the secondary survey.

For the heart to do its job properly, an adequate amount of blood must circulate within the body. As you learned in Chapter 9, this amount is referred to as blood volume. The body can compensate for some decrease in blood volume. Consider what happens when you donate blood. You can lose 500 ml of blood over a 10- to 15-minute period without any real stress to the body. Fluid is reabsorbed from the kidneys, lungs, and intestines to replace lost fluid. The body immediately begins to manufacture the blood's solid components. With severe injuries involving greater or more rapid blood loss, the body may not be able to adjust adequately. Body cells do not receive enough oxygen, and shock occurs. Any significant fluid loss from the body, such as with diarrhea or vomiting, can also precipitate shock.

The blood vessels act as pipelines, transporting oxygen and nutrients to all parts of the body and removing wastes. For the circulatory system to function properly, blood vessels must remain intact to maintain blood volume. Normally, blood vessels decrease or increase the flow of blood to different areas of the body by constricting (decreasing their diameter) or dilating (increasing their diameter). This ability ensures that blood reaches the areas of the body that need it most, such as the vital organs. Injuries or illnesses, especially those that affect the brain and spinal cord, can cause blood vessels to lose this ability to change size, causing a drop in blood volume (Fig. 10-3). Blood vessels can also be affected if the nervous system is damaged by infections, drugs, or poisons.

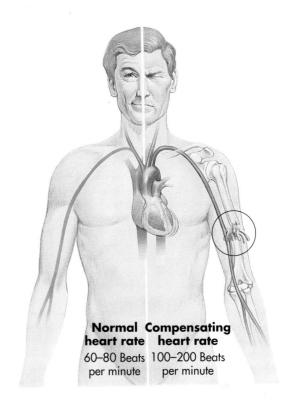

**Normal heart rate**
60–80 Beats per minute

**Compensating heart rate**
100–200 Beats per minute

**Figure 10-2** The heart beats faster to compensate for significant blood loss.

Regardless of the cause, a significant decrease in blood volume affects the function of the heart. The heart will eventually fail to beat rhythmically. The pulse will become irregular or be absent altogether. With some irregular heart rhythms, blood does not circulate at all.

When shock occurs, the body attempts to prioritize its needs for blood by ensuring adequate flow to the vital organs. The body does this by reducing the amount of blood circulating to the less important tissues of the arms, legs, and skin. This is why the skin of a person in shock appears pale and feels cool. When checking capillary refill, you may find it to be slow. In later stages of shock, the skin, especially on the lips and around the eyes, may appear blue from a prolonged lack of oxygen.

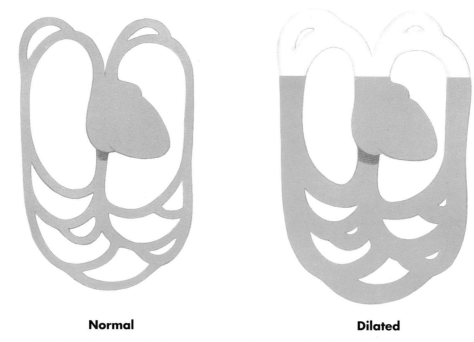

**Normal**                    **Dilated**

**Figure 10-3**  Injuries or medical emergencies that cause blood vessels to dilate cause a serious drop in blood volume.

Increased sweating is also a natural reaction to stress caused by injury or illness. This makes the skin feel moist.

## Signs and Symptoms of Shock

Although you may not always be able to determine the cause, remember that shock is a life-threatening condition. You should learn to recognize its signs and symptoms (Fig. 10-4).

Shock casualties usually show many of the same signs and symptoms. A common one is restlessness or irritability. This is often the first indicator that the body is experiencing a significant problem. More clearly recognizable signs are pale, cool, moist skin; rapid breathing; a rapid and weak pulse; and changes in the level of consciousness. Often, a recognizable symptom is nausea. Conditions that affect blood volume or cause the blood vessels to work improperly can cause significant changes in blood pressure.

If the casualty does not show the telltale signs and symptoms of specific injury or ill-ness, such as the persistent chest pain of heart attack or obvious external bleeding, it can be difficult to know what is wrong. Remember, *you do not have to identify the specific nature of illness or injury to provide care that may help save the casualty's life.* If the signs and symptoms of shock are present, assume there is a potentially life-threatening injury or illness.

## Care for Shock

Care for shock using the emergency action principles. First, do a primary survey by checking the ABCs. The care, such as controlling severe bleeding, that you provide for life-threatening conditions will minimize the effects of shock. If you do not find any life-threatening conditions, perform a secondary survey. During the secondary survey, the signs and symptoms of shock will most likely become evident. Always follow the general care steps you learned in Chapter 5 for any emergency:

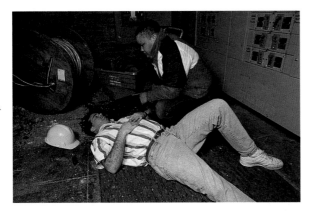

**Figure 10-4**  The signs and symptoms of shock may not be obvious immediately. Be alert for these signs and symptoms in cases of injury or sudden illness.

A 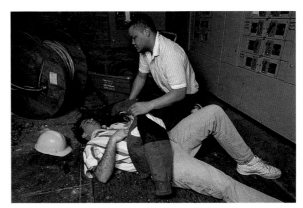 B

**Figure 10-5**  A, Monitor the casualty's ABCs if he or she is in shock. B, Maintain normal body temperature.

- Do no harm.
- Monitor the ABCs and provide care for any airway, breathing, or circulation problem you find (Fig. 10-5, *A*).
- Help the casualty rest comfortably. Helping the casualty rest comfortably is important because pain can intensify the body's stress and accelerate the progression of shock. Helping the casualty rest in a more comfortable position may minimize the pain.
- Help the casualty maintain normal body temperature (Fig. 10-5, *B*).

- Reassure the casualty.
- Provide care for specific conditions.

The general care you provide in any emergency will always help the casualty's body adjust to the stresses imposed by any injury or illness, thus reducing the effects of shock.

You can further help the casualty manage the effects of shock if you—

- Control any external bleeding as soon as possible to minimize blood loss.

# Shock: The Domino Effect

- An injury causes severe bleeding.
- The heart attempts to compensate for the disruption of blood flow by beating faster. The casualty first has a rapid pulse. More blood is lost. As blood volume drops, the pulse becomes weak or hard to find.
- The increased work load on the heart results in an increased oxygen demand. Therefore, breathing becomes faster.
- To maintain circulation of blood to the vital organs, blood vessels in the arms and legs and in the skin constrict. Therefore, the skin appears pale and feels cool. In response to the stress, the body perspires heavily and the skin feels moist.
- Since tissues of the arms and legs are now without oxygen, cells start to die. The brain now sends a signal to return blood to the arms and legs in an attempt to balance blood flow between these body parts and the vital organs.
- Vital organs are now without adequate oxygen. The heart tries to compensate by beating even faster. More blood is lost and the casualty's condition worsens.
- Without oxygen, the vital organs fail to function properly. As the brain is affected, the casualty becomes restless, drowsy, and eventually loses consciousness. As the heart is affected, it beats irregularly, resulting in an irregular pulse. The rhythm then becomes chaotic and the heart fails to pump blood. There is no longer a pulse. When the heart stops, breathing stops.
- The body's continuous attempt to compensate for severe blood loss eventually results in death.

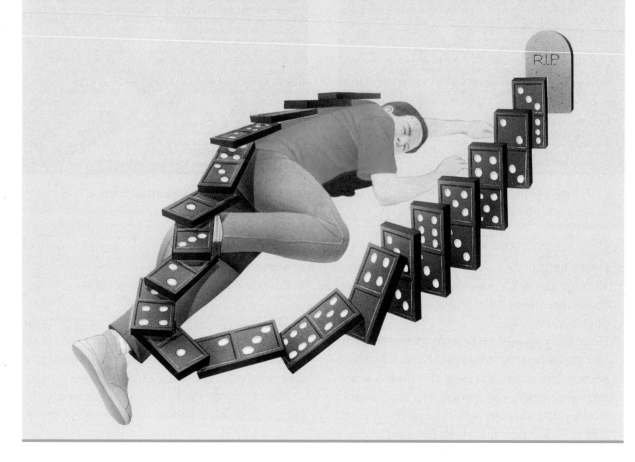

- Administer oxygen if the equipment is available and you are trained to do so.
- Do not give the casualty anything to eat or drink, even though he or she is likely to be thirsty. The casualty's condition may be severe enough to require surgery, in which case, it is better that the stomach be empty.
- Call more advanced medical personnel immediately. Shock cannot be managed effectively by first aid alone. A casualty of shock requires advanced life support as soon as possible.

## ◆ SUMMARY

Do not wait for shock to develop before providing care to a casualty of injury or sudden illness. Always follow the emergency action principles to minimize the effects of shock. Care for life-threatening conditions, such as breathing problems or severe external bleeding, before caring for lesser injuries. Remember that the key to managing shock effectively begins with recognizing a situation in which shock may develop and giving appropriate care.

Remember that shock is a factor in serious injuries and illnesses, particularly if there is blood loss or if the normal function of the heart is interrupted. With serious injuries or illnesses, shock is often the final stage before death. You cannot always prevent shock by administering emergency care, but you can usually slow its progress. Summon more advanced medical personnel immediately if you notice signs and symptoms of shock. Shock can often be reversed by advanced medical care, but only if the casualty is reached in time.

### YOU ARE THE RESPONDER

*You respond to an industrial call and find a casualty seated on the ground, leaning against a wall. You notice a large amount of blood around the casualty. Both of the casualty's wrists have been cut and blood continues to flow from the wounds.*

1. *What signs and symptoms would you look for to indicate shock?*
2. *How would you provide care for this casualty to minimize shock?*

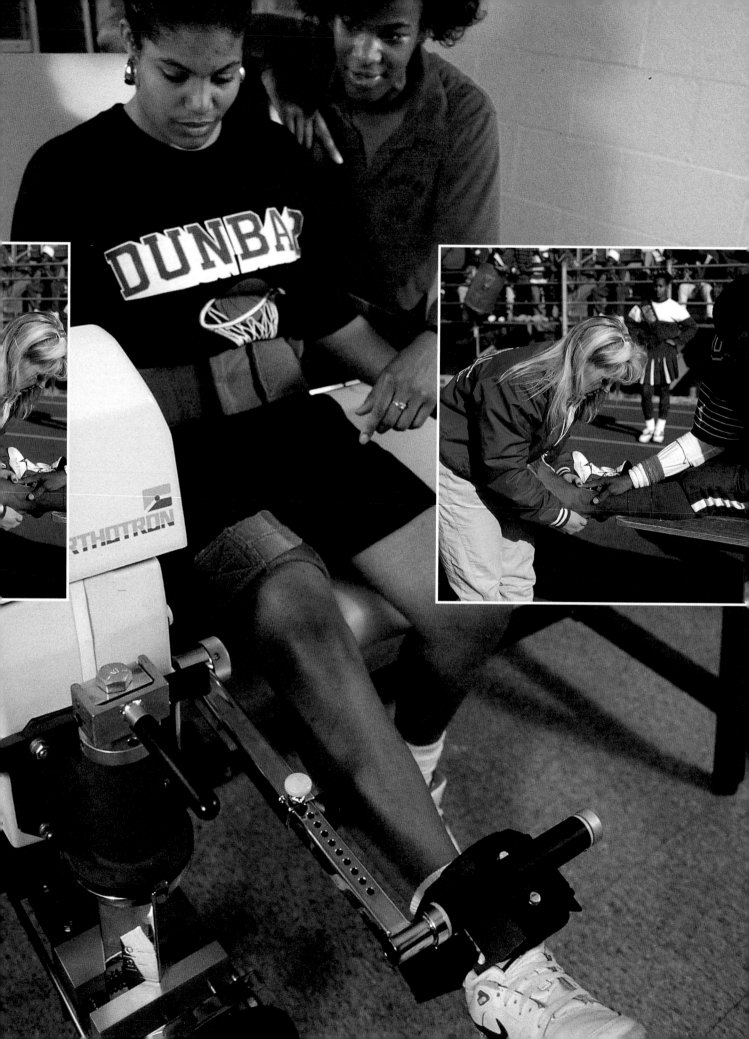

# Part Four

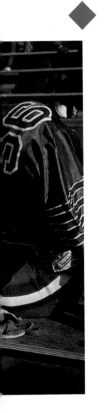

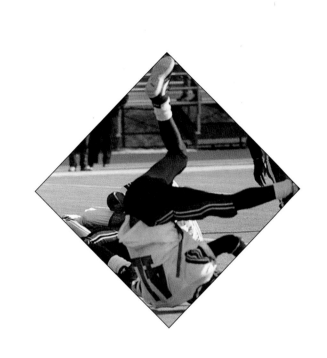

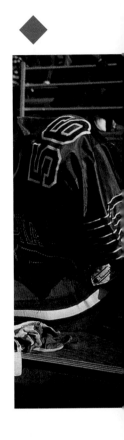

# Injuries

# ◆ INTRODUCTION

*It is nearly the end of a seemingly endless third shift. For some crew members, it has been a double shift. The work has been exhausting as they struggle against the clock to get a new boiler installed before the deadline. The foreman reminds everyone that there is a bonus if they can complete the task on time.*

*The most difficult part, the installation, is complete. Now, a final test is needed to see that everything is working. Paul, one of the crew, notices a leaking pipe and climbs up to tighten a connection. He slips and falls, breaking a pipe. Steam and scalding water spew everywhere, burning his chest and arms.*

*The foreman immediately activates the plant's emergency plan. You, the first responder, arrive quickly and assess the situation. After ensuring the scene is safe for you to approach the casualty, you take steps to cool the crewman's burned skin and administer oxygen. Recognizing that more advanced medical care is needed, you send a co-worker to call the emergency number to request an ambulance.*

*As Paul passes through the hospital's emergency department, his medical records will become part of the statistics that account for one of our nation's most significant health problems—injuries.*

Injury is a leading cause of death and disability in people aged 1 to 44 years. It greatly surpasses all major disease groups (cancer, heart disease, stroke) as a cause of death and disability in this age group. Injury is the leading cause of people contacting physicians and the most common cause of hospitalization among people under 45 years old. Statistics indicate that most people will have a significant injury at some time in their life. Some, because of their chosen professions, are more likely to be injured than others. For example, the International Association of Fire Fighters reports that in 1988, 4 of every 10 fire fighters were injured in the line of duty. Researchers predict that few people will escape the experience of a fatal or permanently disabling injury happening to a relative, co-worker, or friend.

# ◆ INJURIES

## How Injuries Occur

The body has a natural resistance to injury. However, when certain external forms of energy produce forces that the body cannot tolerate, injuries occur. Mechanical forms of energy and the energy from heat, electricity, chemicals, and radiation can damage body tissues and disrupt normal body function. Superficial injuries include minor wounds or burns. Deep injuries include wounds caused by penetrating objects.

Some tissues, such as the soft tissues of the skin, have less resistance and are at greater risk of injury if exposed to trauma than the deeper, stronger tissues of muscle and bone. Some organs, such as the brain, heart, and lungs, are better protected by bones than other organs, such as those in the abdominal cavity. Understanding the forces that cause injury and the kinds of injury that each force can cause will help you recognize certain injuries a casualty may have.

## Mechanical Energy

Mechanical energy produces the following forces: direct, indirect, twisting, and contracting. A direct force is the force of an object striking the body and causing injury at the point of impact. Direct forces can be either blunt or penetrating. For example, a fist striking the chin can break the jaw, or penetrating objects, such as bullets and knives, can injure structures beneath the skin at the point where they penetrate. Direct force can cause internal and external bleeding, head and spinal injuries, fractures, and other problems, such as crushing injuries.

An indirect force travels through the body when a blunt object strikes the body and causes injury to a body part away from the point of impact. For example, a fall on an outstretched hand may result in an injury to the arm, shoulder, or collarbone.

In twisting, one part of the body remains stationary while another part of the body turns. A sudden or severe twisting action can force body parts beyond their normal range of motion, causing injury to bones, tendons, ligaments, and muscles. For example, if a ski and its binding keep the lower leg in one position while the body falls in another, the knee may be forced beyond its normal range of motion. Twisting injuries are not always this complex. They more often occur as a result of simple actions such as stepping off a curb or turning to reach for an out-of-the-way object.

Sudden or powerful muscle contractions often result in injuries to muscles and tendons. These commonly occur in sports activities, such as throwing a ball far or hard without warming up or sprinting when out of shape. However, our daily routines also require sudden and powerful muscle contractions, for example, when we suddenly turn to catch a heavy object, such as a falling child. Although it happens rarely, sudden, powerful muscle contractions can even pull a piece of bone away from the point at which it is normally attached.

Figure IV-1 shows how these forces can result in injuries. These four forces, products of mechanical energy, cause the majority of injuries. Soft tissue injuries and injuries to muscle and bone (musculoskeletal injuries) are most often the result. Soft tissue injuries outnumber musculoskeletal injuries. Combined, they are the major cause of work loss and compensation in the working age group (16 to 65).

## Energy from Heat, Electricity, Chemicals, and Radiation

Together, the energy from heat, electricity, chemicals, and radiation accounts for a significant percent of all injuries. Exposure to any of these can result in burns. Thermal burns, burns caused by heat, are the most common. Sources of electricity, such as common household current or lightning, can penetrate the body, causing external and internal burn damage. Electrical current can also affect the part of the brain that controls breathing and heartbeat. When certain chemicals contact the skin, they cause burns. Solar radiation from the sun's rays causes sunburn. The average citizen is rarely exposed to other forms of radiation.

## Factors Affecting Injury

A number of factors affect the likelihood of injury—among them age, gender, geographic location, economic status, and alcohol use and abuse. The type and frequency of injuries can also be affected by fads and seasonal activities. As certain activities, such as skateboarding, gain and lose popularity or as activities, such as softball or snow skiing, change with the seasons, the injury statistics reflect these changes.

Injury statistics consistently show that—

- Injury rates are higher among people under age 45.
- The highest rate of deaths from injury occur to the elderly and people aged 15 to 24.
- Males are at greater risk than females for any type of injury.
- Motor vehicle crashes are the leading cause of deaths in Canada.

Many factors influence injury statistics. Whether people live in a rural or an urban area, whether a home is built of wood or brick, the type of heat used in the home, and the climate—all affect the degree of risk. Death rates from injury are typically higher in

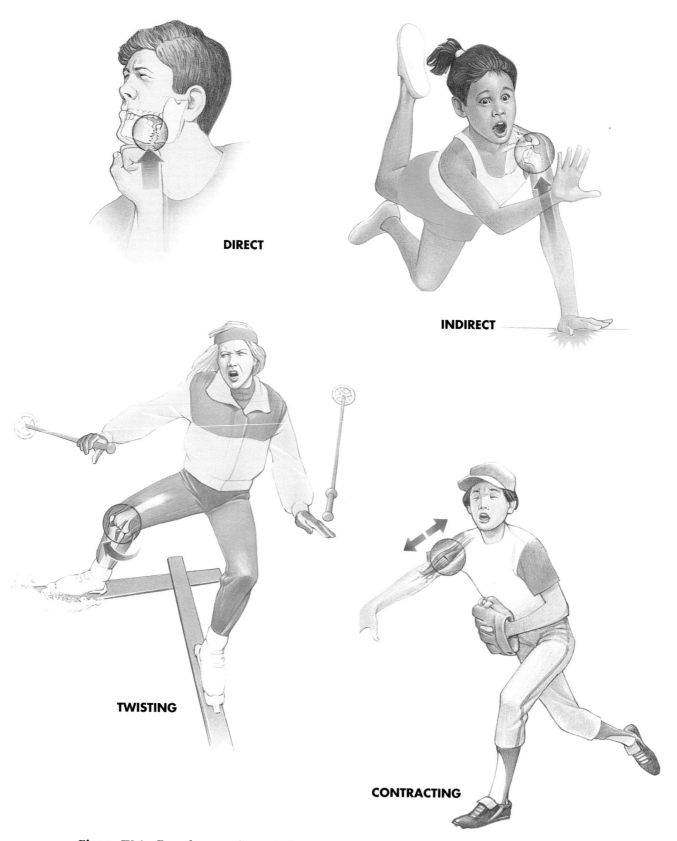

**DIRECT**

**INDIRECT**

**TWISTING**

**CONTRACTING**

**Figure IV-1** Four forces—direct, indirect, twisting, and contracting—cause 76 percent of all injuries.

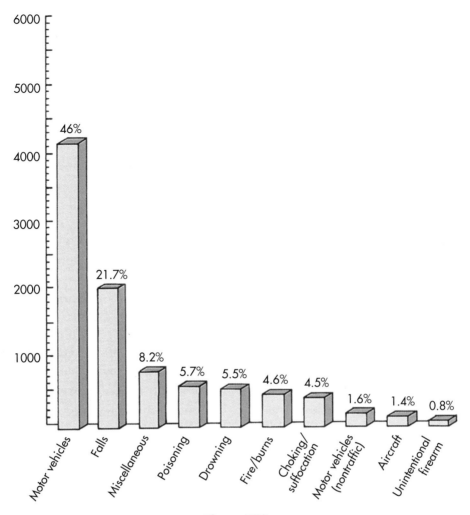

**Figure IV-2**

rural areas. The death rate from injuries is higher in low-income areas than in high-income areas.

The use and abuse of alcohol is a significant factor in many injuries and fatalities, even in young teenagers. The deaths of almost half of all fatally injured drivers involve alcohol, as do those of many adult passengers and pedestrians. Alcohol use also contributes to other injuries. It is estimated that a significant number of casualties who die as a result of falls, drownings, fires, assaults, and suicides have high blood alcohol concentrations.

Figure IV-2 shows the leading causes of death from injuries.

## Injury Prevention

Many people believe that injuries just happen—their targets are unfortunate casualties of circumstance. However, overwhelming evidence exists showing that injury, like disease, does not occur at random. Rather, many injuries are predictable, preventable events resulting from the interaction of people and hazards, whether at home, at work, or during recreation.

Preventing injuries is everyone's responsibility. As a first responder, injury prevention may be part of your job. As an athletic trainer, you are responsible for preventing athletic injuries. As an emergency team member, you may be responsible for ensuring that safety codes and regulations are met. A fire fighter or police officer who supervises or instructs others may be responsible for their safety. In any event, all first responders should take all precautions to ensure their personal safety and to be role models of safe behaviour.

There are three general strategies for preventing injuries:

◆ Persuade people to alter risky behaviour.
◆ Require behaviour change by law and regulation.
◆ Provide automatic protection through product and environmental design.

Laws and regulations that require you to conform to safety measures, such as wearing safety belts when driving and wearing protective clothing when on the job, are only moderately effective. The most successful injury-prevention strategy is the built-in protection of product design. For instance, automatic protection, such as airbags in motor vehicles, does not allow people to make choices (Fig. IV-3).

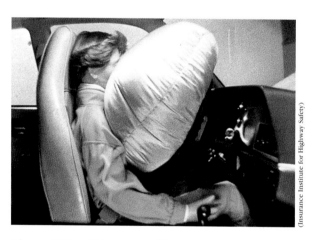

**Figure IV-3**   Airbags provide automatic protection.

(Insurance Institute for Highway Safety)

Typically, people who engage in risky behaviours are the hardest to influence, regardless of whether safer behaviours are required. For example, despite the overwhelming evidence of alcohol-related injuries and fatalities, people still drink when driving and when operating equipment.

Many people view laws or regulations that require certain behaviours as an infringement of their rights—even though these laws and regulations are intended to protect them from injury. Product designs are equally difficult to influence because of manufacturers' reluctance to bear the costs of design changes.

It has been estimated that if everyone worked to prevent injuries, about half of all injuries would not occur. Everyone has a personal responsibility to promote safety, both in his or her own life, as well as in the lives of others. Taking the following three steps could significantly reduce the risk of injury:

◆ *Know your injury risk.*
◆ *Take measures that can make a difference.* Change to behaviours that decrease your risk of injury and the risk of others, both on the job and off.
◆ *Think safety.* Be alert for and avoid potentially harmful conditions or activities that increase your injury risk or that of co-workers. Take precautions, such as wearing appropriate protective clothing—helmets, outer garments, and effective barriers—to prevent disease transmission and buckling up when driving or riding in motor vehicles. Let your representatives in government know that you support legislation that ensures a safer environment for us all.

◆ **NOTES:**

# Soft Tissue Injuries

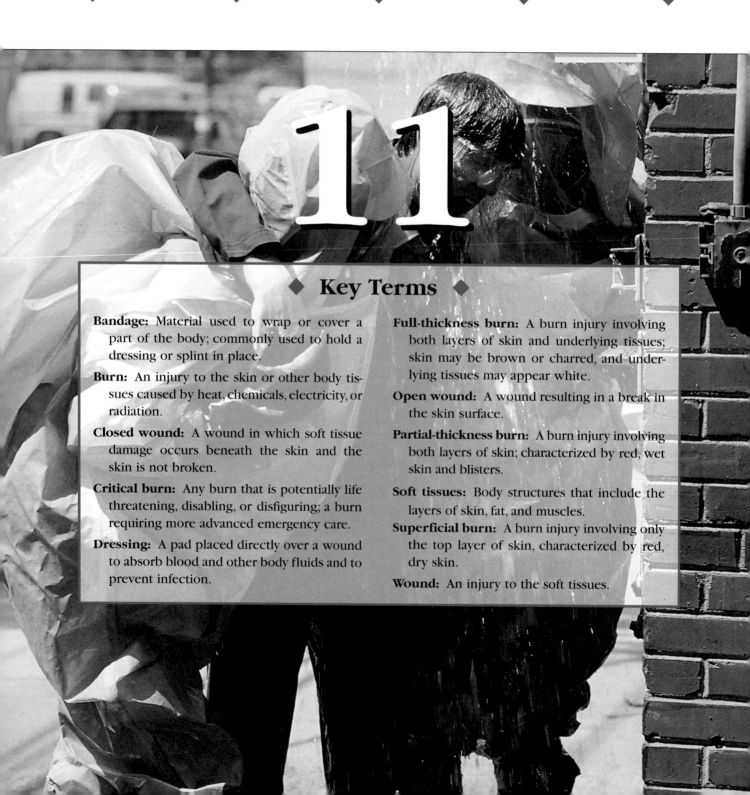

**11**

## ◆ Key Terms ◆

**Bandage:** Material used to wrap or cover a part of the body; commonly used to hold a dressing or splint in place.

**Burn:** An injury to the skin or other body tissues caused by heat, chemicals, electricity, or radiation.

**Closed wound:** A wound in which soft tissue damage occurs beneath the skin and the skin is not broken.

**Critical burn:** Any burn that is potentially life threatening, disabling, or disfiguring; a burn requiring more advanced emergency care.

**Dressing:** A pad placed directly over a wound to absorb blood and other body fluids and to prevent infection.

**Full-thickness burn:** A burn injury involving both layers of skin and underlying tissues; skin may be brown or charred, and underlying tissues may appear white.

**Open wound:** A wound resulting in a break in the skin surface.

**Partial-thickness burn:** A burn injury involving both layers of skin; characterized by red, wet skin and blisters.

**Soft tissues:** Body structures that include the layers of skin, fat, and muscles.

**Superficial burn:** A burn injury involving only the top layer of skin, characterized by red, dry skin.

**Wound:** An injury to the soft tissues.

## ◆ For Review ◆

Before reading this chapter, you should have a basic understanding of the circulatory and integumentary systems and the interrelationship of the body systems (Chapter 3). You should also know how to control bleeding (Chapter 9) and how to care for shock (Chapter 10).

## ◆ INTRODUCTION

*An infant falls and bruises his arm while learning to walk; a toddler scrapes her knee while learning to run; a child needs stitches in his chin after he falls off the "monkey bars" on the playground; an adolescent gets a black eye in a fist fight; a teenager suffers a sunburn after spending a weekend at the beach; and an adult cuts her hand while working in a woodshop. What do these injuries have in common? They are all soft tissue injuries.*

In the course of growing up and in our daily lives, soft tissue injuries occur often and in many different ways. Fortunately, most soft tissue injuries are minor, requiring little attention. Often, only an adhesive bandage or ice and rest are needed. Some injuries, however, are more severe and require immediate medical attention. In this chapter, you will learn how to recognize and care for the most common types of injuries—soft tissue injuries.

## ◆ SOFT TISSUES

The *soft tissues* include the layers of skin, fat, and muscles that protect the underlying body structures (Fig. 11-1). In Chapter 3, you learned that the skin is the largest single organ in the body and that without it the human body could not function. It provides a protective barrier for the body; it helps regulate the body's temperature; and it absorbs information about the environment by way of the nerves in the skin.

The skin has two layers. The outer layer of skin, the **epidermis,** provides a barrier to bacteria and other organisms that can cause infection. The deeper layer, called the **dermis,** contains the important structures of the nerves, the sweat and oil glands, and the blood vessels. Because the skin is well supplied with blood vessels and nerves, most soft tissue injuries are likely to bleed and be painful.

Beneath the skin layers lies a layer of fat. This layer helps insulate the body to help maintain body temperature. The fat layer also stores energy. The amount of fat varies in different parts of the body and in each person.

The muscles lie beneath the fat layer and comprise the largest segment of the body's soft tissues. Most soft tissue injuries involve the outer layers of tissue. However, deep burns or violent forces that cause objects to penetrate the skin can injure all the soft tissue layers. Although the muscles are considered soft tissues, muscle injuries are discussed more thoroughly in the next chapter with other musculoskeletal injuries.

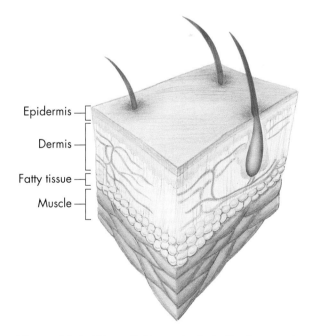

Epidermis —
Dermis —
Fatty tissue —
Muscle —

**Figure 11-1**  The soft tissues include the layers of skin, fat, and muscle.

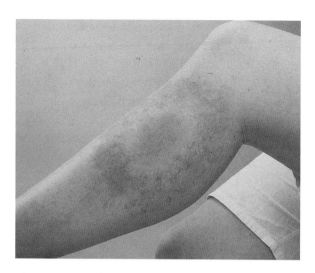

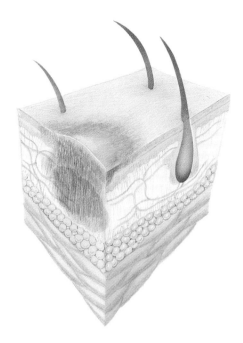

**Figure 11-2**   The simplest closed wound is a bruise.

## Types of Soft Tissue Injuries

An injury to the soft tissues is called a *wound.* Soft tissue injuries are typically classified as either closed or open wounds. A wound is closed when the soft tissue damage occurs beneath the surface of the skin, leaving the outer layer intact. A wound is open if there is a break in the skin's outer layer. Open wounds usually result in external bleeding.

Burns are a special kind of soft tissue injury. A burn occurs when intense heat, caustic chemicals, electricity, or radiation contacts the skin or other body tissues. Burns are classified as either superficial, partial-thickness, or full-thickness. Superficial burns affect only the outer layer of skin. Partial-thickness burns damage both skin layers. Full-thickness burns penetrate the layers of skin and can affect other soft tissues and even bone. Burns are discussed in more detail later in this chapter.

### Closed Wounds

Closed wounds, which occur beneath the surface of the skin, are more common than open wounds. The simplest *closed wound* is a bruise, also called a contusion (Fig. 11-2). Bruises result when the body is subjected to a blunt force, such as when you bump your leg on a table or chair. This usually results in damage to soft tissue layers and blood vessels beneath the skin, causing internal bleeding. When blood and other fluids seep into the surrounding tissues, the area discolours and swells. The amount of discolouration and swelling varies depending on the severity of the injury. At first, the area may only appear red. Over time, more blood may leak into the area, making it appear dark red or purple. Violent forces can cause more severe soft tissue injuries involving larger blood vessels, the deeper layers of muscle tissue, and even organs deep within the body. These injuries can result in profuse internal bleeding. With deeper injuries, a first responder may or may not immediately see bruising.

### Open Wounds

*Open wounds* are injuries that break the skin. These breaks can be as minor as a scrape of the surface layers or as severe as a deep penetration. The amount of bleeding depends on the severity of the injury. Any break in the skin provides an entry point for disease-producing microorganisms. There are four main types of open wounds:

- Abrasions.
- Lacerations.
- Avulsions.
- Punctures.

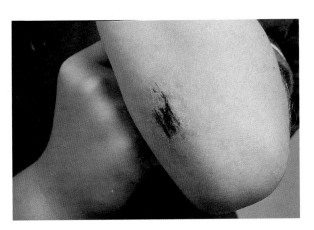

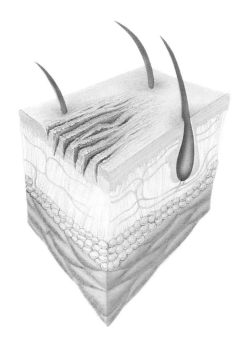

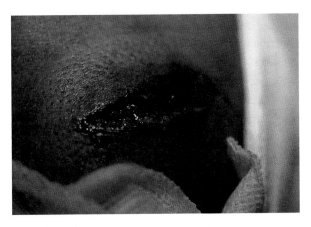

**Figure 11-3**   Abrasions can be painful, but bleeding is easily controlled.

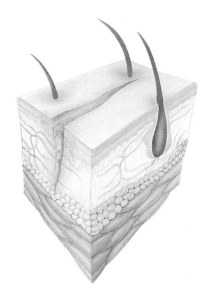

**Figure 11-4**   A laceration may have jagged or smooth edges.

An **abrasion** is the most common type of open wound. It is characterized by skin that has been rubbed or scraped away (Fig. 11-3). This often occurs when a child falls and scrapes his or her hands or knees. An abrasion is sometimes called a *rug burn, road rash,* or *strawberry.* Because the scraping of the outer skin layers exposes sensitive nerve endings, an abrasion is usually painful. Bleeding is easily controlled and not severe, since only the capillaries are affected. Because of the way the injury occurs, dirt and other matter can easily become embedded in the skin, making it especially important to clean the wound.

A **laceration** is a cut, usually from a sharp object. The cut may have either jagged or smooth edges (Fig. 11-4). Lacerations are commonly caused by sharp-edged objects, such as knives, scissors, or broken glass. A laceration can also result when a blunt force splits the skin. This often occurs in areas where bone lies directly under the skin's surface, such as the jaw. Deep lacerations can also affect the layers of fat and muscle, damaging both nerves and blood vessels. Lacerations usually bleed freely and, depending on the structures involved, can bleed profusely. Because the nerves may also

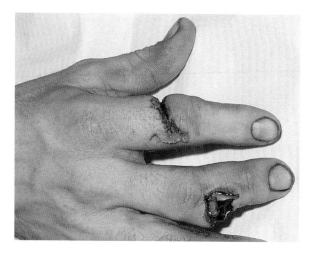

**Figure 11-5** In an avulsion, part of the skin and other soft tissue is torn away.

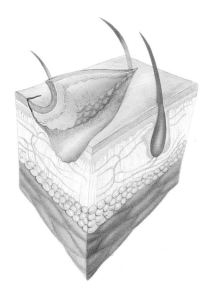

be injured, lacerations are not always immediately painful.

An **avulsion** is an injury in which a portion of the skin and sometimes other soft tissue is partially or completely torn away (Fig. 11-5). A partially avulsed piece of skin may remain attached but hangs like a flap. Bleeding is usually significant because avulsions often involve deeper soft tissue layers. Sometimes a force is so violent that a body part, such as a finger, may be severed. A complete severing of a part is sometimes called an **amputation** (Fig. 11-6). Although damage to the tissue is severe, bleeding is usually not as bad as you might expect. The blood vessels usually

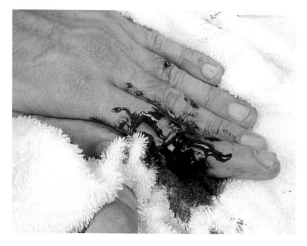

**Figure 11-6** In an amputation, a body part may also be completely severed.

constrict and retract (pull in) at the point of injury, slowing bleeding and making it relatively easy to control with direct pressure. In the past, a completely severed body part could not be successfully reattached. With today's technology, reattachment is often successful, making it important to send the severed part to the hospital with the casualty.

A **puncture** wound results when the skin is pierced with a pointed object, such as a nail, a piece of glass, a splinter, or a knife (Fig. 11-7). A bullet wound is also a puncture wound. Because the skin usually closes around the penetrating object, external bleeding is generally not severe. However, internal bleeding can be severe if the penetrating object damages major blood vessels or internal organs. An object that remains embedded in the open wound is called an **embedded object** (Fig. 11-8). An object also may pass completely through a body part, making two open wounds—one at the entry point and one at the exit point.

Although puncture wounds generally do not bleed profusely, they are potentially more dangerous than wounds that do because they are more likely to become infected. Objects penetrating the soft tissues carry microorganisms that cause infections. Of particular danger is the microorganism that causes tetanus, a severe infection.

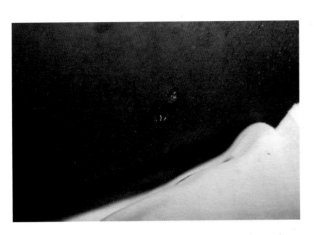

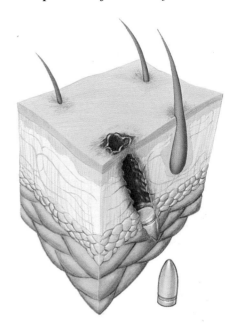

**Figure 11-7** A puncture wound results when skin is pierced by a pointed object.

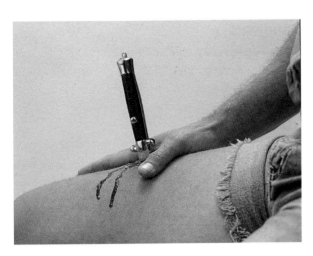

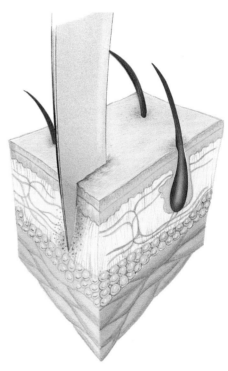

**Figure 11-8** An impaled object is an object that remains embedded in a wound.

## Infection

### Preventing Infection

Injuries causing breaks in the skin carry great risk of infection. Since the skin tends to collect microorganisms, injuries involving breaks in the skin can become infected unless properly cared for.

The best initial defence against infection is to cleanse the area thoroughly. For minor wounds, that is, those that are small and do not bleed severely, wash the area with soap and water. Most soaps are effective in removing harmful bacteria. Do not use alcohol because it can damage tissues. Wounds that require medical attention because of more extensive tissue damage or bleeding need not be washed immediately. These wounds will be cleaned thoroughly in the medical facility as a routine part of the care. It is more important for you to control bleeding.

### Signs of Infection

Sometimes, even the best care for a soft tissue injury is not enough to prevent infection. When a wound becomes infected, the area around the wound becomes swollen and red. The area may feel warm or throb with pain. Some wounds have a pus discharge (Fig. 11-9). Red streaks may develop that progress from the wound toward the heart. More serious infections may cause a casualty to develop a fever and feel ill. Infections require a physician's care.

## Dressings and Bandages

All open wounds need some type of covering to help control bleeding and prevent infection. These coverings are commonly referred to as dressings and bandages. There are many different types of both.

### Dressings

*Dressings* are pads placed directly on the wound to absorb blood and other fluids and to prevent infection. To minimize the chance of infection, dressings should be sterile. Most dressings are porous, allowing air to circulate to the wound to promote healing. Standard dressings include varying sizes of cotton gauze, commonly ranging from 5 to 10 cm (2 to 4 inches) square. Much larger dressings called **universal dressings** are used to cover very large wounds and multiple wounds in one body area (Fig. 11-10). Some dressings have nonstick surfaces to prevent the dressing from sticking to the wound.

A special type of dressing, called an **occlusive dressing,** does not allow air to pass through. Aluminum foil, plastic wrap, and petroleum jelly-soaked gauze are examples of this type of dressing (Fig. 11-11). These dressings are used for certain neck, chest, and abdominal injuries that are discussed in Chapters 13 and 14.

### Bandages

A *bandage* is any material used to wrap or cover any part of the body. Bandages are used to hold dressings in place, to apply pressure to control

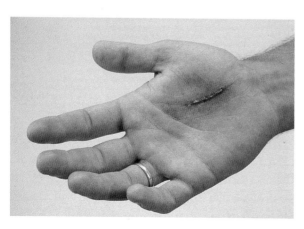

**Figure 11-9**  An infected wound may become swollen and may have a pus discharge.

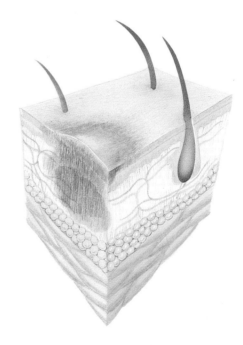

# An Ounce of Prevention . .

A serious infection can cause severe medical problems. One such infection is tetanus, caused by the organism *Clostridium tetani*. This organism, commonly found in soil and faeces of cows and horses, can infect many kinds of wounds. Worldwide, tetanus kills about 50,000 people annually.

Tetanus is introduced into the body through a puncture wound, abrasion, laceration, or burn. Because the organism multiplies in an environment that is low in oxygen, puncture wounds and other deep wounds are at particular risk for tetanus infection. It produces a powerful toxin, one of the most lethal poisons known, that affects the central nervous system and specific muscles. People at risk for tetanus include drug addicts, burn casualties, and people recovering from surgery. Newborn babies can be infected through the stump of the umbilical cord.

Signs and symptoms of tetanus include difficulty swallowing, irritability, headache, fever, and muscle spasms near the infected area. Later, as the infection progresses, it can affect other muscles, such as those in the jaw, causing the condition called "lockjaw." Once tetanus gets into the nervous system, its effects are irreversible.

The first line of defence against tetanus is to thoroughly clean an open wound. Major wounds should be cleaned and treated at a medical facility. Clean a minor wound with soap and water, and apply a clean or sterile dressing. If signs of wound infection develop, seek medical attention immediately. Infected wounds of the face, neck, and head should receive *immediate* medical care, since the tetanus toxin can travel rapidly to the brain. A physician will determine whether a tetanus shot or a booster shot is needed, depending on the casualty's immunization status. Always contact your personal physician if you are unsure how long it has been since you received a tetanus immunization or booster.

The best way to prevent tetanus is to be immunized against it and then receive periodic booster shots. Immunizations assist the natural function of the immune system by building up antibodies, disease-fighting proteins that help protect the body against specific bacteria. Because the effects of immunization do not last a lifetime, booster shots help maintain the antibodies that protect against tetanus. Booster shots are recommended every 5 to 10 years or whenever a wound has been contaminated by dirt or an object, such as a rusty nail, causes a puncture wound. Most children in this country receive an immunization known as *DPT*, which includes the tetanus toxoid.

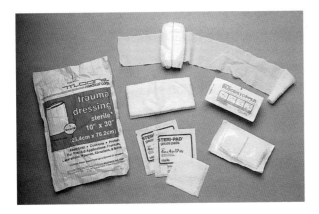

**Figure 11-10**  Dressings come in various sizes.

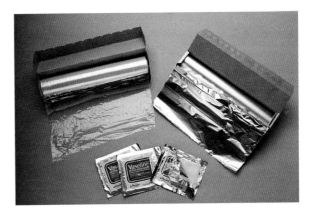

**Figure 11-11**  Special dressings are designed to prevent air from passing through.

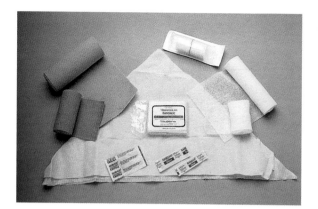

**Figure 11-12** Different types of bandages are used to hold dressings in place, apply pressure to a wound, protect the wound from infection, and provide support to an injured area.

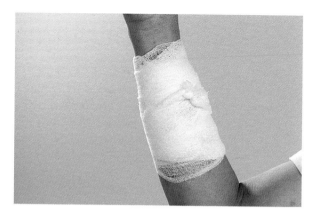

**Figure 11-13** Roller bandages are usually made of gauze and are easy to apply.

bleeding, to help protect a wound from dirt and infection, and to provide support to an injured limb or body part. Many different types of bandages are available commercially (Fig. 11-12). A bandage applied snugly to create pressure on a wound or injury is called a pressure bandage.

A common type of bandage is a commercially made adhesive compress, such as a Band-Aid. Available in assorted sizes, it consists of a small pad of nonstick gauze (the dressing) on a strip of adhesive tape (the bandage) that is applied directly to small injuries. Also available is the **bandage compress,** a thick gauze dressing attached to a gauze bandage. This bandage can be tied in place. Because it is specially designed to help control severe bleeding, the bandage compress usually comes in a sterile package.

A **roller bandage** is usually made of gauze or gauzelike material (Fig. 11-13). Some gauze bandages are made of a self-adhering material that easily conforms to different body parts. Roller bandages are available in assorted widths from 1 to 30 cm (1/2 to 12 inches) and lengths from 5 to 10 metres (or yards). A roller bandage is generally wrapped around the body part, over a dressing, using overlapping turns until the dressing is completely covered. It can be tied or taped in place. A folded strip of roller bandage may also be used as a dressing or compress. In

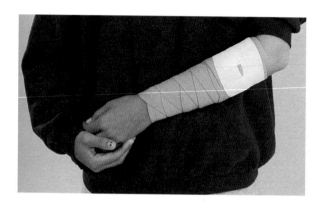

**Figure 11-14** Elastic bandages can be applied to control swelling or support an injured extremity.

the next chapters, you will learn to use roller bandages to hold splints in place.

A special type of roller bandage is an **elastic bandage,** sometimes called Ace bandage or elastic wrap. Roller bandages are designed to keep continuous pressure on a body part (Fig. 11-14). When properly applied, they can effectively control swelling or support an injured limb. Elastic bandages are available in assorted widths from 5 to 15 cm (2 to 6 inches). They are very effective in the management of injuries to muscles, bones, and joints. Elastic bandages are frequently used in athletic environments, and should be used only by individuals who are trained and proficient in their use.

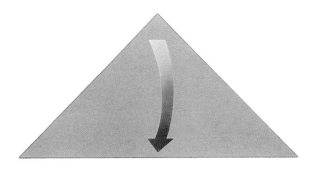

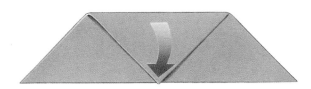

**Figure 11-15** A cravat is made by folding a triangular bandage.

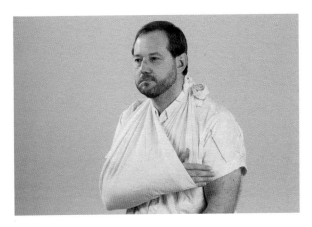

**Figure 11-16** A triangular bandage is commonly used as a sling.

Another commonly used bandage is the **triangular bandage.** Folded, it can hold a dressing or splint in place on most parts of the body (Fig. 11-15). Used as a sling, the triangular bandage can support an injured shoulder, arm, or hand (Fig. 11-16).

### Applying a bandage

To apply a roller bandage, follow these general guidelines:

◆ If possible, elevate the injured body part above the level of the heart.
◆ Secure the end of the bandage in place. Wrap the bandage around the body part until the dressing is completely covered and the bandage extends several inches beyond the dressing. Tie or tape the bandage in place (Fig. 11-17, *A, B,* and *C*).
◆ Do not cover fingers or toes, if possible. By keeping these parts uncovered, you will be able

to tell if the bandage is too tight (Fig. 11-17, *D*). If fingers or toes become cold or begin to turn pale or blue, the bandage is too tight and should be loosened slightly.
◆ If blood soaks through the bandage, apply additional dressings and another bandage. *Do not* remove the blood-soaked ones.
◆ Elastic bandages can easily restrict blood flow if not applied properly. Restricted blood flow is not only painful, but also can cause tissue damage if not corrected. Figure 11-18, *A-D,* shows the proper way to apply an elastic bandage.

## Care for Wounds
### Care for Closed Wounds

Most closed wounds do not require special medical care. Direct pressure on the area decreases bleeding. Elevating the injured part helps to control bleeding and reduce swelling. Cold can be effective in helping control both pain and swelling. When applying ice or a chemical cold pack, place a gauze pad, towel, or other cloth between the ice and the skin to protect the skin (Fig. 11-19).

Do not dismiss a closed wound as "just a bruise." Be aware of possible serious injuries to internal organs or other underlying structures, such as the muscles or bones. Take the time to evaluate how the injury happened and whether

A 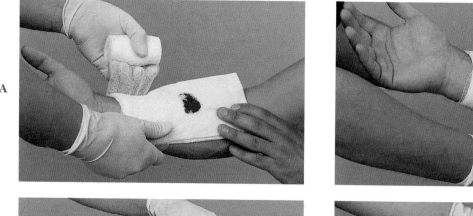 B

C 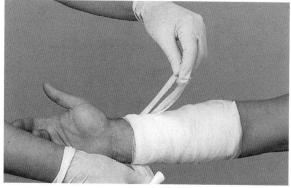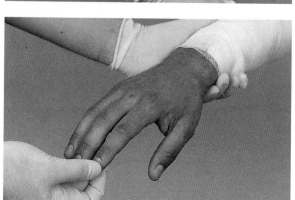 D

**Figure 11-17**  **A,** Start by securing the end of the roller bandage in place. **B,** Use overlapping turns to cover the dressing completely. **C,** Tie or tape the bandage in place. **D,** Check the fingers to ensure the bandage is not too tight.

more serious injuries could be present. If a person complains of severe pain or cannot move a body part without pain, or if you think the force that caused the injury was great enough to cause serious damage, call for more advanced medical attention immediately. Care for these injuries is described in later chapters.

## Care for Major Open Wounds

A major open wound is one with severe bleeding, deep destruction of tissue, or a deeply impaled object. To care for a major open wound, follow these general guidelines:

- *Do not* waste time trying to wash the wound. Remember RED.
- Quickly control bleeding using direct pressure and elevation. Apply direct pressure by placing a sterile dressing over the wound with your gloved hand. If nothing sterile is available, use any clean covering, such as a

towel or a handkerchief. If you do not have a glove and a cloth is not available, have the injured casualty use his or her hand. Use your bare hand only as a last resort.
- Continue direct pressure by applying a pressure bandage.
- Summon more advanced medical care.
- Wash your hands immediately after completing care, even if you wore gloves.

If the casualty has an injury in which a body part has been completely severed, try to retrieve the severed body part. Wrap the part in sterile gauze, if any is available, or in any clean material, such as a washcloth. Place the wrapped part in a plastic bag. If possible, keep the part cool by placing the bag on ice (Fig. 11-20). Be careful to keep the ice from directly contacting the avulsed part so that the part does not freeze. Make sure the part is transported to the medical facility with the casualty.

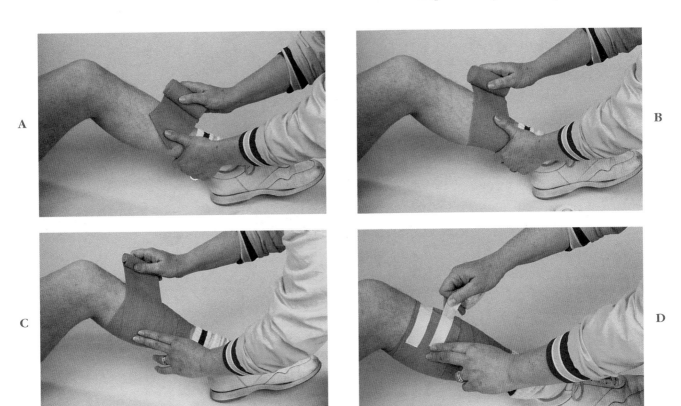

**Figure 11-18**  **A,** Start the elastic bandage at the point furthest from the heart. **B,** Secure the end of the bandage in place. **C,** Wrap the bandage using overlapping turns. **D,** Tape the end of the bandage in place.

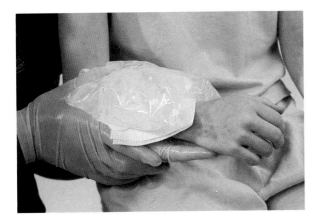

**Figure 11-19**  For a closed wound, apply ice to help control pain and swelling.

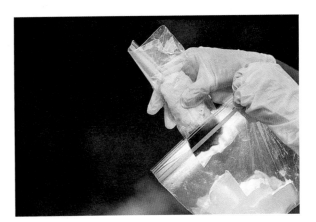

**Figure 11-20**  Wrap a severed body part in sterile gauze, put it in a plastic bag, and put the bag on ice.

If the casualty has an imbedded object in the wound—

♦ *Do not* remove the object unless it involves the cheek or interferes with breathing.

♦ Use bulky dressings to stabilize the object (Fig. 11-21, *A*). Any movement of the object can result in further tissue damage.
♦ Control bleeding by bandaging the dressings in place around the object (Fig. 11-21, *B*).

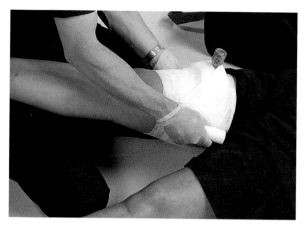

A

B

**Figure 11-21  A,** Use bulky dressings to support an impaled object. **B,** Use bandages over the dressing to control bleeding.

## A Stitch in Time . . .

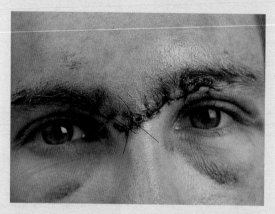

It can be difficult to judge when a wound should be seen by a doctor for stitches. A quick rule of thumb is that stitches are needed when the edges of skin do not fall together or when the wound is more than 2.5 cm (1 inch) long. Stitches speed the healing process, lessen the chances of infection, and improve the look of scars. The wound should be stitched within the first few hours after the injury. The following major injuries may require stitches:

- Bleeding from an artery or uncontrollable bleeding
- Deep cuts or avulsions that show the muscle or bone, involve joints near the hands or feet, gape widely, or involve the thumb or the palm of the hand
- Large or deep punctures
- Large or deeply embedded object
- Human and animal bites
- Wounds that, if left unattended, could leave a conspicuous scar, such as those that involve the lip or eyebrow

If you are caring for a wound and think it may need stitches, it probably does.

## Care for Minor Open Wounds

A minor wound is one, such as an abrasion, in which damage is only superficial and bleeding is minimal. To care for a minor wound, follow these general guidelines:

- Cleanse the wound with soap and water.
- Place a sterile dressing over the wound.
- Apply direct pressure for a few minutes to control any bleeding.
- Apply a new sterile dressing.
- Hold the dressing in place with a bandage or tape.

# Burns

***Burns*** are another type of soft tissue injury, caused primarily by heat. Burns can also occur when the body is exposed to caustic chemicals, electricity, or solar or other forms of radiation.

When burns occur, they first affect the top layer of skin. If the burn progresses, the dermis, the second layer can also be affected. Deep burns can damage underlying tissues. Burns that break the skin can cause infection, fluid loss, and loss of temperature control. Burns can also damage the respiratory system and the eyes.

The severity of a burn depends on the—

- Temperature of the source of the burn.
- Length of exposure to the source.
- Location of the burn.
- Extent of the burn.
- Casualty's age and medical condition.

In general, people under age 5 and over age 60 have thinner skin and often burn more severely. People with acute trauma or chronic medical problems, such as fractures, heart or kidney problems or diabetes, tend to have more complications resulting from burns; the effects of burns in these people may be more severe.

## Degrees of Burns

Burns are classified by their cause, such as heat, chemicals, electricity, or radiation. They are also classified by depth. The deeper the burn, the more severe it is. Generally, three depth classifications are used: superficial (first degree), partial-thickness (second degree), and full-thickness (third degree).

### Superficial burns (first degree)

A ***superficial burn*** involves only the top layer of skin (Fig. 11-22). The skin is red and dry, and

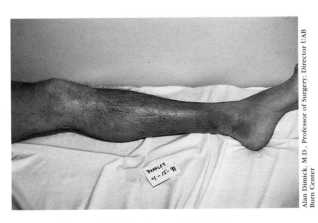

Figure 11-22   A superficial burn.

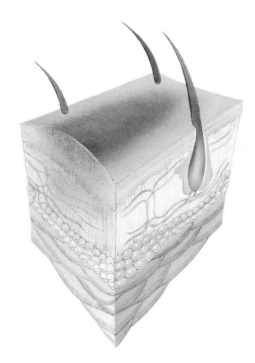

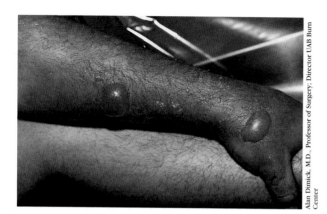

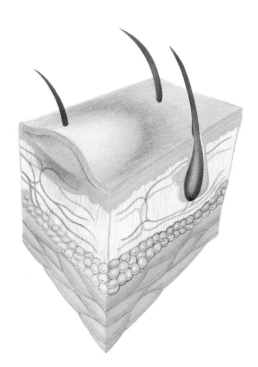

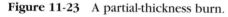

**Figure 11-23**    A partial-thickness burn.

the burn is usually painful. The area may swell. Most sunburns are superficial burns. Superficial burns generally heal in 5 to 6 days without permanent scarring.

### Partial-thickness burns (second degree)

A ***partial-thickness*** burn involves both the epidermis and the dermis (Fig. 11-23). These injuries are also red and have blisters that may open and weep clear fluid, making the skin appear wet. The burned skin may look blotched. These burns are usually painful, and the area often swells. Although the burn usually heals in 3 or 4 weeks, a skin graft may still be necessary. Extensive partial-thickness burns can be serious, requiring more advanced medical care. Scarring may occur from partial-thickness burns.

### Full-thickness burns (third degree)

A ***full-thickness burn*** destroys both layers of skin, as well as any or all of the underlying structures—fat, muscles, bones, and nerves (Fig. 11-24). These burns may look brown or charred (black), with the tissues underneath sometimes appearing white. They can be either extremely painful or relatively painless if the burn destroys nerve endings in the skin. Full-thickness burns are often surrounded by painful partial-thickness burns.

Full-thickness burns can be life threatening. Because the burns are open, the body loses fluid, and shock is likely to occur. These burns also make the body highly prone to infection. Scarring occurs and may be severe. Skin grafts are usually required.

## Identifying Critical Burns

It is important that you be able to identify a critical burn. A ***critical burn*** is one that requires the immediate attention of more advanced medical personnel. Critical burns are potentially life threatening, disfiguring, or disabling.

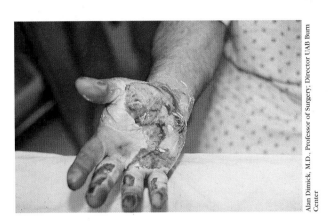

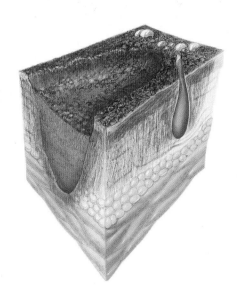

**Figure 11-24** A full-thickness burn.

Knowing whether you should summon more advanced medical personnel for a burn injury can sometimes be difficult. It is not always easy or possible to assess the severity of a burn immediately after injury. Even superficial burns to large areas of the body or to certain body parts can be critical. You cannot judge severity by the pain the casualty feels because nerve endings may have been destroyed. Call for more advanced medical personnel immediately for assistance in caring for the following burns:

◆ Inhalation injury causing breathing difficulty or signs of burns around the mouth and nose.
◆ Flame burns that occurred in a confined space.
◆ Burns covering more than one body part.
◆ Burns to the head, neck, hands, feet, or genitals.
◆ Any partial-thickness or full-thickness burn to a child or an elderly person.

◆ Burns resulting from chemicals, explosions, or electricity.

Expect that burns caused by flames or hot grease will require medical attention, especially if the casualty is under 5 or over 60 years of age. Hot grease is slow to cool and difficult to remove from the skin. Burns that involve hot liquid or flames contacting clothing will also be serious, since the clothing prolongs the heat contact with the skin. Some synthetic fabrics melt and stick to the body. They may take longer to cool than the soft tissues. Although these burns may appear minor at first, they can continue to worsen for a short time.

### Estimating the Extent of Burns

When communicating with more advanced medical personnel about a burned casualty, you may be asked how much of the body is burned. The Rule of Nines is a common method for estimating

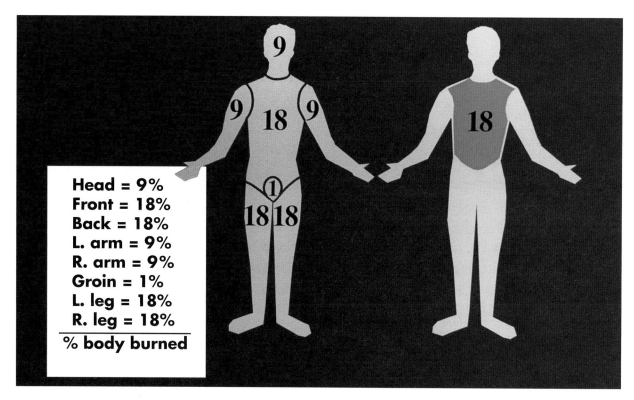

**Head = 9%**
**Front = 18%**
**Back = 18%**
**L. arm = 9%**
**R. arm = 9%**
**Groin = 1%**
**L. leg = 18%**
**R. leg = 18%**
_____
**% body burned**

**Figure 11-25**  The Rule of Nines is one method to help determine how much of the body is burned.

what percentage of the body is affected by burns (Fig. 11-25).

In an adult, the head equals 9 percent of the total body surface. Likewise, each arm also equals 9 percent of the body. Each leg equals 18 percent. This is also true for the front or back of the trunk. For example, if the front of the trunk (18 percent) and one entire arm (9 percent) is burned, you would estimate that 27 percent of the body's surface area has been burned.

If you do not remember the Rule of Nines, simply communicate how the burn occurred, the body parts involved, and the approximate degree of burn. For example, "The casualty was injured when an overheated car radiator exploded. The casualty has partial-thickness burns on her face, neck, chest, and arms."

## Care for Thermal Burns

As you approach the casualty, decide if the scene is safe. Look for fire, smoke, downed electrical wires, and warning signs for chemicals or radiation. If the scene is unsafe and you have not

been trained to manage the situation, summon other specially trained personnel.

If the scene is safe, approach the casualty cautiously. If the source of heat is still in contact with the casualty, take steps to remove and extinguish it. This may require you to smother the flames or extinguish them with water, or to remove smoldering clothing. If the burn is

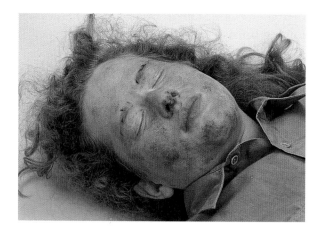

**Figure 11-26**  Burns or soot on the face may signal that air passages or lungs have been burned.

caused by hot tar, cool the area with water but do not attempt to remove the tar.

Do a primary survey. Pay close attention to the casualty's airway. Note soot or burns around the mouth or nose or the rest of the face, which may signal that air passages or lungs have been burned (Fig. 11-26). If the burn occurred in a confined space, the casualty may have an inhalation injury from breathing hot air. If you suspect a burned airway or burned lungs, continually monitor breathing and call for advanced medical personnel immediately. Air passages may swell, impairing or stopping breathing. Oxygen should be administered if available.

As you do a secondary survey, look for additional signs of burn injuries. Look also for other injuries, especially if there was an explosion or electric shock.

If thermal burns are present, follow these three basic care steps:

◆ Cool the burned area.
◆ Cover the burned area.
◆ Minimize shock.

**Cool the burned area**

Even after the source of heat has been removed, soft tissue will continue to burn for minutes afterwards, causing more damage. Therefore, it is essential to cool any burned areas immediately with large amounts of cool water (Fig. 11-27, *A*). Do not use ice or ice water. Ice can cause critical body heat loss. Instead, flush or immerse the area using whatever resources are available—a tub, shower, or garden hose. You can apply soaked towels, sheets, or other wet cloths to a burned face or other area that cannot be immersed. Be sure to keep these compresses cool by adding more water until the site has returned to body temperature.

Allow adequate time for the burned area to cool. If pain continues or if the edges of the burned area are still warm to the touch when the area is removed from the water, continue cooling. With burns over a large body area, be careful not to over-cool the body because of the risk of lowering the body temperature. When the burn is cool, remove any remaining

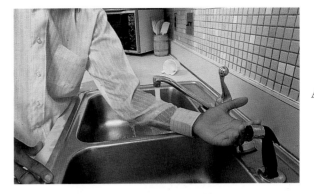

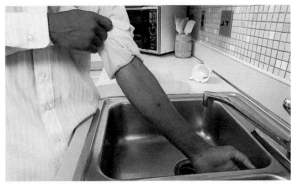

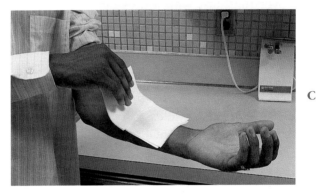

**Figure 11-27 A,** Large amounts of cool water are essential to cool burned areas. **B,** Remove any clothing covering the burned area. **C,** Cover the burned area.

clothing from the area by carefully removing or cutting material away (Fig. 11-27, *B*). Do not try to remove any clothing that is sticking to skin.

In some areas, you may be provided more specific directions for when and how to cool burns. Follow your local protocols.

**Cover the burned area**

Burns often expose sensitive nerve endings. Cover the burned area to keep out air and help reduce pain (Fig. 11-27, *C*). Use dry nonstick or moist sterile dressings if possible, and loosely bandage them in place. The bandage should not put pressure on the burn surface. If the burn covers a large area of the body, cover it with clean, dry sheets or other cloth. Small wounds (under 9% of the body) may be covered with a moist dressing.

Covering the burn helps prevent infection. *Do not* put ointments, butter, oil, or other commercial or home remedies on any burn that will receive medical attention. Oils and ointments seal in heat and do not relieve pain. Other home remedies can contaminate open skin areas, causing infection. Do not break blisters. Intact skin helps prevent infection.

For small superficial burns or small burns with open blisters that are not sufficiently severe or extensive to require medical attention, care for the burned area as an open wound. Wash the area with soap and water. Cover the burn with a dressing and bandage. Tell the casualty to watch for signs of infection.

### Minimize shock

Pain and loss of body fluids from full-thickness and large partial-thickness burns can cause shock. Lay the casualty down unless he or she is having difficulty breathing. Elevate burned areas above the level of the heart, if possible. Burn casualties tend to chill. Help the casualty maintain normal body temperature by protecting him or her from drafts. Administer oxygen if it is available and it is safe to do so.

## Special Situations

### Chemical burns

Chemical burns are common in industrial settings but also occur in the home. Cleaning solutions, such as household bleach, oven or drain cleaners, toilet bowl cleaner, paint strippers, and lawn or garden chemicals, are common sources of caustic chemicals. Caustic chemicals destroy tissues and cause **chemical burns.**

Typically, burns result from chemicals that are strong acids or alkalis. These substances can quickly injure the skin. As with heat burns, the stronger the chemical and the longer the contact, the more severe the burn. The chemical will continue to burn as long as it is on the skin. You must remove the chemical from the skin as quickly as possible and then call for more advanced medical help immediately. If you suspect a chemical burn, also check for a burn to the eye.

With a chemical powder or granules, brush the chemical from the skin before flushing. Whether the substance is liquid, granular, or powder, flush the burn continuously with large amounts of cool, running water (Fig. 11-28). A continuous flow of water will remove a dry substance before the water can activate it. Continue flushing until more advanced medical personnel arrive. Have the casualty remove contaminated clothing if possible. Take steps to minimize shock.

Chemical burns to the eyes can be exceptionally traumatic. If an eye is burned by a chemical, flush the affected eye until more advanced medical personnel arrive (or for at least 20 minutes) (Fig. 11-29). Flush the affected eye from the nose outward to prevent washing the chemical into the unaffected eye.

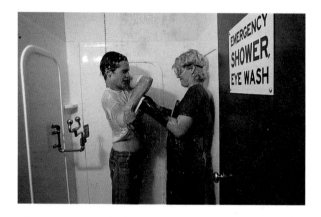

**Figure 11-28** Flush a chemical burn with cool running water.

# Striking Distance

In medieval times, people believed that ringing church bells would dissipate lightning during thunderstorms. It was an unfortunate superstition for the bell ringers. Over 33 years, lightning struck 386 church steeples and 103 bell ringers died.[1]

Church bell ringers have dropped off the list of people most likely to be struck during a thunderstorm, but lightning strikes remain extremely dangerous. Lightning causes more deaths than most other weather hazards. Lightning occurs when particles of water, ice, and air moving inside storm clouds lose electrons. Eventually, the cloud becomes divided into layers of positive and negative particles. Most electrical currents run between the layers inside the cloud. Occasionally, the negative charge flashes toward the ground, which has a positive charge. An electrical current snakes back and forth between the ground and the cloud many times in the seconds that we see a flash crackle down from the sky. Anything tall—a tower, a tree, or a person—becomes a path for the electrical current.

Travelling at speeds up to 500 kilometres (300 miles) per second, a lightning strike can hurl a person through the air, burn his or her clothes off, and sometimes cause the heart to stop beating. The most severe lightning strikes carry up to 50 million volts of electricity, enough to keep 13,000 homes running. Lightning can "flash" over a person's body, or, in its more dangerous path, it can travel through blood vessels and nerves to reach the ground.

Besides burns, lightning can also cause neurologic damage, fractures, and loss of hearing or eyesight. The casualty sometimes acts confused and amnesic and may describe the episode as getting hit on the head or hearing an explosion.

Use common sense around thunderstorms. If you see a storm approaching in the distance, do not wait until you are drenched to seek shelter. If a thunderstorm threatens—

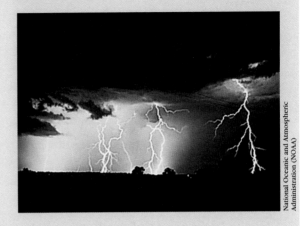

National Oceanic and Atmospheric Administration (NOAA)

- ◆ Go inside a large building or home.
- ◆ Get inside a car and roll up the windows.
- ◆ Stop swimming or boating as soon as you see or hear a storm. Water conducts electricity.
- ◆ Stay away from the telephone, except in an emergency.
- ◆ Stay away from telephone poles and tall trees if you are caught outside.
- ◆ Stay off hilltops; try to crouch down in a ravine or valley.
- ◆ Stay away from farm equipment and small metal vehicles, such as motorcycles, bicycles, and golf carts.
- ◆ Avoid wire fences, clotheslines, metal pipes and rails, and other conductors.
- ◆ Stay several metres apart if you are in a group.

**REFERENCES**

1. Kessler E: *The thunderstorm in human affairs,* Norman, Oklahoma, 1983, University of Oklahoma.
2. Randall T: 50 million volts may crash through a lightning casualty, *The Chicago Tribune,* Section 2D, August 13, 1989.

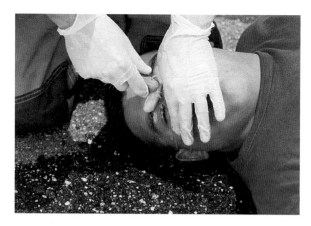

**Figure 11-29** Continuously flush an eye that has been burned by a chemical with cool water.

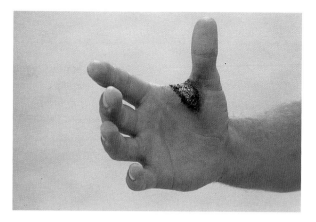

**Figure 11-30** An electrical burn may severely damage underlying tissues.

### Electrical burns

The human body is a good conductor of electricity. When someone comes in contact with an electrical source, such as a power line, a malfunctioning household appliance, or lightning, he or she conducts the electricity through the body. Some body parts, such as the skin, resist the electrical current. Resistance produces heat, which can cause **electrical burns** along the flow of the current (Fig. 11-30). The severity of an electrical burn depends on the type and amount of contact, the current's path through the body, and how long the contact lasted. Electrical burns are often deep. Although these wounds may look superficial, the tissues beneath may be severely damaged. Some electrical burns will be marked by characteristic entry and exit wounds indicating where current has passed through the body. In the secondary survey, look for two burn sites. Cover any burn injuries with a dry nonstick or moist sterile dressing, and give care to minimize shock.

With a casualty of lightning, look and care for life-threatening conditions, such as respiratory or cardiac arrest. The casualty may also have fractures, including spinal fracture, so do not move him or her. Any burns are less of a problem.

### Inhalation injuries

Burns that resulted from a fire in an enclosed, confined space are likely to be associated with

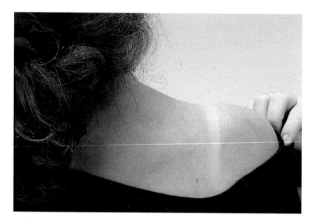

**Figure 11-31** Solar radiation burns can be painful.

inhalation injuries of the airway and lungs. When possible, move the casualty to a well-ventilated place out of the confined area, and provide supplemental oxygen.

### Radiation burns

Both the solar radiation of the sun and other types of radiation can cause **radiation burns.** Solar burns are similar to heat burns. Usually they are mild but can be painful (Fig. 11-31). They may blister, involving more than one *skin layer.* Care for sunburns as you would any other burn. Cool the burn and protect the burned area from further damage by keeping it out of the sun.

People are rarely exposed to other types of radiation unless working in special settings, such as certain medical, industrial, or research sites. If you work in such settings, you will be informed and will be required to take precautions to prevent overexposure.

## ◆ SUMMARY

Caring for wounds is not difficult. You need only follow the basic guidelines to control bleeding and minimize the risk of infection. Remember that with minor wounds your primary concern is to cleanse the wound to prevent infection. With major wounds, you should control the bleeding quickly using direct pressure and elevation and summon more advanced medical professionals. Dressings and bandages, when correctly applied, help control bleeding, reduce pain, and minimize the danger of infection.

Burn injuries damage the layers of the skin and sometimes the internal structures as well. Heat, smoke inhalation, chemicals, electricity, and radiation all cause burn injuries. When caring for a burn casualty, always first ensure your safety. When the scene is safe, approach the casualty and do a primary survey and a secondary survey if necessary.

Once the casualty has been removed from the burn source and is in a well ventilated area, follow the steps of burn care:

◆ Cool the burned area with water to minimize additional tissue destruction.

◆ Keep air away from the burned area by covering it with dry nonstick or moist sterile dressings, clean sheets, or other cloth.

◆ To minimize shock, maintain the casualty's normal body temperature.

◆ Summon more advanced medical personnel for any critical burn.

◆ If inhalation injury is possible, provide supplemental oxygen.

In addition, always check for inhalation injury if the person has a heat or chemical burn involving the face. With electrical burns, check carefully for additional problems, such as breathing difficulty, cardiac problems, and fractures.

In the next chapter, you will learn how to provide care for injuries involving muscles and bones.

### YOU ARE THE RESPONDER

1. You are dispatched to the scene of a house fire. You assist three fire casualties to exit from the burning structure. One elderly gentleman has burns on his arms and chest. Another man has soot on his face, mouth, and nostrils and appears to be having problems breathing. The child does not appear to be burned anywhere. What care would you provide for these casualties?
2. If the child was experiencing difficulty breathing, how would your care change?

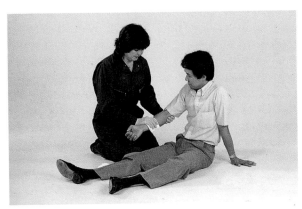

1. Apply direct pressure.

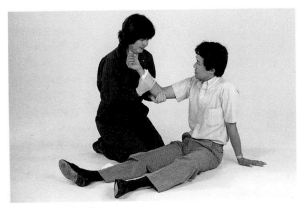

2. Elevate body part.

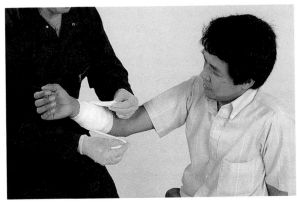

3. Apply pressure bandage.

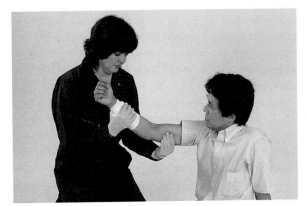

4. Use pressure point if necessary.

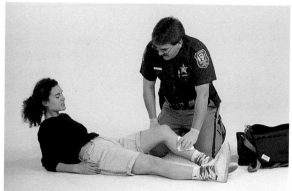

1. Apply direct pressure.

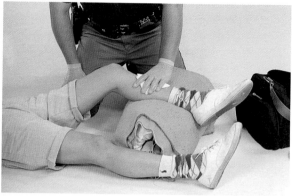

2. Elevate body part.

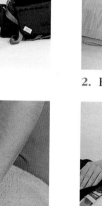

3. Apply pressure bandage.

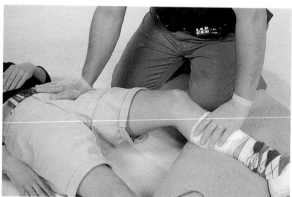

4. Use pressure point if necessary.

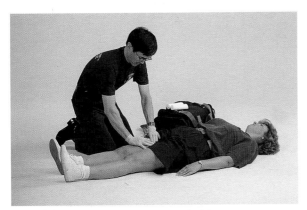

1. Apply direct pressure around object.

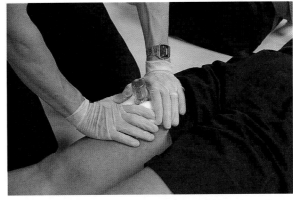

2. Use bulky dressings to support object.

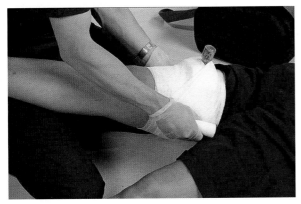

3. Apply pressure bandage.

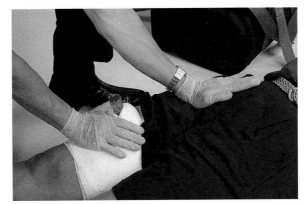

4. Use pressure point if necessary.

# Musculoskeletal Injuries

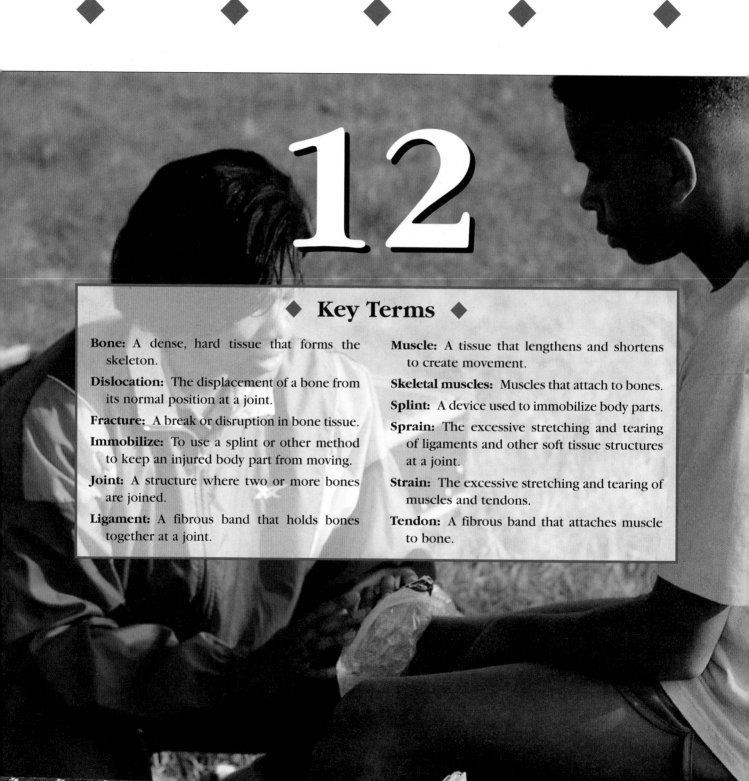

**12**

## ◆ Key Terms ◆

**Bone:** A dense, hard tissue that forms the skeleton.

**Dislocation:** The displacement of a bone from its normal position at a joint.

**Fracture:** A break or disruption in bone tissue.

**Immobilize:** To use a splint or other method to keep an injured body part from moving.

**Joint:** A structure where two or more bones are joined.

**Ligament:** A fibrous band that holds bones together at a joint.

**Muscle:** A tissue that lengthens and shortens to create movement.

**Skeletal muscles:** Muscles that attach to bones.

**Splint:** A device used to immobilize body parts.

**Sprain:** The excessive stretching and tearing of ligaments and other soft tissue structures at a joint.

**Strain:** The excessive stretching and tearing of muscles and tendons.

**Tendon:** A fibrous band that attaches muscle to bone.

## ◆ For Review ◆

Before reading this chapter, you should have a basic understanding of the anatomy and function of the musculoskeletal system and how the musculoskeletal system interacts with the nervous system (Chapter 3). You should also know how to perform a secondary survey (Chapter 5).

## ◆ INTRODUCTION

Injuries to the musculoskeletal system are common. Millions of people at home, at work, or at play injure their muscles, bones, or joints. No age group is immune. An athlete may fall and bruise the muscles of the thigh, making walking painful. Heavy machinery may fall on a worker and break ribs, making breathing difficult. A person who braces a hand against a dashboard in a car crash may injure the bones at the shoulder, disabling the arm. A person who falls while skiing may twist a leg, tearing the supportive tissues of a knee and making it impossible to stand or move.

Although musculoskeletal injuries are almost always painful, they are rarely life threatening. However, when not recognized and taken care of properly, they can have serious consequences and even result in permanent disability or death. In this chapter, you will learn how to recognize and care for musculoskeletal injuries. Developing a better understanding of the structure and function of the body's framework will help you assess musculoskeletal injuries and give appropriate care.

## ◆ MUSCULOSKELETAL SYSTEM

The musculoskeletal system is made up of muscles and bones that form the skeleton, the connective tissues, the tendons, and ligaments. Together, these structures give the body shape, form, and stability. Bones and muscles connect to form various body segments. They work together to provide body movements.

## Muscles

*Muscles* are soft tissues. The body has more than 600 muscles (Fig. 12-1). Most are **skeletal muscles,** which attach to the bones. Skeletal muscles account for most of your lean body weight (body weight without excess fat).

Unlike the other soft tissues, muscles are able to contract (shorten) and relax (lengthen). All body movements result from skeletal muscles contracting and relaxing. Skeletal muscle actions are under your conscious control. Because you move them voluntarily, skeletal muscles are also called voluntary muscles. Skeletal muscles also protect the bones, nerves, and blood vessels.

Most skeletal muscles are anchored to bone at each end by strong, cordlike tissues called **tendons.** Muscles and their adjoining tendons extend across joints. When the brain sends a command to move, electrical impulses travel through the spinal cord and nerve pathways to the individual muscles and stimulate the muscle fibres to move. When a muscle contracts, the muscle fibres shorten, pulling the ends of the muscle closer together. The muscles pull the bones, causing motion at the joint the muscle crosses.

Motion is usually caused by a group of muscles close together pulling at the same time. For instance, the hamstring muscles are a group of muscles at the back of the thigh. When the hamstrings contract, the leg bends at the knee. The quadriceps are a group of muscles at the front of the thigh. When the quadriceps muscles contract, the leg straightens at the knee. Generally, when one group of muscles contracts, another group of muscles on the opposite side of the body part relaxes (Fig. 12-2). Even simple tasks, such as bending to pick up an object from the floor, involve a complex series of movements in which different muscle groups contract and relax.

**FRONT VIEW**

**BACK VIEW**

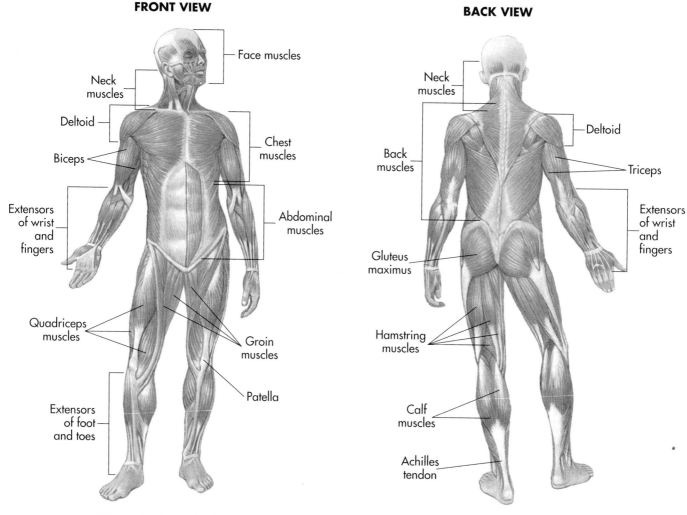

**Figure 12-1**  Skeletal muscles, muscles that attach to bones, comprise the majority of the body's musculature.

Injuries to the brain, the spinal cord, or the nerves can affect muscle control. A loss of muscle control is called paralysis. Injuries to these structures can also affect sensation, the ability to feel. When an isolated injury to a muscle or nerve occurs, the adjacent muscles can sometimes assume the function of the injured muscle (Fig. 12-3).

## Skeleton

The **skeleton** is formed by over 200 bones of various sizes and shapes (Fig. 12-4). These bones shape the skeleton, giving each body part a unique form. The skeleton protects vital organs and other soft tissues. The skull protects the brain (Fig. 12-5, *A*). The ribs protect the heart and lungs (Fig. 12-5, *B*). The spinal cord is protected by the canal formed by the bones that form the spinal column (Fig. 12-5, *C*). Two or more bones come together to form joints. *Ligaments,* fibrous bands that hold bones together at joints, give the skeleton stability and, with the muscles, help maintain posture.

## Bones

*Bones* are hard, dense tissues. Their strong, rigid structure helps them withstand stresses

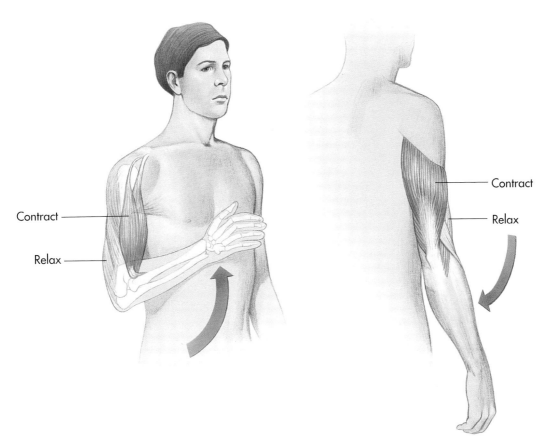

**Figure 12-2**   Movement occurs when one group of muscles contracts and an opposing group of muscles relaxes.

that cause injuries. The shape of bones depends on what the bones do and the stresses on them. For instance, the surfaces of bones at the joints are smooth (Fig. 12-6). Although similar to the bones of the arm, the bones of the leg are much larger and stronger because they carry the body's weight (Fig. 12-7).

Bones have a rich supply of blood and nerves. Some bones store and manufacture red blood cells and supply them to the circulating blood. Bone injuries can bleed and are usually painful. The bleeding can become life threatening if not properly cared for. Bones heal by forming new bone cells. Bone is the only body tissue that can regenerate in this way.

Bones weaken with age. Bones in young children are more flexible than adults' bones, so they are less likely to break. In contrast, elderly people have less dense, brittle bones that are more likely

to give way, even under everyday stresses, which can result in significant injuries. For example, the stress created if an elderly person were to pivot with all the body weight on one leg could break the strongest bone in the body, the thigh bone (femur). The gradual, progressive weakening of bone is called **osteoporosis.**

Bones are classified as long, short, flat, or irregular (Fig. 12-8). Long bones are longer than they are wide. Long bones include the bones of the upper arm (humerus), the forearm (radius, ulna), the thigh (femur), and the lower leg (tibia, fibula). Short bones are about as wide as they are long. Short bones include the small bones of the hand (metacarpals) and feet (metatarsals). Flat bones have a relatively thin, flat shape. Flat bones include the breastbone (sternum), the ribs, the shoulder blade (scapula), and some of the bones that form the skull. Bones that do not

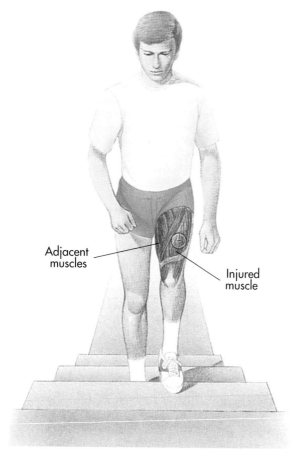

Adjacent muscles

Injured muscle

**Figure 12-3** Adjacent muscles can often assume the function of an injured muscle.

fit in these three categories are called irregular bones. Irregular bones include the vertebrae and the bones of the face. Bones are weakest at the points where they change shape, and fractures usually occur at these points.

## Joints

A *joint* is a structure formed by the ends of two or more bones coming together at one place. Most joints allow motion. However, the bone ends at some joints are fused together, which restricts motion. Fused bones, such as the bones of the skull, form solid structures that protect their contents (Fig. 12-9).

Joints are held together by tough, fibrous, connective tissues called ligaments. Ligaments resist joint movement. Joints surrounded by ligaments

have restricted movement; joints that have few ligaments move more freely. For instance, the shoulder joint, with few ligaments, allows greater motion than the hip joint, although their structure is similar. Joint motion also depends on the bone structure.

Joints that move more freely have less natural support and are therefore more prone to injury. However, all joints have a normal range of movement. When a joint is forced beyond its normal range, ligaments stretch and tear. Stretched and torn ligaments permit too much motion, making the joint unstable. Unstable joints can be disabling, particularly when they are weight-bearing, such as the knee or ankle. Unstable joints are also prone to reinjury and often develop arthritis, an inflamed condition of the joints, in later years.

## Parts of the Skeleton

The bony structures that form the skeleton define the parts of the body. For example, the head is defined by the bones that form the skull, and the chest is defined by the bones that form the rib cage. Prominent bones, bones that can be seen or felt beneath the skin, provide landmarks for locating body parts (Fig. 12-10).

## Injuries to the Musculoskeletal System

Injuries to the musculoskeletal system occur in a variety of ways. They are more commonly caused by forces generated by mechanical forms of energy but can result from heat, chemical, or electrical forms of energy.

## Types of Musculoskeletal Injuries

The four basic types of musculoskeletal injuries are fracture, dislocation, sprain, and strain. Injuries to the musculoskeletal system can be classified according to the body structures that are damaged. Some injuries may involve more than one type of injury. For example, a direct

**FRONT VIEW**     **BACK VIEW**

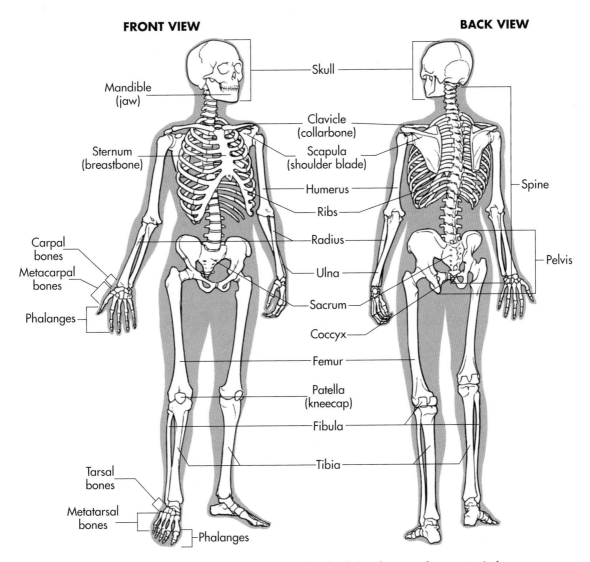

- Skull
- Mandible (jaw)
- Clavicle (collarbone)
- Sternum (breastbone)
- Scapula (shoulder blade)
- Humerus
- Spine
- Ribs
- Carpal bones
- Radius
- Pelvis
- Metacarpal bones
- Ulna
- Phalanges
- Sacrum
- Coccyx
- Femur
- Patella (kneecap)
- Fibula
- Tarsal bones
- Tibia
- Metatarsal bones
- Phalanges

**Figure 12-4**   The bones of the skeleton give the body its shape and protect vital organs.

blow to the knee may injure both ligaments and bones. Injuries are also classified by the nature and extent of the damage.

## Fracture

A *fracture* is a break or disruption in bone tissue. Fractures include chipped or cracked bones, as well as bones that are broken all the way through (Fig. 12-11). Fractures are commonly caused by direct and indirect forces. However, if strong enough, twisting forces and strong muscle contractions can cause a fracture.

Fractures are classified as open or closed. An open fracture involves an open wound. Open fractures often occur when the limb is severely angulated, or bent, causing bone ends to tear the skin and surrounding soft tissues or when an object, such as a bullet, penetrates the skin and breaks the bone. Closed fractures leave the skin unbroken and are more common than open fractures. Open fractures are more serious than closed fractures because of the risks of infection and severe blood loss. Although fractures are rarely an immediate threat to life, any fracture involving a large bone can cause shock, because bones and soft tissue may bleed heavily.

Fractures are not always obvious unless there is a telltale sign, such as an open wound with

# The Breaking Point

Osteoporosis, a degenerative bone disorder usually discovered after the age of 60, affects 30 percent of people over age 65. It will affect one of four women in North America, and it occurs less frequently in men. Fair-skinned women with ancestors from northern Europe, the British Isles, Japan, or China are genetically predisposed to osteoporosis. Inactive people are more susceptible to osteoporosis.

Osteoporosis occurs when there is a decrease in the calcium content of bones. Normally, bones are hard, dense tissues that endure tremendous stresses. Bone-building cells constantly repair damage that occurs as a result of everyday stresses, keeping bones strong. Calcium is a key to bone growth, development, and repair. When the calcium content of bones decreases, bones become frail, less dense, and less able to repair the normal damage they incur.

This loss of density and strength leaves bones more susceptible to fractures. Where once tremendous force was necessary, fractures may now occur with little or no aggravation, especially to hips, vertebrae, and wrists. Spontaneous fractures are those that occur without trauma. The casualty may be taking a walk or washing dishes when the fracture occurs. Some hip fractures thought to be caused by falls are actually spontaneous fractures that caused the casualty's fall.

Osteoporosis can begin as early as age 30 to 35. The amount of calcium absorbed from the diet naturally declines with age, making calcium intake increasingly important. When calcium in the diet is inadequate, calcium in bones is withdrawn and used by the body to meet its other needs, leaving bones weakened.

Building strong bones before age 35 is the key to preventing osteoporosis. Calcium and exercise are necessary to bone building. Many physicians recommend up to 1000 milligrams for women age 19 and over. Three to four daily servings of low-fat dairy products should provide adequate calcium. Vitamin D is also necessary because it aids in calcium absorption. Exposure to sunshine enables the body to make vitamin D. Fifteen minutes of sunshine on the hands and face of a young, light-skinned individual are enough to supply the RDA (recommended daily allowance) of 5 to 10 micrograms of vitamin D per day. Dark-skinned and elderly people need more sun exposure. People who do not receive adequate sun exposure need to consume vitamin D. The best sources are vitamin-fortified milk and fatty fish, such as tuna, salmon, and eel.

Calcium supplements combined with vitamin D are available for those who do not take in adequate calcium. However, before taking a calcium supplement, consult a physician. Many highly advertised calcium supplements are ineffective because they do not dissolve in the body.

Exercise seems to increase bone density and the activity of bone-building cells. Regular exercise may reduce the rate of bone loss by promoting new bone formation and may also stimulate the skeletal system to repair itself.

protruding bone ends or a severely deformed body part. You must always consider the way in which the injury occurred. It is often enough to suggest a possible fracture.

## Dislocation

A *dislocation* is a displacement or separation of a bone from its normal position at a joint (Fig. 12-12). Dislocations are usually caused by severe forces, such as twisting or falls. Some joints, such as the shoulder or fingers, dislocate easily because their bones and ligaments do not provide adequate protection. Others, such as the elbow or the joints of the spine, are well protected and therefore dislocate less easily.

When bone ends are forced far enough beyond their normal position, ligaments stretch and tear. Subsequent dislocations are then more likely to occur. A force violent enough to cause

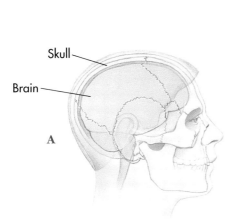

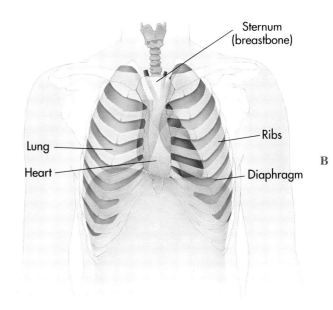

**Figure 12-5** **A,** The immovable bones of the skull protect the brain. **B,** The rib cage protects the lungs and heart. **C,** The vertebrae protect the spinal cord.

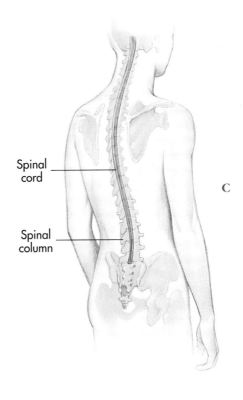

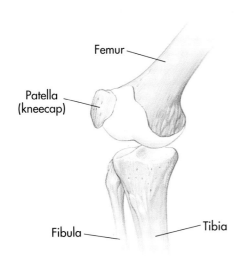

**KNEE**

**Figure 12-6** Bone surfaces at the joints are smooth.

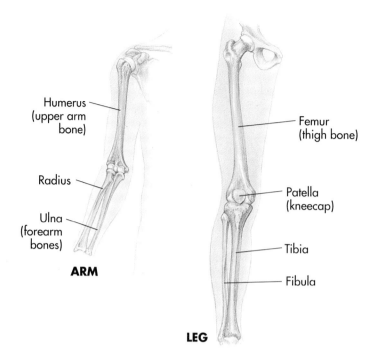

**Figure 12-7** Although similar in shape, the leg bones are larger and stronger than the arm bones because they carry the body's weight.

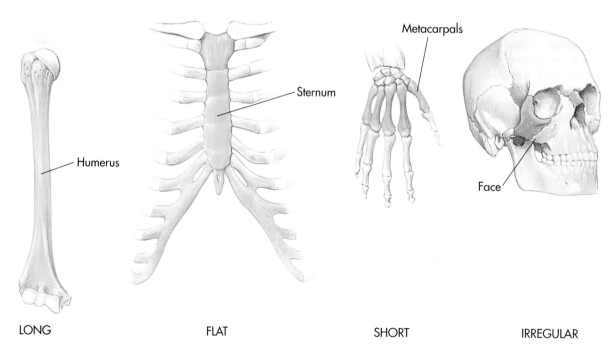

**Figure 12-8** Bones vary in shape and size. Bones are weakest at the points where they change shape and usually fracture at these points.

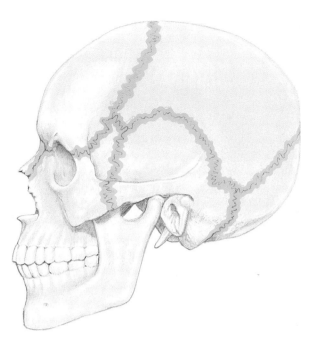

**Figure 12-9** Fused bones, such as the bones of the skull, form solid structures that protect their contents.

a dislocation can also cause a fracture and can damage nearby nerves and blood vessels.

Dislocations are generally more obvious than fractures because the joint appears deformed (Fig. 12-13). The displaced bone end often causes an abnormal lump, ridge, or depression, sometimes making dislocations easier to identify than other musculoskeletal injuries. An injured casualty is also unable to move a joint that is dislocated because the bones are out of place.

### Sprain

A *sprain* is the stretching or tearing of ligaments and other tissues at a joint. A sprain usually results when the bones that form a joint are forced beyond their normal range of motion (Fig. 12-14). The more ligaments that are torn, the more severe the injury. The sudden, violent forcing of a joint beyond its limit can completely rupture ligaments and dislocate the bones. Severe sprains may also involve a fracture of the bones that form the joint.

Mild sprains, which only stretch ligament fibres, generally heal quickly. The casualty

may have only a brief period of pain or discomfort and quickly return to activity with little or no soreness. For this reason, people often neglect sprains, and the joint is often reinjured. Severe sprains or sprains that involve a fracture usually cause pain when the joint is moved or used.

Often, a sprain is more disabling than a fracture. When fractures heal, they usually leave the bone as strong as it was before. It is unlikely that a repeat break would occur at the same spot. On the other hand, once ligaments become stretched or torn, the joint may become less stable if the injury does not receive proper care. A less stable joint makes the injured area more susceptible to reinjury.

### Strain

A *strain* is the excessive stretching and tearing of muscle or tendon fibres. It is sometimes called a "muscle pull" or "tear." Because tendons are tougher and stronger than muscles, tears usually occur in the muscle itself or where the muscle attaches to the tendon. Strains are often the result of overexertion, such as lifting something too heavy or overworking a muscle. They can also result from sudden or uncoordinated movement. Strains commonly involve the muscles in the neck or back, the front or back of the thigh, or the back of the lower leg. Strains of the neck and lower back can be particularly painful and therefore disabling.

Like sprains, strains are often neglected, which commonly leads to reinjury. Strains sometimes reoccur chronically, especially to the muscles of the neck, lower back, and the back of the thigh. Neck and back problems are two of the leading causes of absenteeism from work, accounting for millions of dollars in lost productivity annually.

## Signs and Symptoms of Musculoskeletal Injuries

You identify and care for injuries to the musculoskeletal system during the secondary survey.

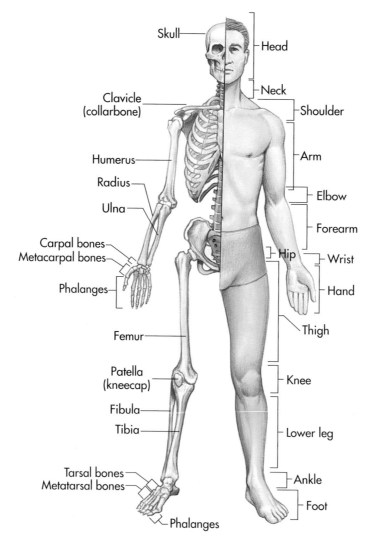

**Figure 12-10** Bones that can be seen and felt beneath the skin provide landmarks for locating parts of the body.

Because they often appear similar, it may be difficult for you to determine exactly what type of injury has occurred. As you do the secondary survey, think about how the body normally looks and feels. Compare the injured side with the uninjured side.

During the interview, ask how the injury happened. The cause of injury is often enough to make you suspect a serious musculoskeletal injury. As the casualty or bystanders explain how the injury occurred, listen for clues, such as a fall from a height or another significant impact to the body that would have the potential to cause a serious injury. Also ask the casualty if any areas are painful.

Then, do a head-to-toe survey of the entire body, beginning with the head. Check each body part. Start with the neck, followed by the shoulders, the chest, and so on. As you conduct the secondary survey, look and listen for clues that may indicate a musculoskeletal injury.

## Common Signs and Symptoms of Musculoskeletal Injuries

Five common signs and symptoms associated with musculoskeletal injuries are—

♦ Pain.
♦ Swelling.
♦ Deformity.

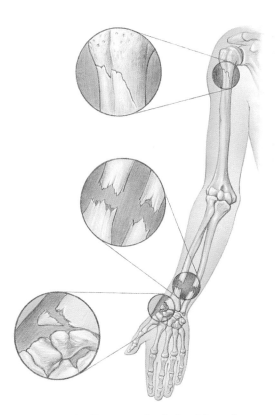

**Figure 12-11**  Fractures include chipped or cracked bones and bones broken all the way through.

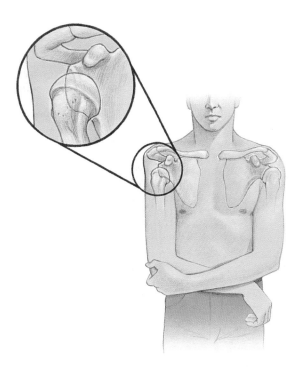

**Figure 12-12**  A dislocation is a displacement or separation of a bone from its normal position at a joint.

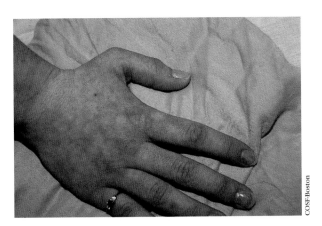

**Figure 12-13**  A dislocation can cause the joint to appear deformed.

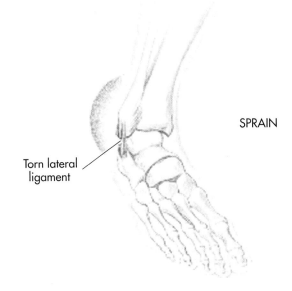

SPRAIN

Torn lateral ligament

**Figure 12-14**  A sprain results when bones that form a joint are forced beyond their normal range of motion, causing ligaments to stretch and tear.

# Sprains and Strains

Spring is the season of flowers, trees, strains, and sprains. Almost as soon as armchair athletes come out of hibernation to become intramural heroes, emergency clinics see an increase in sprained ankles, twisted knees, and strained backs. So what happens when injuries occur? Which do you apply, heat or cold?

The answer is both—first cold, then heat. And it does not matter whether it is a strain or sprain!

### How cold helps initially

When a casualty twists an ankle or strains his or her back, the tissues underneath the skin are injured. Blood and fluids seep out from the torn blood vessels and cause swelling to occur at the site of the injury. Muscles spasm to protect the injured area. This often causes more pain. By keeping the injured area cool, you can help control internal bleeding and reduce pain. Cold causes the broken blood vessels to constrict, limiting the blood and fluid that seep out. Cold reduces pain by numbing the nerve endings, thereby reducing painful muscle spasms.

### How heat helps repair the tissue

A physician will most likely advise applying ice to the injury periodically for up to the first 48 hours or until the swelling goes away. After that, applying heat is appropriate. Heat speeds up chemical reactions needed to repair the tissue. White blood cells move in to rid the body of infections, damaged cells are removed, and other cells begin the repair process. This process enhances proper healing of the injury. If you are unsure whether to use cold or heat on an injured area, always apply cold until you can consult your physician.

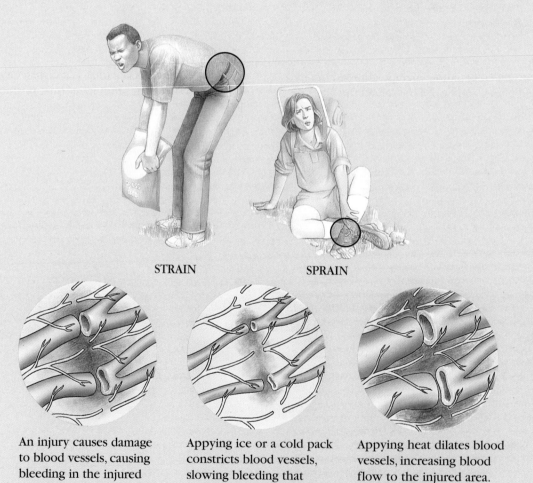

STRAIN          SPRAIN

An injury causes damage to blood vessels, causing bleeding in the injured area. Injury irritates nerve endings, causing pain.

Appying ice or a cold pack constricts blood vessels, slowing bleeding that causes the injury to swell. Cold deadens nerve endings, relieving pain.

Appying heat dilates blood vessels, increasing blood flow to the injured area. Nerve endings become more sensitive.

♦ Discolouration of the skin.
♦ Inability to use the affected part normally.

Pain, swelling, and discolouration of the skin commonly occur with any significant injury. Irritation to nerve endings that supply the injured area causes pain. Pain is the body's signal that something is wrong. The injured area may be painful to touch and to move. Swelling is caused by bleeding from damaged blood vessels and tissues in the injured area. However, swelling is often deceiving. It may appear rapidly at the site of injury, may develop gradually, or may not appear at all. Swelling by itself, therefore, is not a reliable sign of the severity of an injury or of the structures involved. Bleeding may discolour the skin in surrounding tissues. At first, the skin may only look red. As blood seeps to the skin's surface, the area begins to look bruised.

Deformity is also a sign of significant injury (Fig. 12-15). Abnormal lumps, ridges, depressions, or unusual bends or angles in body parts are types of deformities. Marked deformity is often a sign of fracture or dislocation. Comparing the injured part with an uninjured part may help you detect deformity.

A casualty's inability to move or use an injured part may also indicate a significant injury. The casualty may tell you he or she is unable to move or that it is simply too painful to move. Moving or using injured parts can disturb tissues, further irritating nerve endings, which causes or increases pain. Often, the muscles of an affected area will spasm in an attempt to keep the injured part from moving.

Similarly, a casualty often supports the injury in the most comfortable position. To manage musculoskeletal injuries, try to avoid causing additional pain. Avoid any motion or use of an injured body part that causes pain.

## Specific Signs and Symptoms of Serious Musculoskeletal Injuries

In the secondary survey, you may notice certain telltale signs and symptoms that help you determine the type of injury. Often, what the casualty

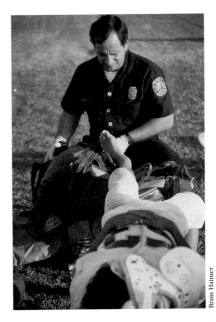

**Figure 12-15** Deformity may be obvious when an injured limb is compared to an uninjured limb.

feels or can recall about the moment of injury provides important clues.

Sprains or strains are fairly easy to tell apart. Because a sprain involves the soft tissues at a joint, pain, swelling, and deformity are usually confined to the joint area. Strains involve the soft tissue structures that, for the most part, stretch between joints. In most strains, pain, swelling, and any deformity are generally in the areas between the joints (Fig. 12-16).

However, it is not always easy to determine if a musculoskeletal injury is serious, requiring more advanced medical care. Always suspect a serious injury when the following signs and symptoms are present:

♦ Significant deformity.
♦ Moderate or severe swelling and discolouration.
♦ Inability to move or use the affected body part.
♦ Bone fragments protruding from a wound.
♦ Casualty feels bones grating or felt or heard a snap or pop at the time of injury.
♦ Loss of circulation or feeling in an extremity.
♦ Cause of the injury suggests the injury may be severe.

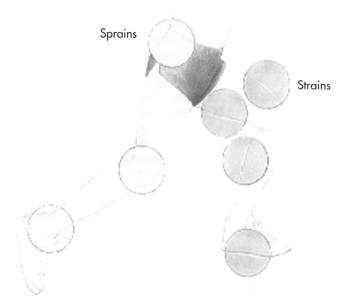

Figure 12-16 Sprains involve the soft tissues at a joint. Strains involve the soft tissues between joints.

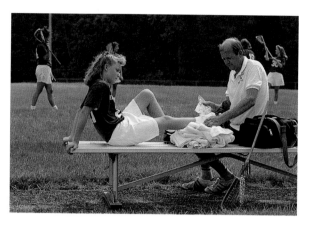

**Figure 12-17** General care for all musculoskeletal injuries is similar. Remember rest, ice, elevation, and immobilization.

# Care for Musculoskeletal Injuries

Some musculoskeletal injuries are obvious because they involve severe deformities, such as protruding bones or bleeding. The casualty also may be in severe pain. Do not be distracted. Such injuries are rarely life threatening. Complete the primary survey and care for any life threatening conditions. Then do the secondary survey and care for any other injuries. When you find a musculoskeletal injury, immediately summon more advanced medical personnel if—

- The injury involves severe bleeding.
- The injury involves the head, neck, or back.
- The injury impairs walking or breathing.
- You see or suspect multiple musculoskeletal injuries.

## General Care

The general care for all musculoskeletal injuries is similar. Just remember the acronym RICE for rest, immobilization, cold, and elevation (Fig. 12-17).

| R – rest |
| I – immobilize |
| C – cold |
| E – elevate |

### Rest

Avoid any movements or activities that cause pain. Help the casualty find the most comfortable position. If you suspect head or spine injuries, leave the casualty lying flat.

### Immobilization

If you suspect a serious musculoskeletal injury, you must immobilize the injured part before giving additional care, such as applying ice or elevating the injured part. To **immobilize**, use a splint or another method to keep the injured part from moving.

The purpose of immobilizing an injury is to—

- Lessen pain.
- Prevent further damage to soft tissues.
- Reduce the risk of serious bleeding.
- Reduce the possibility of loss of circulation to the injured part.
- Prevent closed fractures from becoming open fractures.

If advanced medical personnel have already been summoned, consider that the ground can temporarily immobilize an injured area effectively. However, if necessary, you can further immobilize an injured part by applying a splint, sling, or bandages to keep the injured body part from moving. A **splint** is a device that maintains an injured part in place. To effectively immobilize

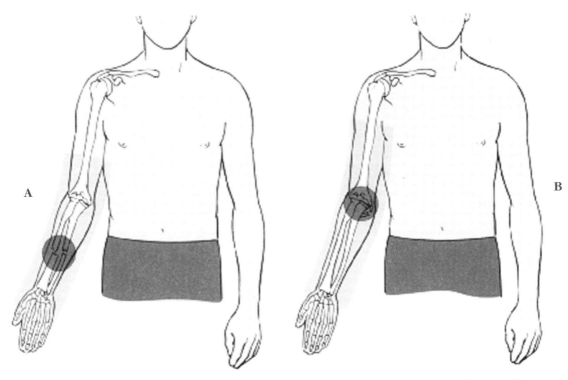

**Figure 12-18**  **A,** To immobilize a bone, splint the joints above and below the fracture. **B,** To immobilize a joint, a splint must include the bones above and below the injured joint.

an injured part, a splint must extend above and below the injury site (Fig. 12-18).

When using a splint, follow these four basic principles:

- Splint only if you can do it without causing more pain and discomfort to the casualty.
- Splint the injured area and the joints above and below the injury site.
- Check for proper circulation and sensation before and after splinting.

If splinting a part causes circulation or sensation to become impaired, loosen the splint and wait for advanced medical help to arrive.

## Types of Splints

Splints, whether commercially made or improvised, are of four general types: soft, rigid, anatomic, and traction. Soft splints include folded blankets, towels, pillows, and a sling or cravat (Fig. 12-19). A blanket can be used to splint an injured ankle (Fig. 12-20). A **sling,** which can be made from a triangular bandage, is tied to support an arm, wrist, or hand (Fig. 12-21). A **cravat** is a folded triangular bandage used to hold dressings or splints in place.

**Rigid splints** include boards, metal strips, and folded plastic or cardboard splints (Fig. 12-22). For example, a padded board can be applied to an injured arm (Fig. 12-23). **Anatomic splints** refer to the use of the body as a splint. You may

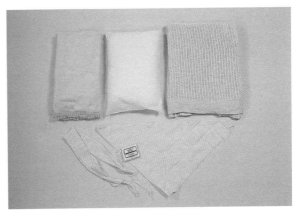

**Figure 12-19**  Soft splints include folded blankets, towels, pillows, and a sling or cravat.

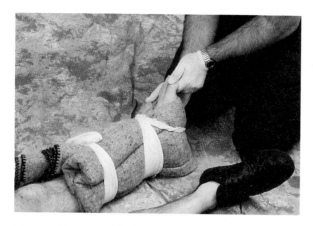

**Figure 12-20** A blanket can be used to splint an injured ankle.

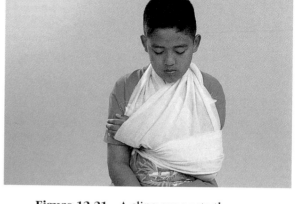

**Figure 12-21** A sling supports the arm.

not ordinarily think of the body as a splint, but it works very well and requires no special equipment. For example, an arm can be splinted to the chest. An injured leg can be splinted to the uninjured leg (Fig. 12-24).

A **traction splint** is a special type of splinting device used primarily to immobilize fractures of the thigh (femur). One end attaches to the hip and the other at the ankle. When traction is engaged, a constant, steady pull is applied against opposite ends of the leg, holding the fractured bone ends in a near-normal position (Fig. 12-25). Each commercial brand of traction splint has its own unique method of application, and rescuers must be thoroughly familiar with and proficient in the

technique of applying the splint being used. It requires two well-trained rescuers working together. Because applying a traction splint requires a special device and two trained rescuers, it is not a device you are likely to use. However, you may be asked to assist more advanced medical personnel in applying a traction splint.

As a first responder, you are likely to have commercially made splints immediately available to you. Commercial splints include padded board splints, air splints, specially designed flexible splints, vacuum splints, and traction splints (Fig. 12-26). You should become familiar with the splinting devices you are likely to have before you use them.

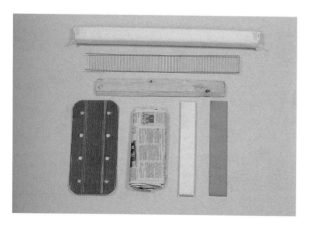

**Figure 12-22** Rigid splints include boards, metal strips, and folded cardboard or plastic.

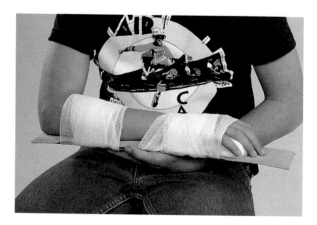

**Figure 12-23** A padded rigid splint can be applied to an injured forearm.

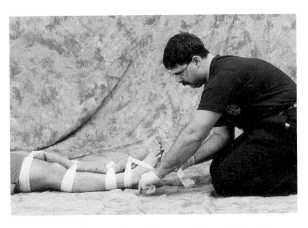

**Figure 12-24** An injured leg can be splinted to the uninjured leg.

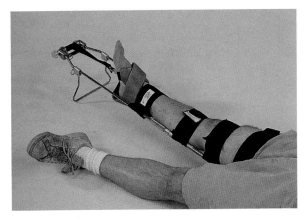

**Figure 12-25** A traction splint is primarily used to immobilize fractures of the femur.

## How to Splint

Whether using a commercially made splint or improvising from available materials, follow these guidelines when splinting an injured body part:

1. Support the injured part. If possible, have the casualty or a bystander help you.
2. Cover any open wounds with a dressing and bandage to help control bleeding and prevent infection.
3. If the injury involves an extremity, check for circulation and sensation at a site below (distal to) the injury. Expose the foot or hand if possible to check for a distal pulse, feel the hand or foot for warmth, or check for capillary refill in the fingers or toes. Ensure that the casualty has feeling in the fingers or toes; compare the injured side with the noninjured side in terms of pulse, skin colour, capillary refill, mobility, and sensation. If the distal pulse is absent, use gentle traction to try to straighten the limb into anatomical alignment.
4. In the case of an angulated fracture, gently straighten the limb into anatomical position. Grasp the limb above and below the site of injury and pull gently. DO NOT attempt this if a joint injury, such as a dislocation, is suspected or you observe firm resistance to movement, a significant increase in pain, or

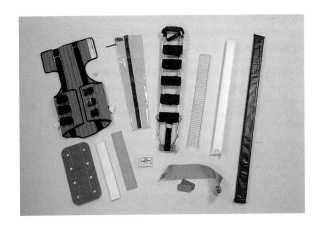

**Figure 12-26** Commercial splints.

the sound or feeling of bone fragments grating.
5. If using a rigid splint or anatomic splint, pad the splint so that it is shaped to the injured part. This will help prevent further injury.
6. Secure the splint in place with folded triangular bandages (cravats), roller bandages (gauze or elastic), or other wide strips of cloth.
7. Recheck circulation below the injury site to ensure that circulation has not been restricted by applying the splint too tightly. Loosen the splint if the casualty complains of numbness or if the fingers or toes discolour (turn blue) or become cold.
8. Elevate the splinted part, if possible.

After the injury has been immobilized, recheck the ABCs and vital signs and take steps to care for shock. Shock is likely to develop as a result of a serious musculoskeletal injury. Help the casualty rest in the most comfortable position, apply ice or a cold pack, maintain normal body temperature, and reassure him or her. Determine what additional care is needed and whether to summon more advanced medical personnel if it has not already been done. Continue to monitor vital signs. Check the casualty's level of consciousness, breathing, pulse, skin colour and temperature, and blood pressure. Be alert for signs and symptoms of shock or other clues that may indicate the casualty's condition is worsening.

### Cold

Regardless of whether the injury is a closed fracture, dislocation, sprain, or strain, apply ice or a cold pack. Cold helps reduce swelling and eases pain and discomfort. Commercial cold packs can be stored in a kit until ready to use, or you can make an ice pack by placing ice in a plastic bag and wrapping it with a towel or cloth. Place a layer of gauze or cloth between the source of cold and the skin to prevent skin damage. Do not apply an ice or cold pack directly over the fracture because doing so would require you to put pressure on the fracture site and could cause discomfort to the casualty. Instead, place cold packs around the site. A general rule for cold application is 15 minutes every hour for the first 24 to 48 hours after the injury.

### Elevation

Elevating the injured area above the level of the heart helps slow the flow of blood, reducing swelling. Elevation is particularly effective in controlling swelling in extremity injuries. However, never attempt to elevate a seriously injured limb area unless it has been adequately immobilized.

## Considerations for Transporting a Casualty

Some musculoskeletal injuries are obviously minor. The casualty may choose not to get emergency medical care. Others are more serious, requiring more advanced care. Summon more advanced medical personnel immediately if you suspect an injury involving severe bleeding, injuries to the head or spine, an injury that impairs breathing, or if you see or suspect multiple musculoskeletal injuries. Fractures of large bones can cause severe bleeding and are likely to result in shock.

Some situations may require you to move the casualty before an ambulance arrives. If possible, always splint the injury before moving the casualty. Follow the general rule: "When in doubt, splint." If you are in a position where you must transport the casualty to a medical facility, have someone drive so that you can continue to provide care.

## ◆ SUMMARY

The musculoskeletal system has four main structures—bones, muscles, tendons, and ligaments. Sometimes it is difficult to tell whether an injury is a fracture, dislocation, sprain, or strain. Since you cannot be sure which injury a casualty might have, always care for the injury as if it were serious. If more advanced medical personnel are on the way, do not move the casualty. Control any bleeding first. Take steps to minimize shock and monitor the ABCs and vital signs. If you are going to transport the casualty to a medical facility, be sure to first immobilize the injury before moving the casualty.

Chapters 13 through 15 discuss recognition of and care for specific injuries, starting with the head and progressing downward, much like the sequence of the secondary survey.

## YOU ARE THE RESPONDER

1. A basketball player leaps for a rebound. She and another player collide and fall to the ground. What signs and symptoms would you look for that suggest a serious injury?
2. The same player complains of pain in her lower leg and ankle and says that she cannot support her weight. You note a deformity, swelling, and discolouration. Describe how you might provide care for this casualty.

# Applying a Rigid Splint

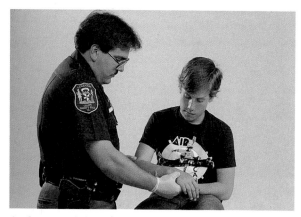

1. Support injured area.

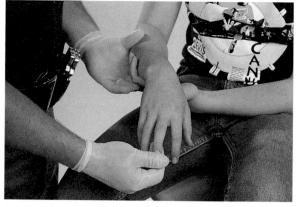

2. Check circulation and sensation below injured area.

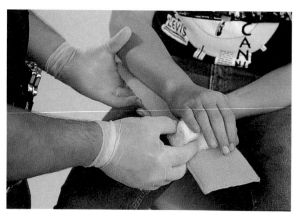

3. Position splint.

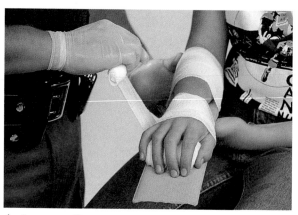

4. Secure splint.

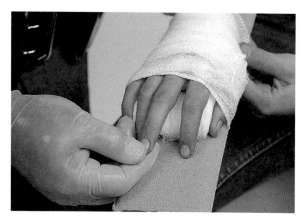

5. Recheck circulation sensation.

# Applying a Sling and Binder

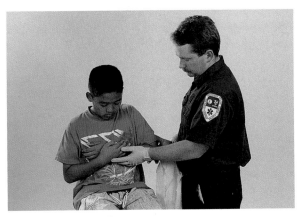

1. Support injured area.

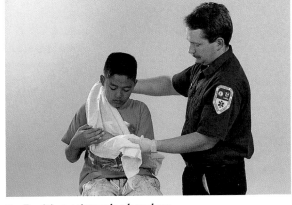

2. Position triangular bandage.

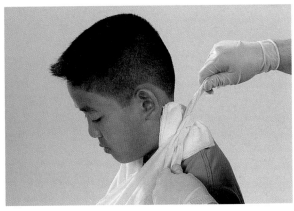

3. Tie ends.

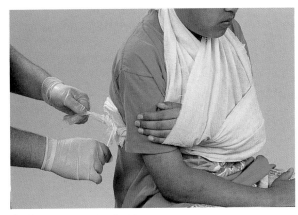

4. Secure arm to chest.

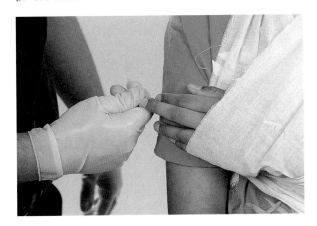

5. Recheck circulation and sensation.

# Applying an Anatomic Splint

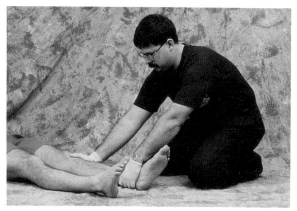

1. Support injured area.

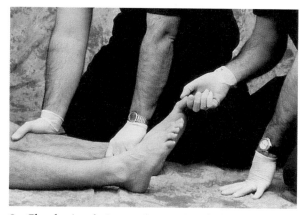

2. Check circulation and sensation below injured area.

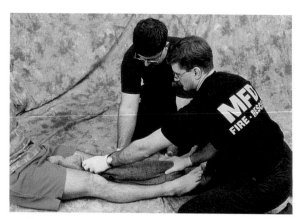

3. Move uninjured limb next to injured limb.

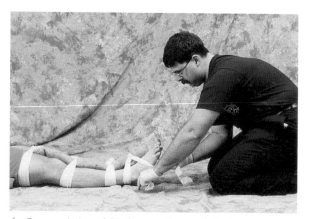

4. Secure injured limb to uninjured limb.

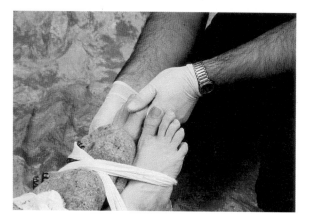

5. Recheck circulation and sensation.

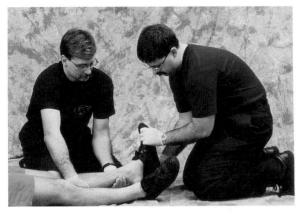

1. Support injured area.

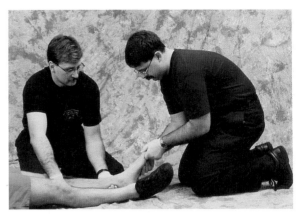

2. Check circulation and sensation below injured area.*

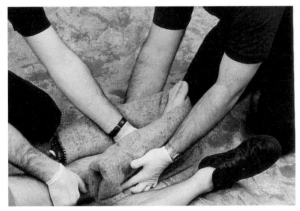

3. Position splint.

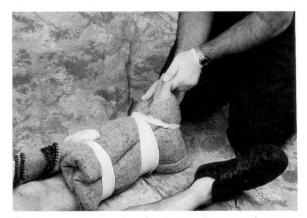

4. Secure splint and recheck circulation and sensation.

*It may not be possible to check circulation in an injured foot, ankle, or leg if a sock or a shoe is in place. Also, a recheck may not be possible if the soft splint is particularly bulky.

# Injuries to the Head and Spine

# 13

## ◆ Key Terms ◆

**Cervical collar:** A rigid device positioned around the neck to limit movement of the head and neck.

**In-line stabilization:** A technique used to minimize movement of the casualty's head and neck.

**Spinal column:** The series of vertebrae extending from the base of the skull to the tip of the tailbone (coccyx).

**Spinal cord:** A bundle of nerves extending from the base of the skull to the lower back, protected by the spinal column.

**Vertebrae:** The 33 bones of the spinal column.

## ◆ For Review ◆

Before reading this chapter, you should have a basic understanding of the nervous system and its relationship to other body systems (Chapter 3), how to care for soft tissue injuries (Chapter 11), and how to care for musculoskeletal injuries (Chapter 12).

## ◆ INTRODUCTION

*It's summer vacation at the beach. High school and college students are having fun in the sun. The weather is great, the water refreshing. The day is perfect for a game of touch football on the beach.*

*Later in the day, the tide comes in and the game becomes more aggressive. Players lunge into the surf to catch passes and runners. As the game is about to end, the quarterback throws a long pass. The receiver has the chance to score the winning touchdown, or the defender can intercept the pass to guarantee victory. They both run into the surf and dive headfirst at the ball. As they strike the water, a wave crashes over them, forcing them underwater and into a sandbar. Both players strike their heads on the sandy bottom. The result? Both are pulled from the surf by their friends and by lifeguards summoned to the scene. One player is lucky and escapes with only a concussion. The other, not so lucky, suffers a broken neck and is paralysed for life.*

Although injuries to the head and spine account for only a small percentage of all injuries, they cause more than half the fatalities. Each year, tens of thousands of Canadians suffer a head or spine injury serious enough to require medical care. Most of these casualties are males between the ages of 15 and 30. Motor vehicle collisions account for about half of all head and spinal injuries. Other causes include falls, sports and recreational activities, and violent acts, such as assault.

Besides those who die each year from head and spinal injury, thousands of casualties become permanently disabled. Today there are many thousands of permanently disabled casualties of head or spinal injuries in Canada. These survivors have a wide range of physical and mental impairments, including paralysis, speech and memory problems, and behavioural disorders.

Fortunately, prompt, appropriate care can help minimize the damage from most head and spinal injuries. In this chapter, you will learn how to recognize when a head or spinal injury may be serious. You will also learn how to provide the appropriate care to minimize injuries to the head and spine.

## ◆ PREVENTING HEAD AND SPINAL INJURIES

Injuries to the head and spine are a major cause of death, disability, and disfigurement. However, many such injuries can be prevented. By using safety practices in all areas of your life, you can help reduce risks to you and to others around you.

Safety practices that can help prevent injuries to the head and spine include—

- Wearing seat belts.
- When appropriate, wearing approved helmets, eyewear, faceguards, and mouthguards.
- Preventing falls.
- Obeying rules in sports and recreational activities.
- Avoiding inappropriate use of drugs.
- Inspecting work and recreational equipment periodically.
- Thinking and talking about safety.

### Wearing Seat Belts

Always wear seat belts, including shoulder restraints, when driving or riding in an automobile. Be sure all passengers also wear them.

Airbags, available in some cars, provide additional protection. All small children riding in a car must be in approved safety seats correct for the child's age and weight.

## Wearing Helmets and Eyewear

Helmets can prevent many needless injuries to the head and spine. They are designed for different purposes, with varying degrees of protection, and offer protection only for their intended use (Fig. 13-1). For example, the industrial work helmet called a "hard hat" provides adequate protection against falling debris but does not offer the proper protection for riding a motorcycle.

Any open form of transportation, such as a motorcycle, moped, or all-terrain vehicle, exposes the head and spine to injury. Wearing a helmet can help reduce such injuries. The ideal helmet, sometimes called a "full-face helmet," protects the lower face and jaw and has a large, clear or tinted face shield. In all cases, the helmet should be the correct size and fit comfortably and securely.

Eyewear can help prevent many needless injuries that result in loss of sight. Anytime you operate machinery or perform an activity that may involve flying particles or splashing chemicals, you should wear protective eyewear, such as goggles.

## Safeguarding Against Falls

Although most falls occur at home and involve young children and the elderly, falls can and do occur in the workplace. You can take precautions to prevent falls. Floor surfaces should be made of nonslip material. Stairs should have nonslip treads and hand rails. Rugs should be secured to the floor with double-sided tape. Clean up any spills promptly. The bathroom should be safe for all those using it. If necessary, install hand rails by the bathtub and toilet.

## Taking Safety Precautions in Sports and Recreation

Participants in sports or recreational activities should know their physical limitations. Proper protective equipment is necessary for any activity in which serious injury may occur. In all sports involving physical contact, participants should wear mouthpieces. Most important, everyone must know and follow the rules. Rules not only make the activity fair, they also help prevent injuries. The coach, athletic trainer, or a

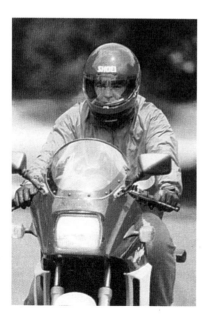
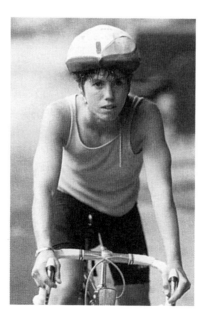
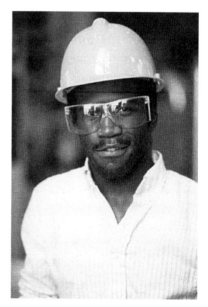

**Figure 13-1** Wearing a helmet helps protect against head and spine injuries.

more experienced participant may impose additional rules for the safety of newcomers. Never participate in a new activity until you know the rules and risks involved.

## Avoiding Inappropriate Use of Drugs

Alcohol and other drugs used inappropriately cause or contribute to many serious motor vehicle collisions and water-related incidents that involve head and spinal injuries. Drugs impair judgment and reflexes, causing the body to respond abnormally. Drugs can give the user a feeling of false confidence. Certain prescription and common drugstore medications also have side effects, such as drowsiness, that can make driving or operating machinery dangerous. Follow your physician's directions and the directions and warnings on medication labels.

## Inspecting Equipment

Inspect mechanical equipment, sports equipment, and ladders periodically to ensure good working order. Check for worn or loose parts that could break and cause a mishap. Before climbing a ladder, place its legs on a firm, flat surface and have someone anchor it while you climb.

## Thinking and Talking Safety

People too often neglect thinking about safety in their daily lives, yet we are most vulnerable to injury at work, during recreational activities, or while travelling. Take the time to inspect and think about your daily environment. Evaluate your habits. Answer the following five questions:

◆ Are there things that you could do in your workplace or home to help prevent injuries to you or others?
◆ Are you taking unnecessary risks in any activities?
◆ Do you follow rules meant for your safety?
◆ Do you frequently check the tires on your motor vehicle(s)?

◆ Do you ever attempt any activity without being in the physical condition that would allow you to do it without injury?

Talk with others about preventing injuries at work, at home, and in recreation. Everyone needs to know about safety. Seek guidance to help prevent injuries that could permanently affect your life or the lives of others. Discuss safety when using mechanical devices or equipment or when approaching a potentially dangerous scene.

## ◆ RECOGNIZING SERIOUS HEAD AND SPINAL INJURIES

Injuries to the head or spine can damage both bone and soft tissue, including brain tissue and the spinal cord. It is usually difficult to determine the extent of damage in head and spinal injuries. In most cases, the only way to assess the damage is by having x-ray films taken in an emergency department. Since you have no way of knowing exactly how severe an injury is, *always* provide initial care as if the injury is serious.

## The Brain

Injuries to the head can affect the brain. Blood from a ruptured vessel in the brain can accumulate in the skull (Fig. 13-2). Because there is very little empty space in the skull, bleeding can build up pressure that can cause further damage to brain tissue.

Bleeding in the skull can occur rapidly or slowly over a period of days. This bleeding will affect the brain, causing changes in consciousness. An altered level of consciousness is often the first and most important sign of a serious head injury.

## The Spine

The spine is a strong, flexible column that supports the head and the trunk and encases and protects the spinal cord. The *spinal column,* which extends from the base of the skull to

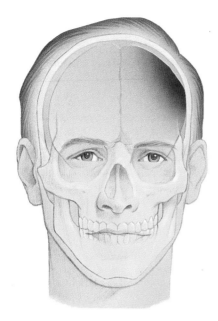

**Figure 13-2** Injuries to the head can rupture blood vessels in the brain. Pressure builds within the skull as blood accumulates, causing brain injury.

the tip of the tailbone, consists of small bones, *vertebrae,* with circular openings. The vertebrae are separated from each other by cushions of cartilage called disks (Fig. 13-3, *A*). This **cartilage,** an elastic tissue, acts as a shock absorber when a person is walking, running, or jumping. The **spinal cord,** a bundle of nerves extending from the base of the skull to the lower back, runs through the hollow part of the vertebrae. Nerve branches extend to various parts of the body through openings on the sides of the vertebrae.

The spine is divided into five regions: the cervical or neck region, the thoracic or mid-back region, the lumbar or lower back region, the sacrum, and the coccyx, the small triangular bone at the lower end of the spinal column. Injuries to the spinal column include fractures and dislocations of the vertebrae, sprained ligaments, and compression or displacement of the disks between the vertebrae.

Injuries to the spine can fracture the vertebrae and sprain the ligaments. These injuries usually heal without problems. With severe injuries, however, the vertebrae may shift and compress

or sever the spinal cord. This can cause temporary or permanent paralysis, even death. The extent of the paralysis depends on which area of the spinal cord is damaged (Fig. 13-3,*B*).

## Mechanism of Injury

Consider the mechanism of injury to help you determine whether a casualty has suffered a head or spinal injury. Survey the scene and think about the forces involved in the injury. Strong forces are likely to cause severe injury to the head and spine. For example, a driver whose head breaks a car windshield in a crash may have a serious head and spinal injury. A diver who hits his or her head on the bottom of a swimming pool may also have a serious head or spinal injury. Evaluate the scene for clues as to whether a serious head or spinal injury has occurred.

## Injury Situations

You should consider the possibility of a serious head or spinal injury in a number of situations. These include—

◆ A fall from a height greater than the casualty's height.
◆ Any diving mishap.
◆ Unconsciousness of unknown cause.
◆ Any injury, involving severe blunt force to the head or trunk.
◆ Any injury, such as a gunshot wound, that penetrates the head or trunk.
◆ Any motor vehicle crash.
◆ Any casualty thrown from a motor vehicle.
◆ Any injury in which a casualty's helmet is broken.
◆ Any incident involving a lightning strike.

## Signs and Symptoms of Head and Spinal Injuries

You also may notice certain signs and symptoms that indicate a head or spinal injury. These

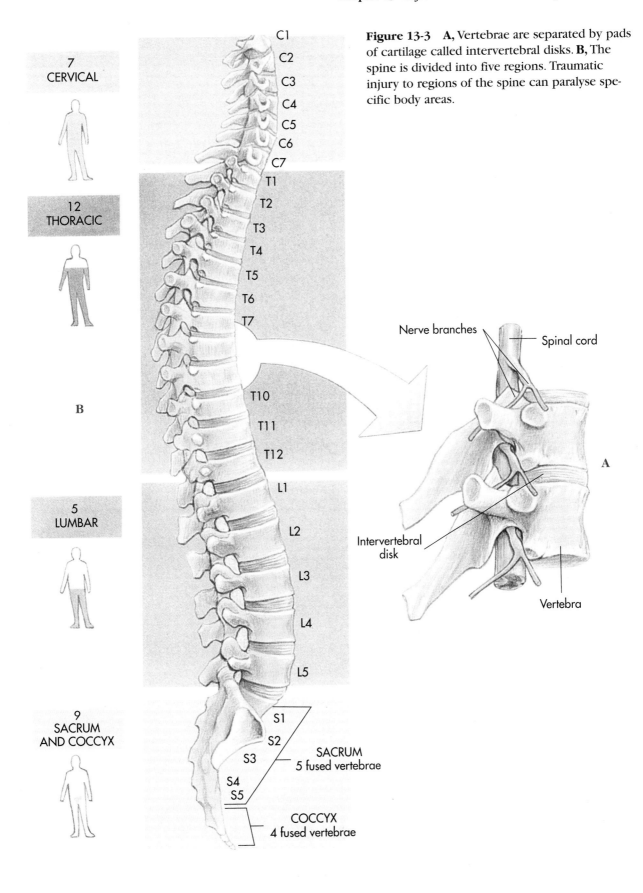

**Figure 13-3** **A,** Vertebrae are separated by pads of cartilage called intervertebral disks. **B,** The spine is divided into five regions. Traumatic injury to regions of the spine can paralyse specific body areas.

7
CERVICAL

12
THORACIC

B

5
LUMBAR

9
SACRUM
AND COCCYX

C1
C2
C3
C4
C5
C6
C7
T1
T2
T3
T4
T5
T6
T7
T10
T11
T12
L1
L2
L3
L4
L5
S1
S2
S3
S4
S5

SACRUM
5 fused vertebrae

COCCYX
4 fused vertebrae

Nerve branches

Spinal cord

Intervertebral
disk

A

Vertebra

# Typical Diving Injuries

Who is the average spinal cord injury casualty?

- Male, 17 to 22 years old, and athletic
- No formal training in diving
- First-time visitor to the location
- Making his first dive in the location
- Was not warned, by word or sign, about dangers
- Had been using alcohol and/or drugs

How does a diving injury occur?

- Diving into shallow water (95%)
- Diving from a deck or adjacent structure into an in-ground pool
- Diving without supervision or training from starting blocks into shallow water

What is the situation?

- There is no lifeguard on duty.
- Water depth where the casualty hit the bottom is less than 1.5 metres.
- The water is cloudy or murky.
- The bottom has no markings.
- No warning signs prohibit diving.

What happens then?

- Your head hits the bottom, and you stop instantly with an injured spinal cord.
- Even if you're conscious, you may be unable to move and may drown before someone reaches you.
- Even if someone reaches you, he or she may not know how to move you, and any movement of your head may worsen the injury.
- Even if you're rescued and reach the emergency room, you have just begun to suffer. Your life is saved, but you are paralyzed.

Imagine living the rest of your life unable to move your arms and legs or control when you go to the bathroom.

Imagine how your relationships with friends and family will change.

Now think:

- Is it worth it to make one careless dive?
- Is it worth it to allow your friends to dive recklessly?

may be obvious right away or may develop later. These signs and symptoms include—

- Changes in the level of consciousness.
- Severe pain or pressure in the head or spine.
- Tingling or loss of sensation in the extremities (arms and legs).
- Partial or complete loss of movement of any body part.
- Unusual bumps or depressions on the head or spine.
- Blood or other fluids draining from the ears or nose.
- Profuse external bleeding of the head or spine.
- Seizures.
- Impaired breathing or vision as a result of injury.
- Nausea or vomiting.
- Persistent headache.
- Loss of balance.
- Bruising of the head, especially around the eyes and behind the ears.

These signs and symptoms alone do not always suggest a head or spinal injury, but they may when combined with the cause of the injury. Regardless of the situation, always summon more advanced medical personnel when you suspect a head or spinal injury.

## ◆ CARE FOR SERIOUS HEAD AND SPINAL INJURIES

Head and spinal injuries can become life-threatening emergencies. A serious injury can cause a casualty to stop breathing. Care for serious head and spinal injuries also involves supporting the respiratory, circulatory, and nervous systems. Provide the following care while waiting for more advanced medical personnel to arrive:

- Minimize movement of the head and spine.
- Maintain an open airway.
- Control any external bleeding.
- Monitor vital signs.
- Maintain normal body temperature.
- Administer oxygen if available.

## Minimize Movement

Caring for a head or spinal injury is similar to caring for any other serious soft tissue or musculoskeletal injury. You should immobilise the injured area and control any bleeding. Because movement of an injured head or spine can damage the spinal cord irreversibly, keep the casualty as still as possible until you can obtain more advanced care. To minimize movement of the head and neck, use a technique called *in-line stabilization.*

With this technique, you place your hands on both sides of the casualty's head, gently position it, if necessary, in line with the body, and support it in that position. You can do this in various ways, depending on the condition in which you find the casualty (Fig. 13-4). This skill is simple to perform but can be important to the casualty's outcome. Keeping the head in this anatomically normal position helps prevent further damage to the spinal column. If a second rescuer is available, that person can give care for any other conditions while you keep the head and neck stable.

There are, however, some circumstances in which you would *not* move the casualty's head in line with the body. These include—

- When the casualty's head is severely angled to one side.
- When the casualty complains of pain, pressure, or muscle spasms in the neck when you begin to align the head with the body.
- When the rescuer feels resistance when attempting to move the head in line with the body.

In these circumstances, support the casualty's head in the position in which you found it except when the casualty's airway cannot be maintained open in that position.

After the casualty's head is stabilized, as previously described, a rigid *cervical collar* should be applied (Fig. 13-5). This collar helps minimize movement of the head and neck and keeps the head in line with the body. Applying a cervical collar requires two rescuers. While one rescuer maintains in-line stabilization, another carefully applies an appropriately sized

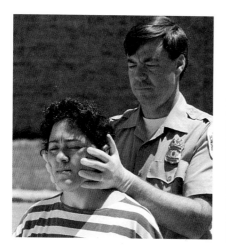
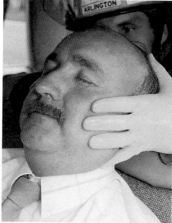
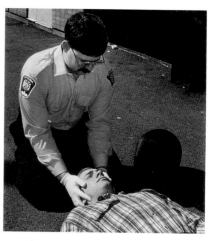

**Figure 13-4**  Support the casualty's head in line with the body using in-line stabilization.

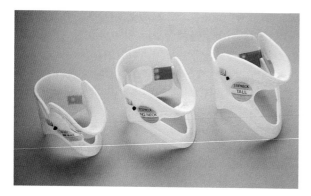

**Figure 13-5**  There are a variety of rigid cervical collars available.

cervical collar (Fig. 13-6). An appropriately sized collar is one that fits securely, with the casualty's chin resting in the proper position and the head maintained in line with the body. Some cervical collars come with specific manufacturer's instructions for proper sizing.

## Immobilise the Casualty

Once the cervical collar has been applied and in-line stabilization maintained, the casualty's entire body should be immobilised. This can be done using the following equipment:

- ◆ Rigid splint, such as a backboard.
- ◆ Large towel or blanket.
- ◆ Straps or triangular bandage(s) folded into a cravat(s).

If you do not have a backboard available, support the casualty in the position you found him or her until more advanced medical personnel arrive.

Once the cervical collar is in place, the casualty is positioned on a backboard. This is done by "log-rolling" the casualty onto the board. This technique keeps the head in line with the body. It requires a minimum of two rescuers: one to maintain in-line stabilization and another to position the backboard and roll the casualty's body (Fig. 13-7, *A*). However, it is highly preferable to have three rescuers available to perform this technique. With three rescuers, one can

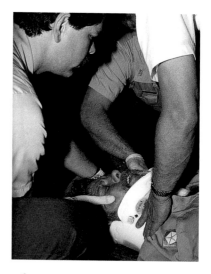

**Figure 13-6**  Apply a cervical collar that fits securely, with the chin resting in the designated position and the head held in line with the body.

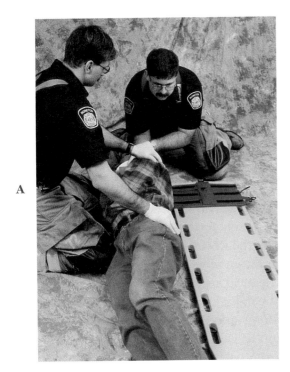

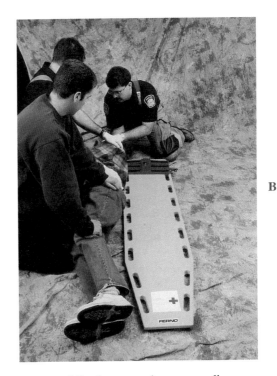

A

B

**Figure 13-7** **A,** One rescuer maintains in-line stabilization while the second rescuer rolls the casualty's body and positions the backboard. Visually assess the casualty's back for injury before repositioning the casualty on the backboard. **B,** A third rescuer can help log-roll the casualty and position the backboard.

provide in-line stabilization and the second and third can log-roll the casualty and position the backboard (Fig. 13-7, *B*).

Once the casualty is on the board, use several straps or cravats to secure the casualty's body to the backboard (Fig. 13-8). There are several different configurations that can be used to strap the casualty onto the board. A common one is that of securing the chest by crisscrossing the straps. Regardless of which method is used, the straps should be snug but not so tight as to restrict movement of the chest during breathing. With the remaining straps, secure the casualty's hips, thighs, and legs. If necessary, secure the hands in front of the body.

Once the casualty's body is secured to the backboard, secure the casualty's head. If the casualty's head does not appear to be resting in line with the body, you may need to place a small amount of padding, such as a small folded towel, to support the head. Normally, approximately 2.5 centimetres (1 inch) of padding is all that is needed to keep the head in line with the

body, while at the same time providing comfort for the casualty. Next, place a folded or rolled blanket in a horseshoe shape around the head and neck of the casualty (Fig. 13-9). Use a cravat or tape to secure the forehead.

You may have a commercially made head-immobilisation device available (Fig. 13-10). Many of these use Velcro straps to secure the head. You should follow the manufacturer's directions when using these devices. Sandbags,

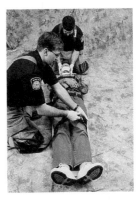

**Figure 13-8** Secure the casualty to the backboard.

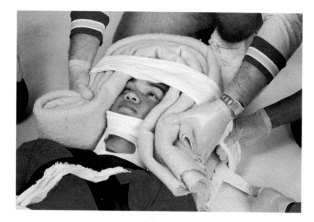

**Figure 13-9** To secure the head, place a rolled blanket around the head and neck, and use a cravat to secure the forehead.

once traditionally used to secure the casualty's head, are no longer recommended. This is because of the force they exert on a casualty's neck if the casualty must be turned on his or her side to clear the airway while secured to the backboard.

### Use of the Kendrick Extrication Device (KED)

You might be called upon to assist EMTs or paramedics to immobilise a casualty with a KED. The steps are as follows (Fig. 13-11):

1. After manual in-line stabilization and the application of a rigid cervical collar, the KED short spine board device is placed behind

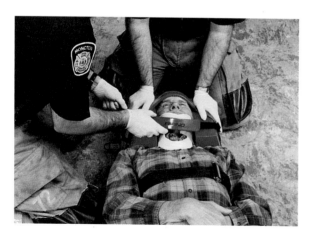

**Figure 13-10** A commercial device may be used in place of a blanket and cravat to stabilize the head.

the casualty. It should be positioned snugly beneath the casualty's armpits to prevent it from moving up the torso.

2. The upper and middle torso is immobilised by fastening the upper, middle, and lower chest straps. The upper strap can be relatively tight without impairing chest movement. The middle and lower straps should be snug so that fingers cannot be slipped beneath the straps.

3. Each groin strap is positioned and fastened separately, forming a loop. These straps prevent the KED from moving up and the lower end from moving laterally.

4. The head is padded and secured to the KED.

5. The casualty is carefully moved as a unit to a long spine board by rotating the casualty and KED onto the board. The legs are held proximal to the knees and lifted during the transition.

6. The casualty is centred on the long spine board, the leg straps are loosened, and the legs are slowly lowered to an in-line position.

7. The casualty and KED are secured to the long spine board, maintaining a neutral in-line position with the long axis of the body. Then the KED chest straps are loosened.

## Maintain an Open Airway

As you learned in earlier chapters, you do not always have to roll the casualty onto his or her back to check breathing. A cry of pain, regular chest movement, or the sound of breathing tells you the casualty is breathing. If the casualty is breathing, support the casualty in the position in which you found him or her. If the casualty begins to vomit, position the casualty onto one side to keep the airway clear. Ask other rescuers to help move the casualty's body while you maintain in-line stabilization.

## Monitor Vital Signs

After immobilising the casualty, monitor the vital signs. Pay close attention to the casualty's level

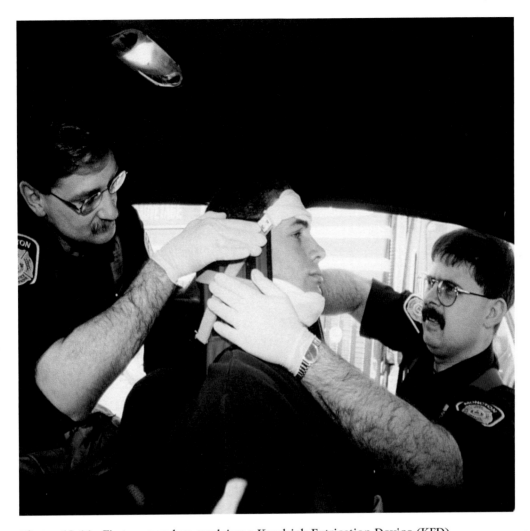

**Figure 13-11**  First responders applying a Kendrick Extrication Device (KED).

of consciousness and breathing. A serious head injury will often cause changes in consciousness. The casualty may give inappropriate responses when asked name, time, place, or what happened or may speak incoherently. The casualty may be drowsy, appear to fall asleep, and may then suddenly awaken or lose consciousness completely. Breathing may become rapid or irregular. Because injury to the head or spine can paralyse chest nerves and muscles, breathing can stop. If this happens, perform rescue breathing. Casualties of serious head or spinal injury need supplemental oxygen. Administer oxygen if it is available.

## Control External Bleeding

Some head and neck injuries include soft tissue damage. Because there are many blood vessels in the head and two major arteries—the carotid arteries—in the neck, the casualty can lose large amounts of blood quickly. If there is external bleeding, control it promptly.

## Maintain Normal Body Temperature

A serious injury to the head or spine can disrupt the body's normal heating or cooling mechanism. When this happens, a casualty is more susceptible to shock. For example, a casualty suffering a serious head or spinal injury while outside on a cold day will be more likely to suffer from hypothermia, a life-threatening cooling of the body. This is because the normal shivering response to rewarm the body may not work. It is always important to minimize shock by maintaining normal body temperature.

## Special Situation—Removing a Helmet

There may be a time when someone wearing a helmet, such as a motorcyclist or an athlete, suffers a serious head injury. Since most helmets fit snugly to the head, it is difficult to remove one without moving the head and neck. Fortunately, there is rarely a time when the helmet needs to be removed. If the helmet has a face piece, such as a mask or visor, that interferes with normal breathing, maintaining an open airway, or performing rescue breathing, remove the mask or visor only (Fig. 13-12). Usually, you can remove the face piece by unsnapping, unscrewing, or cutting it.

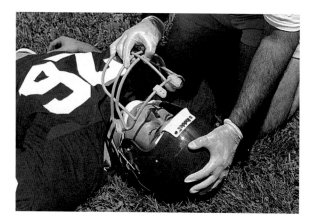

**Figure 13-12** When removing a face mask, unscrew or cut the straps and expose the face.

The only time you should remove a helmet is if it interferes with the care you are providing, such as stabilizing the head in line with the body or performing rescue breathing. In these rare situations, two rescuers should carefully remove the helmet.

To remove a helmet, first remove the chinstrap. Next, as one rescuer supports the head by holding the jaw with one hand while the other hand supports the back of the head (occipital region), a second rescuer spreads the sides of the helmet to clear the ears. While the first rescuer continues to support the head, the second rescuer slides the helmet off, causing as little motion of the head as possible. The rescuer who removed the helmet then maintains in-line stabilization. Figure 13-13 shows how to remove a helmet.

## ◆ CARE FOR SPECIFIC HEAD INJURIES

The head is easily injured because it lacks the padding of muscle and fat that are in other areas of the body. You can feel bone just beneath the surface of the skin over most of the head, including the chin, cheekbones, and scalp (Fig. 13-14).

## Concussion

Any significant force to the head can cause a concussion, a temporary impairment of brain function. A concussion usually does not result in permanent physical damage to brain tissue. In most cases, the casualty only loses consciousness for an instant and may say that he or she "blacked out" or "saw stars." Sometimes, a concussion causes a loss of consciousness for a longer period. Other times, a casualty may be confused or have amnesia (memory loss). Anyone suspected of having a concussion should be examined by a physician.

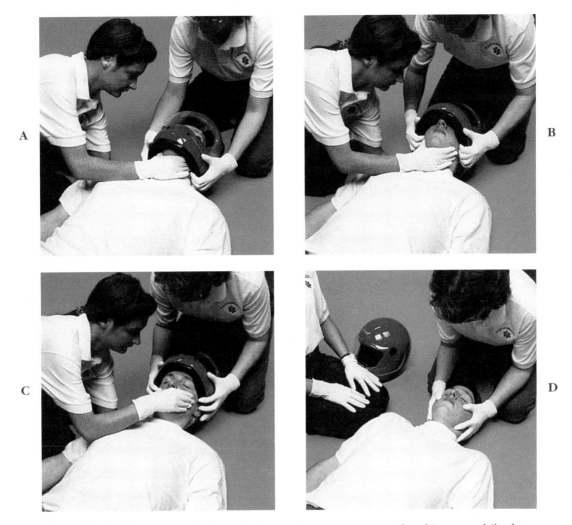

**Figure 13-13**   To remove a helmet, **A,** the first rescuer removes the chinstrap while the second rescuer holds the head in line with the body. The first rescuer then grasps the casualty's mandible by placing the thumb at the angle of the mandible on one side and two fingers at the angle on the other side. The first rescuer's other hand is placed under the neck at the base of the skull, producing in-line immobilization of the casualty's head. **B,** While the first rescuer supports the head, the second rescuer spreads the sides of the helmet. **C,** The second rescuer slides the helmet off the casualty. **D,** Once the helmet is removed, the second rescuer applies in-line stabilization.

## Scalp Injury

Scalp bleeding can be minor or severe. The bleeding is usually easily controlled with direct pressure. Because the skull may be injured, be careful to press gently at first. If you feel a depression, a spongy area, or bone fragments, do not put direct pressure on the wound. Attempt to control bleeding with pressure on the area around the wound (Fig. 13-15). Examine the injured area carefully because

the casualty's hair may hide part of the wound. If you are unsure about the extent of a scalp injury, summon more advanced medical personnel. They will be better able to evaluate the injury.

If the casualty has only an open wound, control the bleeding with direct pressure. Apply several dressings and hold them in place with your hand (Fig. 13-16, *A*). Secure the dressings with a roller bandage (Fig. 13-16, *B*).

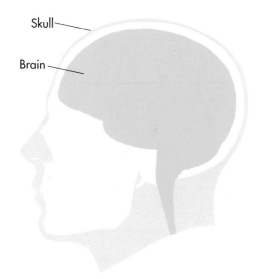

**Figure 13-14** The head is easily injured because it lacks the padding of muscle and fat found in other areas of the body.

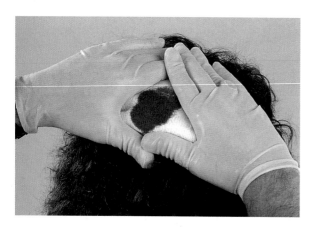

**Figure 13-15** To avoid putting pressure on a deep scalp wound, apply pressure around the wound.

## Cheek Injury

Injury to the cheek often involves soft tissue only. Control bleeding from the cheek in the same way as other soft tissue bleeding. The only difference is that you may have to control bleeding on either the outside or the inside of the cheek or in both places. Begin by examining both the outside and inside of the cheek. Bleeding from inside may result from a blow that caused the teeth to cut the inside of the cheek or from a laceration or puncture wound outside. To control bleeding, place several folded dressings inside the mouth,

against the cheek. If possible, have the casualty hold them in place. If external bleeding is also present, place dressings on the outside of the cheek and apply direct pressure with your hand or a pressure bandage (Fig. 13-17, *A* and *B*).

If an object passes completely through the cheek and becomes embedded, you may have to remove it to control bleeding and keep the airway open. This circumstance is the only exception to the general rule of not removing embedded objects from the body. An embedded object in the cheek cannot be easily stabilized, makes control of bleeding more difficult, and may become dislodged and obstruct the airway. You can remove the object by pulling it out the same way it entered. If doing this is difficult or is painful to the casualty, leave the object in place and stabilize it with bulky dressings and bandages.

If you remove the object, fold or roll several dressings and place them inside the mouth. Be sure not to obstruct the airway. Apply dressings to the outside of the cheek also. The casualty may not be able to hold these in place, so you may have to hold them. Bleeding inside the cheek can cause the casualty to swallow blood. If the casualty swallows enough blood, nausea or vomiting could result, which would complicate the situation. When possible, place the casualty in a seated position, leaning slightly forward so that blood will not drain into the throat. As with any situation involving serious bleeding or an embedded object, summon more advanced medical personnel.

## Nose Injury

Nose injuries are usually caused by a blow from a blunt object. The result is often a nosebleed. High blood pressure or changes in altitude can also cause nosebleeds. In most cases, you can control bleeding by having the casualty sit with the head slightly forward while pinching the nostrils together (Fig. 13-18). Other methods of controlling bleeding include applying an ice pack to the bridge of the nose or putting pressure on the upper lip just beneath the nose.

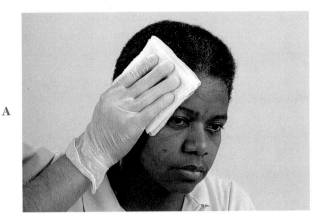
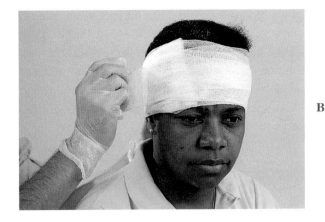

**Figure 13-16** Apply pressure to control bleeding from a scalp wound. **A,** Hold several dressings against the wound with your hand. **B,** Then secure the dressings with a bandage.

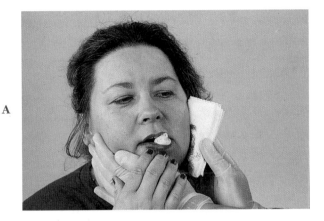
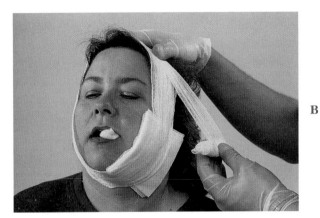

**Figure 13-17 A,** Control bleeding inside the cheek by placing a rolled dressing inside the mouth against the wound. Control external bleeding of the cheek using a dressing to apply pressure directly to the wound. **B,** Apply a pressure bandage.

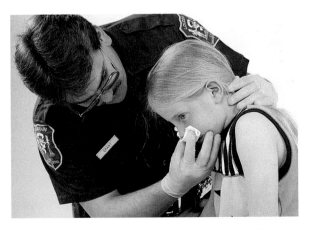

**Figure 13-18** To control a nosebleed, have the casualty lean forward and pinch the nostrils together until bleeding stops.

Once you have controlled the bleeding, tell the casualty to avoid rubbing, blowing, or picking the nose, since this could restart the bleeding. Later, the casualty may apply a little petroleum jelly inside the nostril to help keep it moist.

You should summon more advanced medical personnel if the bleeding cannot be controlled, if it stops and then recurs, or if the casualty says the bleeding is the result of high blood pressure. If the casualty loses consciousness, place the casualty on his or her side to allow blood to drain from the nose.

If you think an object is in the nostril, look into the nostril. If you see the object and can easily grasp it with your fingers, then do so. However, do not probe the nostril with your finger. Doing so may push the object farther into the nose and cause bleeding or make it more difficult to remove later. If the object cannot be removed easily, the casualty should receive medical care.

## Eye Injury

Injuries to the eye can involve the eyeball, the bone, and the soft tissue surrounding the eye. Blunt objects, like a fist or a baseball, may injure the eye and surrounding area, or a smaller object may penetrate the eyeball. Care for open or closed wounds *around* the eye as you would for any other soft tissue injury.

Injury to the eyeball requires different care. Injuries that penetrate the eyeball or cause the eye to be removed from its socket are very serious and can cause blindness. Never put direct pressure on the eyeball. Instead, follow

these guidelines when providing care for an eye in which an object has been embedded:

1. Place the casualty on his or her back.
2. Do not attempt to remove any object embedded in the eye.
3. Place a sterile dressing around the object (Fig. 13-19, *A*).
4. Stabilize any embedded object in place as best you can. You can do this by placing a paper cup to support the object (Fig. 13-19, *B*).
5. Apply a bandage (Fig. 13-19, *C*).

Foreign bodies that get in the eye, such as dirt, sand, or slivers of wood or metal, are irritating and can cause significant damage. The eye immediately produces tears in an attempt to flush out such objects. Pain is often severe. The casualty may have difficulty opening the eye because light further irritates it.

First, try to remove the foreign body by telling the casualty to blink several times. Then try gently flushing the eye with water (Fig. 13-20).

A

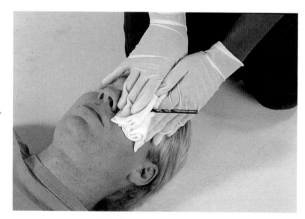

B

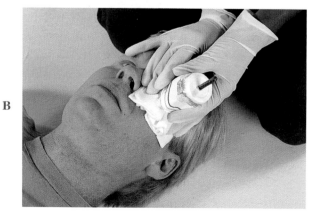

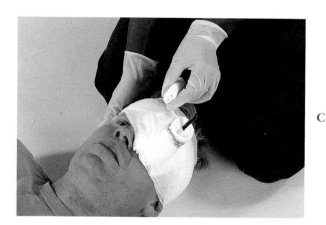

C

**Figure 13-19 A,** Place sterile dressings around an object impaled in the eye. **B,** Support the object with a paper cup. **C,** Carefully bandage the cup in place.

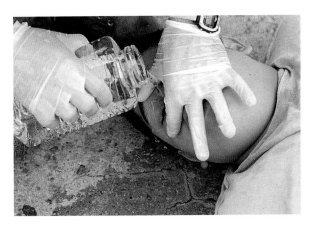

**Figure 13-20**  If a foreign body is in the eye, flush the eye gently with water.

If the object remains, the casualty should receive professional medical attention.

Flushing the eye with water is also appropriate if the casualty has any chemical in his or her eye. The eye should be continuously flushed until more advanced medical personnel arrive.

## Ear Injury

Ear injuries are common. Either the soft tissue of the outer ear or the eardrum within the ear may be injured. Open wounds, such as lacerations or abrasions, can result from recreational injuries, for example, being struck by a racquetball or falling off a bike. An avulsion of the ear may occur when a pierced earring catches on something and tears the earlobe. You can control bleeding from the soft tissues of the ear by applying direct pressure to the affected area.

If the casualty has a serious head or spinal injury, blood or other fluid may be in the ear canal or draining from the ear. *Do not* attempt to stop this drainage with direct pressure. Instead, just cover the ear lightly with a sterile dressing, stabilize the head and spine, and summon more advanced medical personnel.

The ear can also be injured internally. A direct blow to the head may rupture the eardrum. Sudden pressure changes, such as those caused by an explosion or a deep-water dive, can also injure the ear internally. The casualty may lose hearing

or balance or experience inner ear pain. These injuries require more advanced medical care.

A foreign object, such as dirt, an insect, or a piece of cotton, can easily become lodged in the ear canal. If you can easily see and grasp the object, remove it. Do *not* try to remove any object by using a pin, toothpick, or any sharp item. You could force the object farther back or puncture the eardrum. Sometimes you can remove the object if you pull down on the earlobe, tilt the head to the side, and shake or gently strike the head on the affected side. If you cannot easily remove the object, the casualty should be seen by a physician.

## Mouth, Jaw, and Neck Injuries

Your primary concern for any injury to the mouth, jaw, or neck is to ensure an open airway. Injuries in these areas may cause breathing problems if blood or loose teeth obstruct the airway. A swollen or fractured trachea may also obstruct breathing.

If the casualty is bleeding from the mouth and you do not suspect a serious head or spinal injury, place the casualty in a seated position with the head tilted slightly forward. This will allow any blood to drain from the mouth. If this position is not possible, place the casualty on his or her side to allow blood to drain from the mouth.

For injuries that penetrate the lip, place a rolled dressing between the lip and the gum. You can place another dressing on the outer surface of the lip. If the tongue is bleeding, apply a dressing and direct pressure. Applying cold to the lips or tongue can help reduce swelling and ease pain. If the bleeding cannot be controlled, summon more advanced medical personnel.

If the injury knocked out one or more of the casualty's teeth, control the bleeding and save any teeth so that they can be reinserted. To control the bleeding, roll a sterile dressing and insert it into the space left by the missing tooth. Have the casualty bite down to maintain pressure (Fig. 13-21).

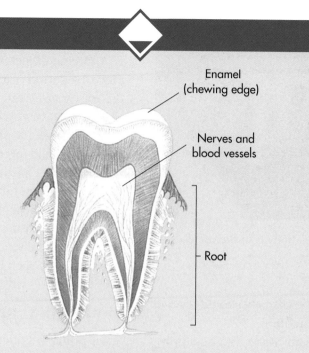

Enamel
(chewing edge)

Nerves and
blood vessels

Root

A tooth must be replaced so that periodontal fibres will reattach.

# Now Smile

Knocked-out teeth no longer spell doom for pearly whites. Most dentists can successfully replant a knocked-out tooth if they can do so quickly and if the tooth is properly cared for.

Replanting a tooth is similar to replanting a tree. On each tooth, tiny root fibres called periodontal fibres attach to the jawbone to hold the tooth in place. Inside the tooth, a canal filled with bundles of blood vessels and nerve ends runs from the tooth into the jawbone and surrounding tissues.

When these fibres and tissues are torn from the socket, it is important that they be replaced within an hour. Generally, the sooner the tooth is replanted, the greater the chance it will survive. The knocked-out tooth must be handled carefully to protect the fragile tissues. Be careful to pick up the tooth by the chewing edge (crown), not the root. Do not rub or handle the root part of the

tooth. It is best to preserve the tooth by placing it in a closed container of cool, fresh milk until it reaches the dentist. Milk is not always available at an injury scene; water may be substituted.

A dentist or emergency room doctor will clean the tooth, taking care not to damage the root fibres. The tooth is then placed back into the socket and secured with special splinting devices. The devices keep the tooth stable for 2 to 3 weeks while the fibres reattach to the jaw-bone. The bundles of blood vessels and nerves grow back within 6 weeks.

### REFERENCES

Bogert J, DDS, Executive Director, American Academy of Pediatric Dentists: Interview, April 1990.

Medford H, DDS: Acute care of an avulsed tooth, *Ann Emerg Med* 11:559, October 1982.

Opinions vary as to how a tooth should be saved. One thought is to place the dislodged tooth or teeth in the casualty's mouth. This, however, is not always the best approach, since a crying child could aspirate the tooth. Also, the

tooth could be swallowed with blood or saliva. You also may need to control serious bleeding in the mouth. Because of these concerns, it is best to place the tooth in a cup of milk. If milk is not available, the tooth can be placed in water.

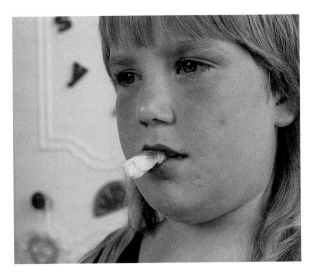

**Figure 13-21** If a tooth is knocked out, place a sterile dressing in the space left by the tooth. Tell the casualty to bite down.

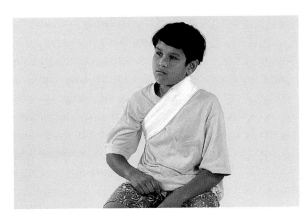

**Figure 13-22** Apply a pressure bandage to the neck so that it does not restrict blood flow.

If the injury is severe enough for you to summon more advanced medical personnel, give the tooth to them when they arrive. If the injury is not severe, the casualty should immediately seek a dentist who can replant the tooth. Time is a critical factor if the tooth is to be successfully replanted. Ideally, the tooth should be replanted within an hour after the injury.

Injuries serious enough to fracture or dislocate the jaw can also cause other head or spinal injuries. Be sure to maintain an open airway. Check inside the mouth for bleeding. Control bleeding as you would for other head injuries. Minimize movement of the head and neck. Summon more advanced medical personnel.

A soft tissue injury of the neck can cause severe bleeding and swelling that may obstruct the airway. Because the spine also may be involved, care for a neck injury as you would a possible serious spinal injury. If the casualty struck his or her neck on an object, such as a steering wheel, or was struck in the neck by an object, such as a stick, the injury could be devastating.

This type of injury can fracture the trachea, causing an airway obstruction that requires immediate advanced medical attention. While waiting for more advanced medical personnel, try to keep the casualty from moving and encourage him or her to breathe slowly. Control any external bleeding with direct pressure. Be careful not to apply pressure that constricts both carotid arteries or that interferes with breathing. Apply a pressure bandage so that it does not restrict blood flow (Fig. 13-22).

## ◆ SUMMARY

In this chapter, you have learned how to recognize and care for serious head and spinal injuries and specific injuries to the head and neck. To decide whether an injury is serious, you must consider its cause. Often the cause is the best indicator of whether an injury to the head or spine should be considered serious. If you have any doubts about the seriousness of an injury, summon more advanced medical personnel.

Like injuries elsewhere on the body, injuries to the head and spine often involve both soft tissues and bone. Control bleeding as necessary, usually with direct pressure on the wound. With scalp injuries, be careful not to apply pressure to a possible skull fracture. With eye injuries, remember not to apply pressure on the eyeball.

If you suspect that the casualty may have a serious head or spinal injury, minimize movement of the injured area when providing care. This is best accomplished by using in-line stabilization. Administer oxygen if it is available. Secure the casualty to a backboard if you must move the casualty.

As you read the next chapter about how to care for injuries to the chest and abdomen, remember the principles of care for head and spinal injuries. Serious injuries of the chest and abdomen can also affect the spine.

## YOU ARE THE RESPONDER

*You respond to an industrial accident involving a casualty who has fallen from a height of approximately 3 metres. You arrive to find a male casualty lying on his side. He is conscious, but disoriented. He states he "blacked out" when he struck the ground. He also states that he has a tingling feeling in his legs and feet. Do you consider his injury serious? How would you provide care?*

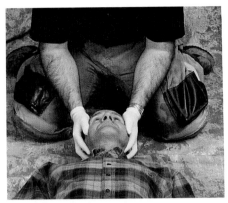

1. Apply in-line stabilization.

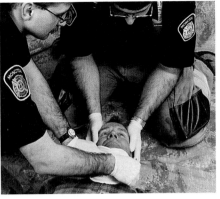

2. Apply cervical collar.

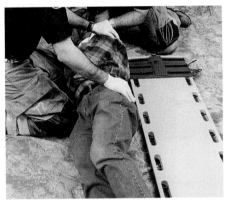

3. Log-roll casualty onto backboard and visually check back.

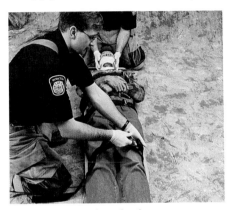

4. Secure casualty's body.

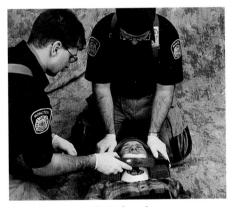

5. Secure casualty's head.

# Injuries to the Chest, Abdomen, and Pelvis

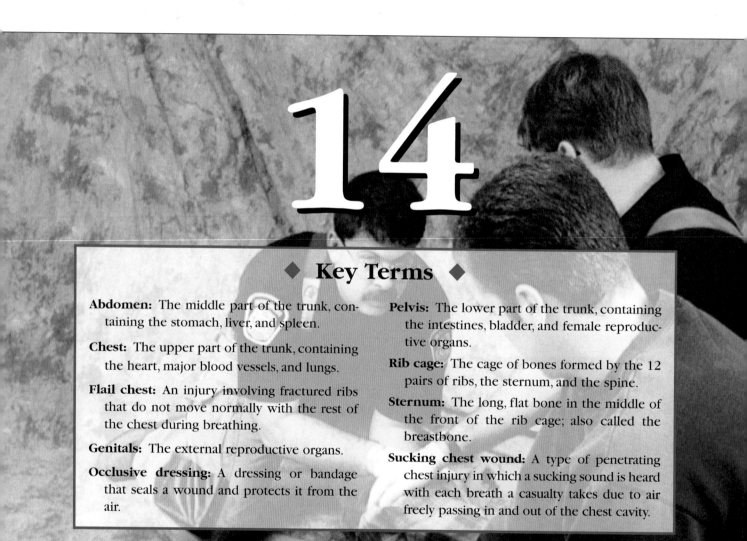

## 14

### ◆ Key Terms ◆

**Abdomen:** The middle part of the trunk, containing the stomach, liver, and spleen.

**Chest:** The upper part of the trunk, containing the heart, major blood vessels, and lungs.

**Flail chest:** An injury involving fractured ribs that do not move normally with the rest of the chest during breathing.

**Genitals:** The external reproductive organs.

**Occlusive dressing:** A dressing or bandage that seals a wound and protects it from the air.

**Pelvis:** The lower part of the trunk, containing the intestines, bladder, and female reproductive organs.

**Rib cage:** The cage of bones formed by the 12 pairs of ribs, the sternum, and the spine.

**Sternum:** The long, flat bone in the middle of the front of the rib cage; also called the breastbone.

**Sucking chest wound:** A type of penetrating chest injury in which a sucking sound is heard with each breath a casualty takes due to air freely passing in and out of the chest cavity.

## ◆ For Review ◆

Before reading this chapter, you should have a basic understanding of how to care for shock (Chapter 10), soft tissue injuries (Chapter 11), and musculoskeletal injuries (Chapter 12).

## ◆ INTRODUCTION

Most injuries to the chest and abdomen involve only soft tissues. Often these injuries, like those elsewhere on the body, are only minor cuts, scrapes, and bruises. Occasionally, severe injuries occur, such as fractures to the ribs or pelvic bones or organ injuries, that cause severe bleeding or impair breathing. Fractures and lacerations often occur in motor vehicle collisions to occupants not wearing safety belts. Falls, penetration by objects such as bullets, and other forms of trauma may also cause such injuries.

Injuries to the pelvis may be minor soft tissue injuries or serious bone and internal structure injuries. The pelvis includes a group of large bones that forms a protective girdle around the organs inside. A great force is required to cause serious injury to the pelvis.

Because the chest, abdomen, and pelvis contain many organs important to life, injury to these areas can be fatal. You may recall that a force that can cause severe injury in these areas may also cause injury to the spine. Care for these injuries includes—

◆ Controlling external bleeding.
◆ Limiting movement.
◆ Minimizing shock.
◆ Administering oxygen if available.
◆ Monitoring vital signs.
◆ Calling for more advanced medical personnel.

This chapter describes the signs and symptoms of and care for injuries to the chest, abdomen, and pelvis. In all cases, follow the emergency action principles. Care for all life-threatening injuries first. *All injuries described in this chapter are serious enough that you should always summon more advanced medical personnel immediately.*

## ◆ INJURIES TO THE CHEST

The **chest** is the upper part of the trunk, containing the heart, major blood vessels, and lungs. It is formed by 12 pairs of ribs, 10 of which attach to the **sternum** (breastbone) in front and to the spine in back. The other 2 pairs attach only to the spine in the back and are sometimes called "floating" ribs. The **rib cage** is the cage of bones formed by the 12 pairs of ribs, the sternum, and the spine. It protects vital organs, such as the heart, major blood vessels, and the lungs (Fig. 14-1). Also in the chest are the esophagus, the trachea, and the muscles of respiration.

Chest injuries are the second leading cause of trauma deaths each year. Many traffic fatalities involve chest injuries. Injuries to the chest also may result from a wide variety of other causes, such as falls, sports mishaps, and crushing or penetrating forces (Fig. 14-2).

Chest wounds are either open or closed. Open chest wounds occur when an object, such as a knife or bullet, penetrates the chest wall. Fractured ribs may break through the skin to cause an open chest injury. A chest wound is closed if the skin is not broken. Closed chest wounds are generally caused by a blunt object, such as a steering wheel.

### Signs and Symptoms of Chest Injury

You should know the signs and symptoms of serious chest injury. These may occur with both open and closed wounds. You will recognize some of these signs and symptoms from Chapter 6. They include—

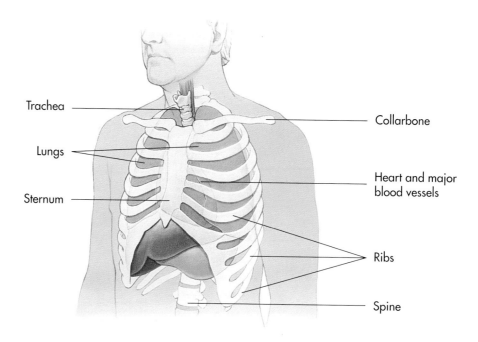

Trachea

Collarbone

Lungs

Heart and major blood vessels

Sternum

Ribs

Spine

**Figure 14-1** The rib cage surrounds and protects several vital organs.

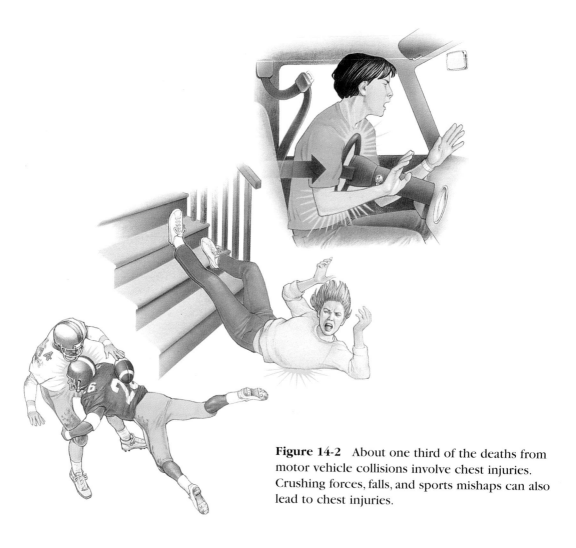

**Figure 14-2** About one third of the deaths from motor vehicle collisions involve chest injuries. Crushing forces, falls, and sports mishaps can also lead to chest injuries.

- Difficulty breathing.
- Pain at the site of the injury that increases with deep breathing or movement.
- Obvious deformity, such as that caused by a fracture.
- Flushed, pale, or bluish discolouration of the skin.
- Coughing up blood.

## Specific Types of Chest Injuries
### Rib Fractures

Rib fractures are usually caused by a forceful blow to the chest (Fig. 14-3). Although painful, a simple rib fracture is rarely life threatening. A casualty with a fractured rib often breathes shallowly because normal or deep breathing is painful. The casualty will usually attempt to ease the pain by leaning toward the side of the fracture and pressing a hand or arm over the injured area. Therefore, pain in the rib area, shallow breathing, and holding the area are signs and symptoms of possible rib fracture.

However, serious rib fractures can be life threatening. In severe blows or crushing injuries, multiple ribs can fracture in multiple places. This can produce a loose section of ribs that does not move normally with the rest of the chest during breathing. Usually, the loose section will move in the opposite direction

from the rest of the chest. The portion of chest wall lying between the fractures is called *flail chest.* When a flail chest involves the breastbone (sternum), the breastbone is separated from the rest of the ribs. In flail chest there may be paradoxical movement, in which the fractured section moves in the opposite direction to the rest of the chest during breathing.

### Care for rib fractures

If you suspect a fractured rib(s), have the casualty rest in a position that will make breathing easier. You can use an object, such as a pillow or rolled blanket, to help support and immobilize the injured area. Serious fractures often cause severe bleeding and difficulty breathing; shock is likely to develop. Administer oxygen if it is available and continue to monitor the vital signs.

### Care for flail chest

Have the casualty rest in a position that makes breathing easier, usually a semi-reclining position. Feel the chest area gently to locate the area of the flail segment, and apply bulky dressings several inches thick. Bandage the dressings in place with long strips of tape. If bulky dressings are not available, use a small pillow or other lightweight material. Do not try to bind, strap, or tape the flail section itself.

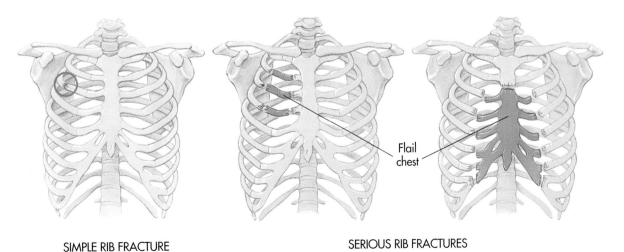

SIMPLE RIB FRACTURE          Flail chest          SERIOUS RIB FRACTURES

**Figure 14-3**  Forceful blows to the chest can fracture the ribs.

## Puncture Injuries

Puncture wounds to the chest range in severity from minor to life threatening. Stab and gunshot wounds are examples of puncture injuries. A forceful puncture may penetrate the rib cage and allow air to enter the chest through the wound (Fig. 14-4). This prevents the lungs from functioning normally. The penetrating object can injure any structure within the chest, including the lungs, heart, or major arteries or veins.

### Care for puncture injuries

Puncture wounds cause varying degrees of internal or external bleeding. If the injury penetrates the rib cage, air can pass freely in and out of the chest cavity and the casualty cannot breathe normally. With each breath the casualty takes, you may hear a sucking sound coming from the wound. This is the primary sign of a penetrating chest injury called a ***sucking chest wound.***

Without proper care, the casualty's condition will worsen quickly. The affected lung or lungs will fail to function, and breathing will become more difficult. Your main concern is the breathing problem. To care for a sucking chest wound, cover the wound with an ***occlusive dressing***—one that does not allow air to pass through it. A plastic bag, a plastic or latex glove, or a piece of plastic wrap or aluminum foil folded several times and placed over the wound can be substituted if a sterile occlusive dressing is not available. Tape the dressing in place, except for one corner that remains loose (Fig. 14-5). This

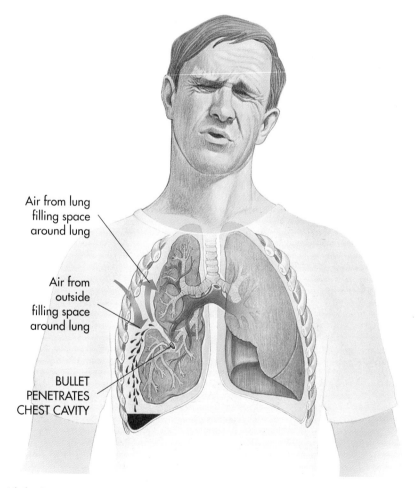

Air from lung filling space around lung

Air from outside filling space around lung

BULLET PENETRATES CHEST CAVITY

**Figure 14-4**  A puncture wound that penetrates the lung or the chest cavity surrounding the lung allows air to go in and out of the cavity.

keeps air from entering the wound during inhalation but allows it to escape during exhalation. If none of these materials are available, use a folded cloth or, as a last resort, your gloved hand. Administer oxygen if available, and take steps to minimize shock.

# ◆ INJURIES TO THE ABDOMEN

The ***abdomen*** is the area immediately under the chest and above the pelvis. It is easily injured because it is not surrounded by bones. It is protected at the back by the spine. The upper abdomen is only partially protected in front by the lower ribs. The muscles of the back and abdomen also help protect the internal organs, many of which are vital (Fig. 14-6). Most important are the organs that are easily injured or tend to bleed profusely when injured, such as the liver, spleen, and stomach.

The liver is rich in blood. Located in the upper right quadrant of the abdomen, this organ is protected somewhat by the lower ribs. However, it is delicate and can be torn by blows from blunt objects or penetrated by a fractured rib. The resulting bleeding can be severe and can quickly be fatal. A liver, when injured, can also leak bile into the abdomen, which can cause severe infection.

The **spleen** is located in the upper left quadrant of the abdomen behind the stomach and is protected somewhat by the lower left ribs. Like the liver, this organ is easily damaged. The spleen may rupture when the abdomen is struck forcefully by a blunt object. Since the spleen stores blood, an injury can cause a severe loss of blood in a short time and can be life threatening.

The **stomach** is one of the main digestive organs. The upper part of the stomach changes shape depending on its contents, the stage of digestion, and the size and strength of the stomach muscles. It is lined with many blood vessels and nerves. The stomach can bleed severely when injured, and food contents may empty into the abdomen and possibly cause infection.

## Signs and Symptoms of Abdominal Injury

The signs and symptoms of serious abdominal injury include—

+ Severe pain.
+ Bruising.
+ External bleeding.

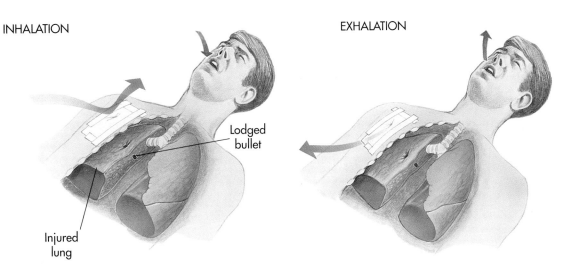

INHALATION             EXHALATION

Lodged bullet

Injured lung

**Figure 14-5** A special dressing that is considerably larger than the wound itself, with one loose corner, keeps air from entering the wound during inhalation and allows air to escape during exhalation. This helps keep the injured lung from collapsing.

FRONT VIEW                                              BACK VIEW

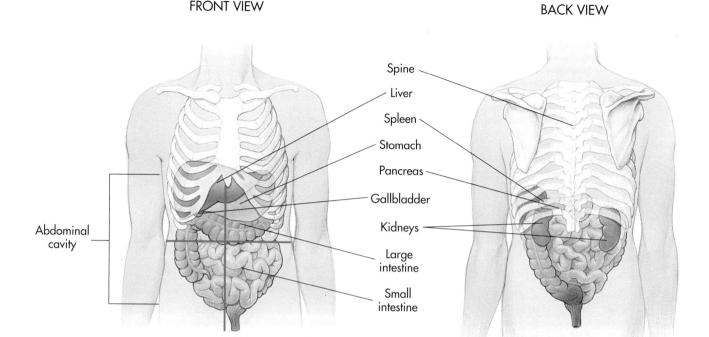

**Figure 14-6** Unlike the organs of the chest or pelvis, organs in the abdominal cavity are relatively unprotected.

◆ Nausea and vomiting (sometimes vomit containing blood).
◆ Pale, moist skin.
◆ Weakness.
◆ Thirst.
◆ Pain, tenderness, or a tight feeling in the abdomen.
◆ Organs possibly protruding from the abdomen.

## Care for Abdominal Injuries

Like a chest injury, an injury to the abdomen is either open or closed. Even with a closed wound, the rupture of an organ can cause serious internal bleeding that can quickly result in shock. Injuries to the abdomen can be extremely painful. Serious reactions can occur if organs leak blood or other contents into the abdomen.

With a severe open injury, abdominal organs sometimes protrude through the wound (Fig. 14-7, *A*). To care for an open wound in the abdomen, follow these steps (Fig. 14-7, *B, C,* and *D*):

◆ Carefully position the casualty on the back.
◆ *Do not* apply direct pressure.
◆ *Do not* push organs back in.
◆ Remove clothing from around wound.
◆ Apply moist, sterile dressings loosely over wound. (Warm tap water can be used.)
◆ Cover dressings loosely with plastic wrap if available.
◆ Cover dressings lightly with a folded towel to maintain warmth.
◆ Maintain normal body temperature.
◆ Administer oxygen if available.
◆ Summon more advanced medical personnel.

To care for a closed abdominal injury—

◆ Carefully position the casualty on the back.
◆ *Do not* apply direct pressure.
◆ Bend the casualty's knees slightly. This allows the muscles of the abdomen to relax. Place rolled-up blankets or pillows under the casualty's knees. If the movement of the casualty's legs causes pain, leave the legs straight.
◆ Administer oxygen if it is available.

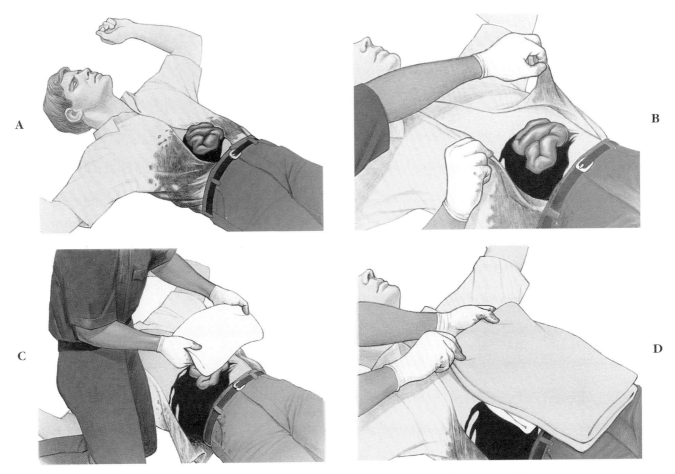

**Figure 14-7 A,** Severe injuries to the abdominal cavity can result in protruding organs. **B,** Carefully remove clothing from around the wound. **C,** Apply a large, moist sterile dressing over the wound and cover it with plastic wrap. **D,** Place a folded towel or other cloth over the dressing to maintain warmth.

◆ Take steps to minimize shock.
◆ Summon more advanced medical personnel.

## ◆ INJURIES TO THE PELVIS

The *pelvis* is the lower part of the trunk and contains the bladder, female reproductive organs, and the lower portion of the large intestine, including the rectum. Arteries and nerves pass through the pelvis. The organs within the pelvis are well protected on the sides and back but not in front (Fig. 14-8). Injuries to the pelvis may include fractures to the pelvic bone and damage to structures within. Fractured bones may puncture or lacerate internal organs. These organs can also be injured when struck by forceful blows from blunt or penetrating objects.

## Signs and Symptoms of Pelvic Injury

Signs and symptoms of injury to the pelvis are very similar to those of abdominal injury. Certain pelvic injuries may also cause loss of sensation in the legs or inability to move them. This may indicate an injury to the lower spine.

## Care for Pelvic Injuries

Care for pelvic injuries in the same way as for abdominal injuries. Do not move the casualty unless necessary. If possible, keep the casualty

# Organ Donation

Many years ago, organ transplants were an experimental procedure—but not any more. Over 200,000 people have received organ transplants, and in most cases their lives were saved by this surgery. Organ transplantation has become an accepted, even routine, medical practice with very high success rates.

Some 25 different organs and body tissues are now being transplanted. Most people have heard about lifesaving heart and liver transplants. Other organs and tissues transplanted include kidneys, lungs, pancreas, skin, bone, and corneas. Organ donations not only save many lives but also greatly improve the quality of life for others for whom no other treatment is available.

Despite this medical success story, there is a significant problem with organ donation: far more people need organ donations than there are organs available. About 30,000 people in North America are currently waiting for transplants. Many of these are children with their whole lives ahead of them. Every 18 minutes another name is added to the list of people waiting. Yet because there are not enough organs available for transplantation, 8 people a day die while waiting.

Donated organs come from people in good health who have died suddenly, often because of a fatal injury. Although the brain dies and the person cannot recover, the vital organs can be kept alive for transplantation. Organ donors can range from infants to senior citizens.

The shortage of organs for donation occurs because too few people volunteer to donate their organs, or those of family members, after death. Some people simply may never think about becoming a donor, while others seem to avoid thinking about death at all. After the sudden death of a loved one, family members may not want to think or talk about donation, or health care workers may be uncomfortable discussing donation with family members. For these and other reasons, the organs of too few donors are available for transplant.

We can all help solve this problem. With an organ donor card, you can make your wishes known to donate your organs after death. This card makes it easier for family members to give consent for donation if death suddenly occurs. It also makes it easier for health care professionals to initiate the process of requesting donation. Organ donor cards are available from many provincial offices, physicians, hospitals, and pharmacies. There is no charge for the card or for donating organs. You can give this gift of life for free. When you consider that you or your loved ones could someday need an organ transplant to stay alive, can there be any good reason not to give this gift?

---

lying flat. If not, help him or her become comfortable. Control any external bleeding and cover any protruding organs. Always call for more advanced medical personnel, administer oxygen if available, and take steps to minimize shock.

An injury to the pelvis sometimes involves the **genitals,** the external reproductive organs. Genital injuries are either closed wounds, such as a bruise, or open wounds, such as an avulsion or laceration. Any injury to the genitals is extremely painful. Care for a closed wound as you would for any closed wound. If the injury is an open wound, apply a sterile dressing and direct pressure with your hand or the casualty's hand. If any parts are avulsed, wrap them appropriately and make sure they are transported with the casualty.

Injuries to the genital area can be embarrassing for both the casualty and the rescuer. Explain briefly what you are going to do and do it. Do not act in a timid or hesitant manner. This will only make the situation more difficult for you and the casualty.

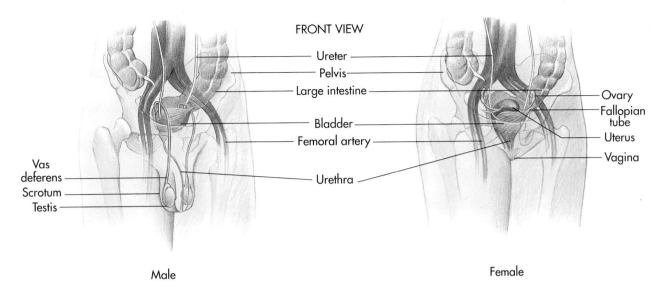

**Figure 14-8** The internal structures of the pelvis are well protected on the sides and back but not on the front.

## ◆ SUMMARY

Injuries to the chest, abdomen, or pelvis can be serious. They can damage soft tissues, bones, and internal organs. Although many injuries are immediately obvious, some may be detected only as the casualty's condition worsens over time. Watch for the signs and symptoms of serious injuries that require medical attention.

Care for any life-threatening condition, such as respiratory distress, then give any additional care needed for specific injuries. For open wounds to the chest, abdomen, or pelvis, control bleeding. If you suspect fracture, immobilize the injured part. Use special dressings for sucking chest wounds and open abdominal wounds when these materials are available. Always summon more advanced medical personnel as soon as possible, administer oxygen if it is available, and take steps to minimize shock. This gives the casualty of a serious injury the best chance for survival and full recovery.

In the next chapter, you will learn about injuries to the extremities (arms and legs), which, like injuries described in this chapter, are often caused by trauma.

**YOU ▸ ARE THE RESPONDER**

*You are in a local convenience store late Saturday night when a robbery occurs. The store clerk is beaten and stabbed. There is blood on the front of his shirt. He is conscious but in considerable pain and having difficulty breathing. You hear an abnormal sucking sound when he breathes. What care would you provide for this casualty?*

# Injuries to the Extremities

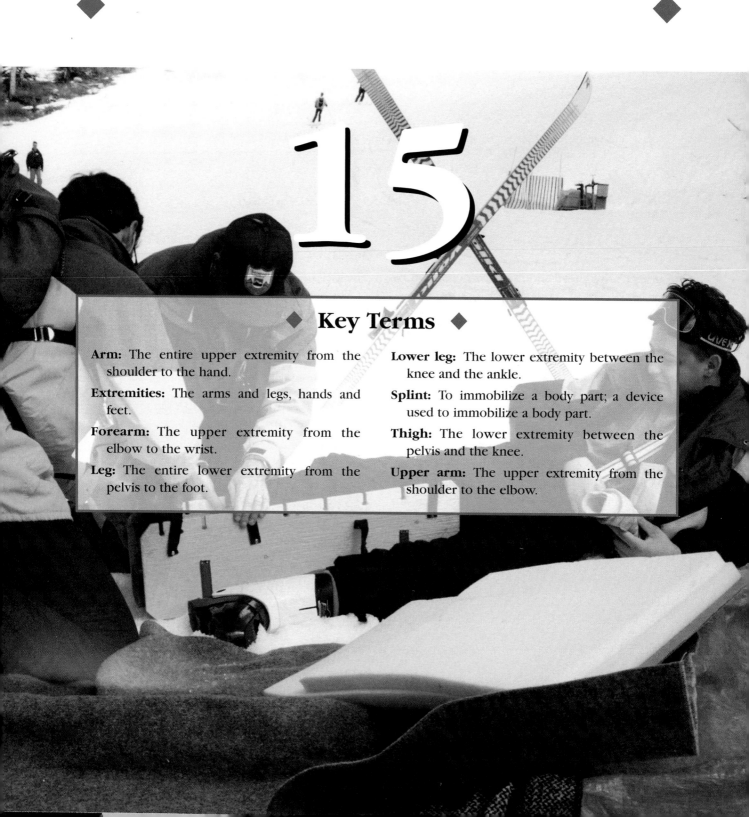

15

◆ **Key Terms** ◆

**Arm:** The entire upper extremity from the shoulder to the hand.

**Extremities:** The arms and legs, hands and feet.

**Forearm:** The upper extremity from the elbow to the wrist.

**Leg:** The entire lower extremity from the pelvis to the foot.

**Lower leg:** The lower extremity between the knee and the ankle.

**Splint:** To immobilize a body part; a device used to immobilize a body part.

**Thigh:** The lower extremity between the pelvis and the knee.

**Upper arm:** The upper extremity from the shoulder to the elbow.

◆ **For Review** ◆

Before reading this chapter, you should have a basic understanding of how to control bleeding (Chapter 9) and how to care for soft tissue and musculoskeletal injuries (Chapters 11 and 12).

## ◆ INTRODUCTION

Injuries to the *extremities,* the arms and legs, hands and feet, are quite common. They range from simple bruises to open fractures, where bone protrudes through the skin. With any injury to the extremities, the prompt care you give can help prevent further pain and damage.

As you will learn in this chapter, care for soft tissue and musculoskeletal injuries involving the extremities is like the care for other parts of the body. In general, control bleeding first. Then support the injured body part to allow it to rest and apply ice or a cold pack. If you suspect a serious injury, always immobilize the injured body part using whatever devices are available. Elevate the area if doing so does not cause pain. If necessary, summon more advanced medical personnel. Continue to monitor vital signs. Minimize shock by maintaining normal body temperature, administering oxygen if it is available, and helping the casualty into the most comfortable position.

## ◆ SIGNS AND SYMPTOMS OF SERIOUS EXTREMITY INJURIES

The extremities consist of bones, soft tissues, blood vessels, and nerves. They are subject to a variety of both soft tissue and musculoskeletal injuries.

Signs and symptoms of a serious extremity injury include—

- ◆ Pain.
- ◆ Tenderness.
- ◆ Moderate or severe swelling.
- ◆ Discolouration.
- ◆ Significant deformity of the limb.
- ◆ Inability to move or use the affected part.
- ◆ Severe external bleeding.

## ◆ UPPER EXTREMITY INJURIES

The **upper extremities** are the arms and hands. The bones of each upper extremity include the **collarbone (clavicle), shoulder blade (scapula),** bones of the upper arm **(humerus)** and **forearm (radius and ulna),** and bones of the **hand (carpals and metacarpals)** and **fingers (phalanges).** Figure 15-1 shows the major structures of the upper extremities.

The upper extremities are commonly the most injured area of the body. Injuries to the upper extremities occur in many different ways. The most frequent cause is falling on the hand of an outstretched arm. Since the hands are rarely protected, abrasions occur easily. A falling casualty instinctively tries to break the fall by extending the arms and hands, so these areas receive the force of the body's weight. This can cause a serious injury to the hand, forearm, upper arm, or shoulder, such as a severe sprain, fracture, or dislocation (Fig. 15-2).

When caring for serious upper extremity injuries, minimize any movement of the injured part. If an injured casualty is holding the arm securely against the chest, do not change the position. Holding the arm against the chest is an effective method of **immobilization,** keeping an injured body part from moving. Allow the casualty to continue to support the arm in this manner. You can further assist him or her by binding the injured arm to the chest. This eliminates the need for special splinting equipment and still provides an effective method of immobilization.

Injuries to the upper extremity may also damage blood vessels, nerves, and other soft

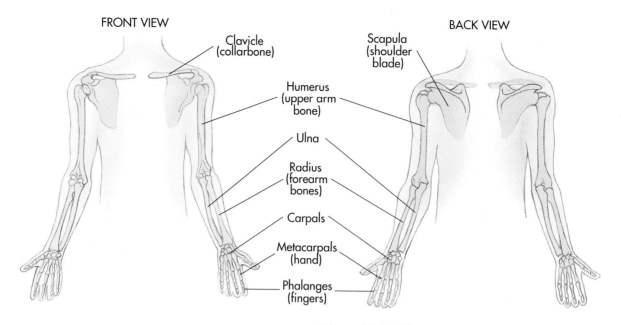

Figure 15-1 labels:

FRONT VIEW  BACK VIEW

Clavicle (collarbone)
Scapula (shoulder blade)
Humerus (upper arm bone)
Ulna
Radius (forearm bones)
Carpals
Metacarpals (hand)
Phalanges (fingers)

**Figure 15-1** The upper extremities include the bones of the arms and hands, nerves, and blood vessels.

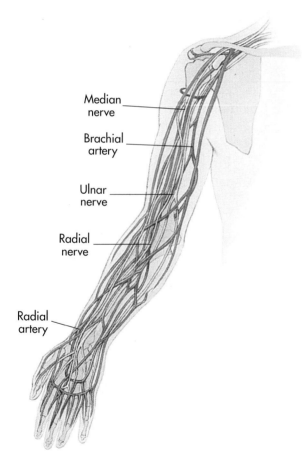

Median nerve
Brachial artery
Ulnar nerve
Radial nerve
Radial artery

tissues. It is particularly important to ensure that blood flow and nerve function have not been impaired. Always check for circulation and sensation below the injury site, both before and after splinting. Sometimes when a splint is applied too tightly, blood flow may be impaired. If this occurs, loosen the splint. If you suspect that either the blood vessels or the nerves have been damaged, minimize movement of the area and summon more advanced emergency personnel immediately.

## Shoulder Injuries

The shoulder consists of three bones that meet to form the shoulder joint. These bones are the clavicle, scapula, and humerus. The most common shoulder injuries are sprains. However, injuries of the shoulder may also involve a fracture or dislocation of one or more of these bones.

The most frequently injured bone of the shoulder is the clavicle, injured more commonly in children than adults. Typically, the clavicle is fractured as a result of a fall. The casualty usually feels pain in the shoulder area.

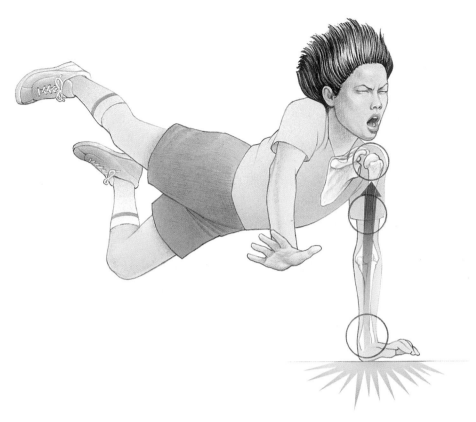

**Figure 15-2**  A fall can cause a serious injury to the hand, arm, or shoulder.

The pain may radiate down the arm. A person with a fractured clavicle usually attempts to ease the pain by holding the arm against the chest. Since the clavicle lies directly over major blood vessels and nerves to the arm, it is important to immobilize the injured area to prevent injury to these structures.

Scapula fractures are not common. A fracture of the scapula typically results from violent force. The signs and symptoms of a fractured scapula are the same as for any other extremity fracture, although you are less likely to see deformity of the scapula. The most significant signs and symptoms are extreme pain and the inability to move the arm.

It takes great force to break the scapula, so you must consider that the force may have been great enough to injure the ribs or internal organs in the chest. If this is the case, a casualty may have difficulty breathing.

A dislocation is another common type of shoulder injury. Like fractures, dislocations often result from falls. This happens frequently in contact sports, such as football and rugby. A player may attempt to break a fall with an outstretched arm or may land on the tip of the shoulder, forcing the arm against the joint formed by the scapula and clavicle. This can result in ligaments tearing, causing the end of the clavicle to displace. Dislocations also occur at the joint where the humerus meets the socket formed by the scapula. For example, when an arm in a throwing position is hit, it forces the arm to rotate backward. Ligaments tear, causing the upper end of the arm to dislocate from its normal position in the shoulder socket.

Shoulder dislocations are painful and can often be identified by the deformity present. As with other shoulder injuries, the casualty often tries to minimize the pain by holding the arm in the most comfortable position.

## Care for Shoulder Injuries

To care for shoulder injuries, first control any external bleeding with direct pressure. Apply a pressure bandage using a figure-eight pattern

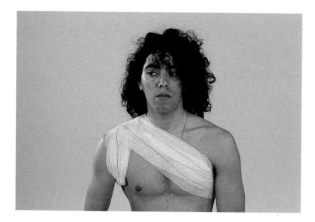

**Figure 15-3** Use a figure-eight pattern to apply a pressure bandage to the shoulder.

(Fig. 15-3). Allow the casualty to continue to support the arm in the position in which he or she is holding it (usually the most comfortable position), and if possible splint it in that position. If the casualty is holding the arm away from the body, use a pillow, rolled blanket, or similar object to fill the gap between the arm and chest to provide support for the injured area. Check for circulation and sensation in the hand and fingers. Then **splint** the arm in place. This can be done by merely binding the arm to the chest or by placing the arm in a sling and binding the arm to the chest with a cravat (Fig. 15-4). Recheck for circulation and sensation. Apply cold to the injured area to help minimize pain and reduce swelling. Take steps to minimize shock.

# Upper Arm Injuries

The bone of the **upper arm,** the part of the extremity between the shoulder and the elbow, is the humerus. It is the largest bone in the **arm,** the upper extremity from the shoulder to the wrist. This bone can be fractured at any point, although it is usually fractured at the upper end near the shoulder or in the middle of the bone. The upper end of the humerus often fractures in the elderly and in young children as a result of a fall. Breaks in the middle of the bone occur mostly in young adults.

When the humerus is fractured, there is danger of damage to the blood vessels and nerves supplying the entire arm. Most humerus fractures are very painful and prevent the casualty from using the arm. A fracture can cause considerable arm deformity.

## Care for Upper Arm Injuries

To care for a serious upper arm injury, immobilize the upper arm from the shoulder to the elbow. This can be done in the same way as for shoulder injuries. Control any external bleeding with direct pressure. Place the arm in a sling and bind it to the chest with cravats. You can use a short splint, if one is available, to give more support to the upper arm (Fig. 15-5). Apply cold in the best way possible. Always check for circulation and sensation in the hand and fingers before and after immobilizing the injured area.

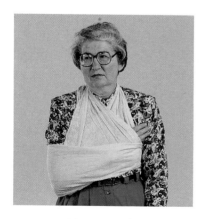 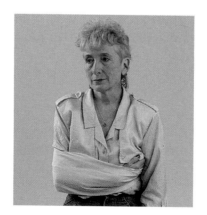 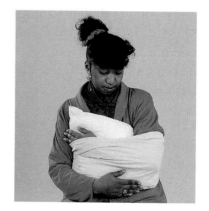

**Figure 15-4** Splint the arm against the chest in the position the casualty is holding it, using a sling, cravats, and a small pillow or a rolled blanket when necessary.

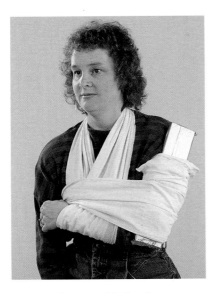

**Figure 15-5** A short, padded splint can provide additional support for an injury to the upper arm.

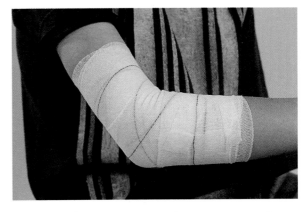

**Figure 15-6** Use a figure-eight pattern to apply a pressure bandage to the elbow.

## Elbow Injuries

Like other joints, the elbow can be sprained, fractured, or dislocated. Injuries to the elbow can cause permanent disability, since all the nerves and blood vessels to the forearm and hand go through the elbow. Therefore, take elbow injuries seriously. Injuries to a joint like the elbow can be made worse by movement.

### Care for Elbow Injuries

If the casualty says that he or she cannot move the elbow, do not try to move it. Control any external bleeding with direct pressure and a pressure bandage using a figure-eight pattern (Fig. 15-6). Check for circulation and sensation. Support the arm and immobilize it from the shoulder to the wrist.

Immobilize the elbow in the position in which you find it. Place the arm in a sling and secure it to the chest, as shown in Figure 15-4. If this is not possible, immobilize the elbow with a splint and two cravats. If the elbow is bent, apply the splint diagonally across the underside of the arm (Fig. 15-7, *A*). The splint should extend beyond both the upper arm and the wrist. If the elbow is straight, apply the splint along the arm. Secure the splint at the wrist and upper arm with cravats or roller bandages (Fig. 15-7, *B*).

A

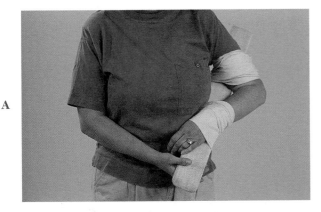

B

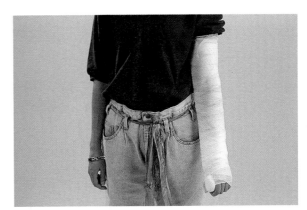

**Figure 15-7** **A,** If the elbow is bent, apply a splint diagonally across the underside of the arm. **B,** If the arm is straight, apply a splint along the underside of the arm.

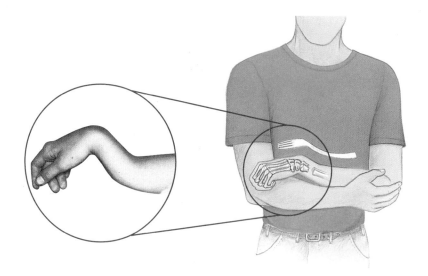

**Figure 15-8** Fractures of both forearm bones often have a characteristic s-shaped deformity. This is sometimes called a "silver-fork" deformity.

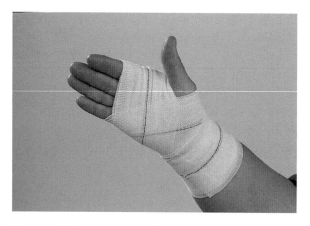

**Figure 15-9** A pressure bandage for the palm of the hand.

Recheck for circulation and sensation. Summon more advanced medical personnel. Apply ice or a cold pack and take steps to care for shock.

## Forearm, Wrist, and Hand Injuries

The *forearm* is the upper extremity from the elbow to the wrist. Fractures of the two forearm bones, the radius and ulna, are more common in children than adults. If a person falls on an outstretched arm, both bones may break, but not always in the same place. With forearm fractures, the arm may look s-shaped (Fig. 15-8). This characteristic shape is why it is sometimes

A

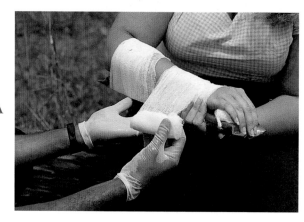

B

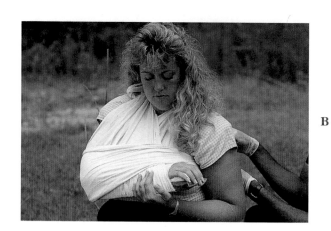

**Figure 15-10 A,** If the forearm is fractured, place a splint under the forearm and secure it. **B,** Put the arm in a sling and secure it to the chest with cravats.

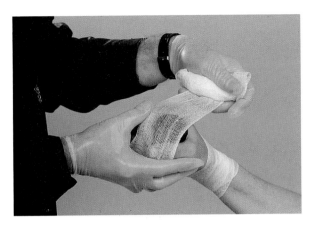

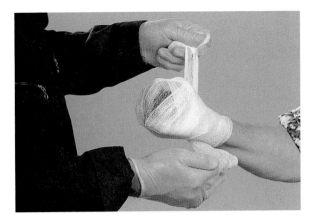

**Figure 15-11**  A soft splint is an effective splint for a hand or finger injury.

called a "silver-fork" deformity. Because the radial artery and nerve are near these bones, a fracture may cause severe bleeding or a loss of movement in the wrist and hand. The wrist is also a common site of sprains.

Because the hands are used in so many daily activities, they are very susceptible to injury. Most injuries to the hands and fingers involve only minor soft tissue damage. However, a serious injury may damage nerves, blood vessels, and bones. Home, recreational, and industrial mishaps often produce lacerations, avulsions, burns, and fractures of the hands. Because the hand structures are delicate, deep lacerations can cause permanently disabling injuries.

### Care for Forearm, Wrist, and Hand Injuries

Begin by controlling any external bleeding with direct pressure. To bandage the hand, apply a pressure bandage using a figure-eight pattern (Fig. 15-9). Check for circulation and sensation, then care for the injured forearm, wrist, or hand by immobilizing the injured part. When using a rigid splint, support the injured part by placing a splint underneath the forearm. Extend the splint beyond both the hand and elbow. Place a roll of gauze or a similar object in the palm to keep the palm and fingers in a normal position. Then secure the splint with cravats or roller gauze (Fig. 15-10, *A*). Recheck circulation and sensation. Then put the arm in a sling and secure it to the chest (Fig. 15-10, *B*).

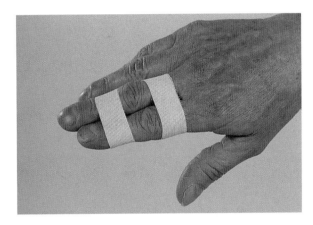

**Figure 15-12**  An injured finger can be splinted to an adjacent finger.

You can immobilize hand and finger injuries using a soft splint made of a roll of gauze or rolled up cloth and bandages (Fig. 15-11). You can splint an injured finger to an adjacent finger with tape (Fig. 15-12). *Do not* attempt to put displaced finger or thumb bones back into place. Always apply ice or a cold pack to forearm, wrist, and hand injuries, and elevate the injured area.

## ◆ LOWER EXTREMITY INJURIES

Injuries to the *leg,* the entire lower extremity, can involve both soft tissue and musculoskeletal damage. The major bones of the *thigh* (between the pelvis and the knee) and *lower leg* (between the knee and the ankle) are large and strong enough to carry the body's weight.

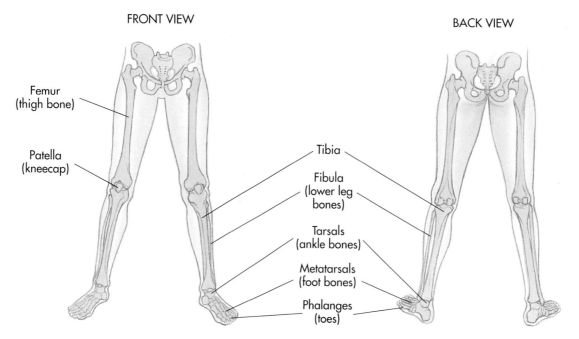

FRONT VIEW                BACK VIEW

Femur (thigh bone)

Patella (kneecap)

Tibia

Fibula (lower leg bones)

Tarsals (ankle bones)

Metatarsals (foot bones)

Phalanges (toes)

**Figure 15-13** The lower extremities.

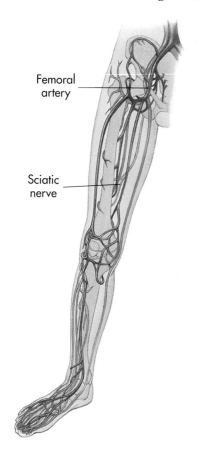

Femoral artery

Sciatic nerve

Bones of the leg include the one in the thigh **(femur),** the kneecap **(patella),** the two bones in the lower leg **(tibia and fibula),** the bones of the **foot (tarsals and metatarsals),** and the bones of the **toes (phalanges).** Because of the size and strength of the bones in the thigh and lower leg, a significant amount of force is required to cause a fracture.

The **femoral artery** is the major supplier of blood to the legs and feet. If it is damaged, which may happen with a fracture of the femur, the blood loss can be life threatening.

Figure 15-13 shows the major structures of the lower extremities. When caring for lower extremity injuries, follow the same general principles of care described in Chapter 12. Serious injury to the lower extremities can result in their inability to bear weight. Since the casualty may be unable to walk, you should summon more advanced medical personnel.

## Thigh and Lower Leg Injuries

The femur is the largest bone in the body. Because it bears most of the weight of the body, it is most important in walking and running.

Thigh injuries range from bruises and torn muscles to severe injuries, such as fractures. The upper end of the femur meets the pelvis at the hip joint (Fig. 15-14). Most femur fractures involve the upper end of the bone. Even though the hip joint itself is not involved, such injuries are often called hip fractures.

A fracture of the femur usually produces a characteristic deformity. When the fracture occurs, the thigh muscles contract. Because the thigh muscles are so strong, they pull the broken bone ends together, causing them to overlap. This may cause the injured leg to be noticeably shorter than the other leg. The injured leg may also be turned outward (Fig. 15-15). Other signs and symptoms of a fractured femur may include severe pain and swelling and inability to move the leg.

A fracture in the lower leg may involve one or both bones. Often both are fractured simultaneously. However, a blow to the outside of the lower leg can cause an isolated fracture of the smaller bone (fibula). Because these two bones lie just beneath the skin, open fractures are common (Fig. 15-16). Lower leg fractures may cause a severe deformity in which the lower leg is bent at an unusual angle (angulated). These injuries are painful and result in

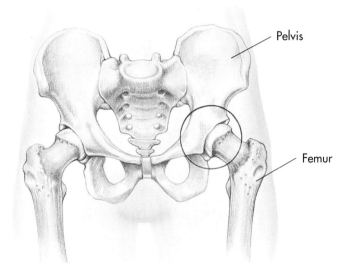

**Figure 15-14** The upper end of the femur meets the pelvis at the hip joint.

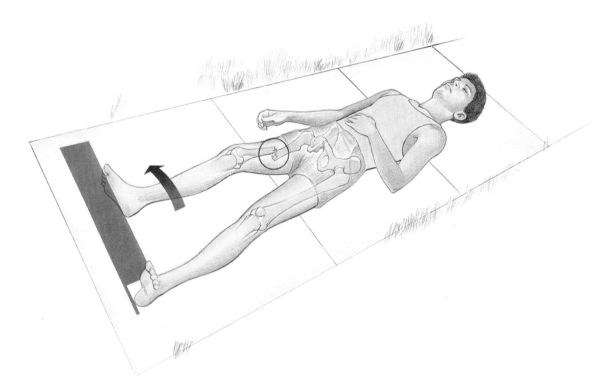

**Figure 15-15** A fractured femur often produces a characteristic deformity. The injured leg is shorter than the uninjured leg and may be turned outward.

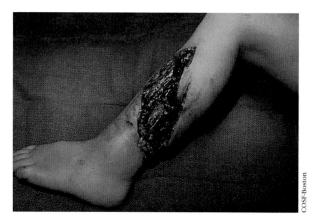

**Figure 15-16** Open fractures of the lower leg are common.

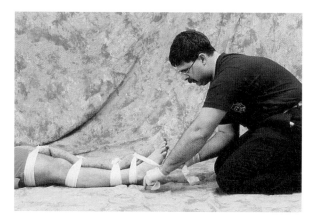

**Figure 15-17** To splint an injured leg, secure the injured leg to the uninjured leg with cravats. A pillow or rolled blanket can be placed between the legs.

an inability to move the leg. However, fractures of the fibula, and some very small fractures of the tibia, may not cause any deformity and the casualty may be able to continue to use the leg.

### Care for Thigh and Lower Leg Injuries

Initial care for the casualty with a serious injury to the thigh or lower leg is to stop any external bleeding, immobilize the injured area, and help the casualty rest in the most comfortable position. Summon more advanced medical personnel immediately. They are much better prepared to care for and transport a casualty with a serious leg injury. Consider that the ground can adequately immobilize the legs, if the surface is relatively flat and firm, until more professional medical personnel arrive.

However, there may be situations, such as moving the casualty, in which you will need to splint an injured leg. Securing the injured leg to the uninjured leg with several wide cravats is one simple method. If available, place a pillow or rolled blanket between the legs and bind the legs together in several places above and below the site of the injury (Fig. 15-17). If rigid splints are available, apply one long splint to the outside of the injured leg, extending above the hip and beyond the foot. Place a shorter padded splint to the inside of the leg,

also extending beyond the foot. Secure the splints to the leg with cravats (Fig. 15-18). Other commercial splints, such as air splints or vacuum splints, can also be used if available. Regardless of the type of splint applied, always check and recheck circulation and sensation of the foot. Apply ice or a cold pack to reduce pain and swelling.

A fractured femur can injure the femoral artery, and serious bleeding can result. The likelihood of shock is great. Therefore, take steps to minimize shock. Keep the casualty lying down and try to keep him or her calm. Maintain normal body temperature, administer oxygen if it is available, and make sure that more advanced

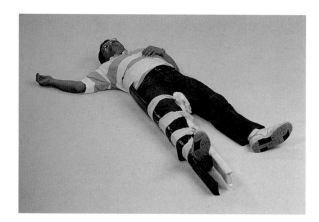

**Figure 15-18** Rigid splints can also be used to splint an injured leg.

# Quick Recovery

The train tracks that once criss-crossed the injured knees of Olympic skiers, professional football players, and arthritis sufferers have almost disappeared. Both the scars and the trauma of knee surgery have been diminished with the advent of a new medical technique, arthroscopy.

Arthroscopy has aided thousands of athletes cursed with bad knees. It put Chicago Bears defensive tackle Dan Hampton back on the football field countless times and saved the careers of gymnast Mary Lou Retton and marathon runner Joan Benoit just before the 1984 Olympics. Their recoveries were remarkable, considering that 15 years ago, knee surgery meant a 5-day hospital stay, a cast, and 3 to 4 months of rehabilitation. With arthroscopic surgery, many athletes leave the hospital the same day and begin rehabilitation within days of the procedure.

The most agile of joints, the knee is also the most vulnerable. It joins the two longest bones of the body. Four ligaments attach to the bones and hold the knee together. Two cartilage disks serve as shock absorbers on the ends of the bones. Repeated and excessive shocks to the knee will splinter the cartilage pads and stretch or fray ligaments.

The arthroscope, a thin, steel, 25-centimetre (10-inch) telescope for surgeons, allows physicians to perform delicate joint surgery without cutting muscles and ligaments and without lifting the kneecap to get to the injured area. After injecting a saline solution to distend the knee joint, the surgeon inserts the arthroscope through small puncture wounds into the space of the knee joint. By projecting magnified images inside the knee onto a screen, the arthroscope allows orthopaedic surgeons to use microsurgical instruments to smooth arthritic surfaces, remove chipped bones and cartilage, and sew up torn ligaments.

The procedure is not limited to rich and famous knees. Thousands of people undergo arthroscopic surgery each year. Arthroscopes, some less than 1.7 millimetres in diameter, are being used to repair shoulders, ankles, wrists, and even jaws. Not all joint problems can be repaired with arthroscopy, but most surgeons would agree that advances in arthroscopy have had a profound impact on the lives of people who might otherwise be incapacitated.

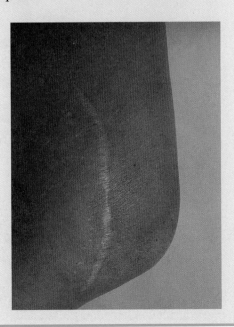

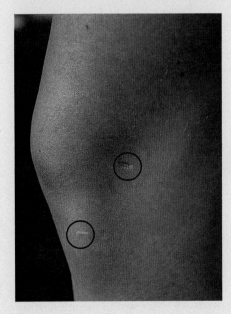

medical personnel have been summoned. Monitor the ABCs and vital signs specifically for changes in the casualty's level of consciousness.

Some fractures of the femur may require traction splinting. Traction helps prevent broken bone ends from causing further injury and helps to reduce pain and minimize shock. However, not all emergency responders are trained to use traction splints. If you are not trained or if you are alone, wait for more advanced medical personnel. Immobilize the injured leg in the best way possible, and provide care until these personnel arrive. Figure 15-19 shows the basic steps for assisting in the application of a traction splint.

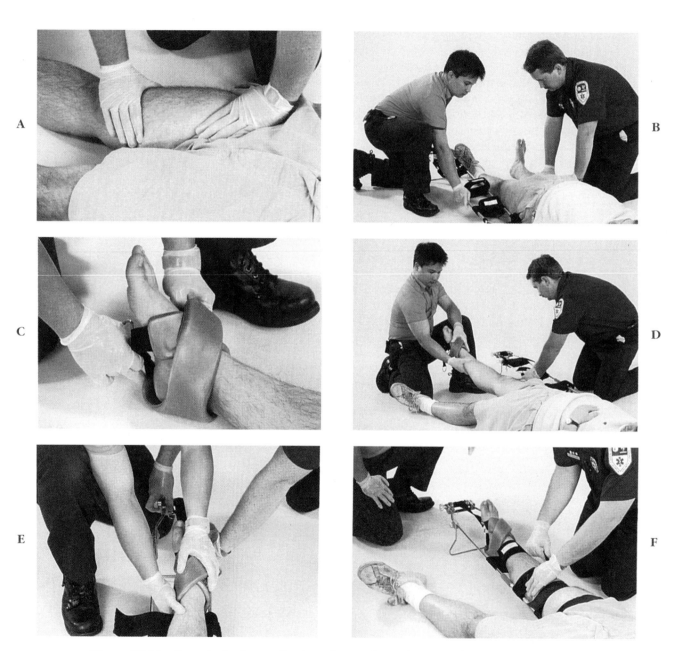

**Figure 15-19** To assist in the application of a traction splint, **A,** stabilize the leg and check the distal pulse. **B,** Measure the splint to extend below the foot. **C,** Apply the ankle hitch. **D,** Apply the traction splint. **E,** Engage traction. **F,** Secure the splint and check the distal pulse again.

# Knee Injuries

The knee joint is very vulnerable to injury. The knee includes the lower end of the femur, the upper ends of the tibia and fibula, and the patella (kneecap). The kneecap is a free-floating bone that moves on the lower front surface of the thigh bone. Knee injuries range from cuts and bruises to sprains, fractures, and dislocations. Deep lacerations in the area of the knee can later cause severe joint infections. Sprains, fractures, and dislocations of the knee are common in athletic activities that involve quick movements or exert unusual force on the knee.

The kneecap is unprotected in that it lies directly beneath the skin. This part of the knee is very vulnerable to bruises and lacerations, as well as dislocations. Violent forces to the front of the knee, such as those caused by hitting the dashboard of a motor vehicle or by falling and landing on bent knees, can fracture the kneecap.

## Care for Knee Injuries

To care for an injured knee, first control any external bleeding. Apply a pressure bandage using a figure-eight pattern (Fig. 15-20). If the knee is bent and cannot be straightened without pain, support it in the bent position (Fig. 15-21). If the knee is straight or can be straightened without pain, splint the leg as you would for an injury of the thigh or lower leg or apply a long rigid splint to the leg. Other commercial splints can also be used if available. Apply ice or a cold pack. Help the casualty to rest in a comfortable position. Summon more advanced medical personnel.

# Ankle and Foot Injuries

Ankle and foot injuries are commonly caused by twisting forces. Injuries range from minor sprains with little swelling and pain that heal with a few days' rest to fractures and dislocations. As with other joint injuries, you cannot always distinguish between minor and severe injuries. You should initially care for all ankle and foot injuries as if they are serious. As with other lower extremity injuries, if the ankle or foot is painful to move, if it cannot bear weight, or if the foot or ankle is swollen, a physician should evaluate the injury. Foot injuries may also involve the toes. Although these injuries are painful, they are rarely serious.

Fractures of the feet and ankles can occur when a casualty forcefully lands on the heel. With any great force, such as falling from a height and landing on the feet, fractures are possible. The force of the impact may also be transmitted up the legs. This can result in an injury elsewhere in the body, such as the thigh, pelvis, or spine.

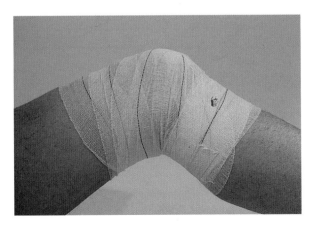

**Figure 15-20** A figure-eight pattern is used to apply a pressure bandage to the knee.

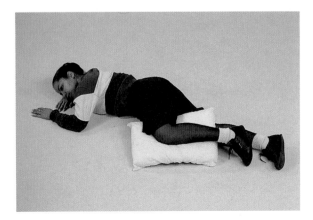

**Figure 15-21** Support a knee injury in the bent position if the casualty cannot straighten the knee.

## Care for Ankle and Foot Injuries

Care for ankle and foot injuries by controlling external bleeding and immobilizing the ankle and foot in the best way possible. Some commercial splints are specifically designed for this area. If you must improvise, you can use a soft splint, such as a pillow or folded blanket. Secure the splint to the injured area with two or three cravats or a roller bandage. Once it is splinted, elevate the injured ankle or foot to help reduce the swelling. Apply ice or a cold pack. Suspect that any casualty who has fallen or jumped from a height may have additional injuries. Call more advanced emergency personnel. Keep the casualty from moving until they arrive.

## ◆ SUMMARY

Injuries are a leading health problem in Canada. When the body experiences violent forces, many kinds of injuries can occur. As you have learned in Chapters 11 through 15, injuries may affect soft tissues, nerves, muscles, bones, ligaments, and tendons. These injuries can have permanent, disabling effects on the body and can even be life threatening.

The musculoskeletal system and the soft tissues are complex groups of structures that provide protection, support, and movement for the body. You can care for serious musculoskeletal and soft tissue injuries to the extremities by focusing on minimizing pain, shock, and further damage to the injured area. You can do this by—

* Managing airway or breathing problems.
* Controlling any external bleeding.
* Checking circulation and sensation below the site of injury before and after immobilizing.
* Immobilizing the injured area of the body.
* Applying ice or a cold pack to the injured area.
* Limiting movement of or by the casualty.
* Calming and reassuring the casualty.
* Maintaining normal body temperature.
* Summoning more advanced medical personnel

### YOU ▼ ARE THE RESPONDER

1. You arrive on the scene to find a man who has fallen down a steep flight of stairs. He is clutching his right arm to his chest. He says his shoulder hurts and he cannot move his arm. How would you care for this injury?
2. You arrive on the scene to find that a child has fallen from a bicycle onto the pavement, landing on her elbow. The elbow is bent and the girl says she cannot move it. How would you care for this injury?

**NOTES:**

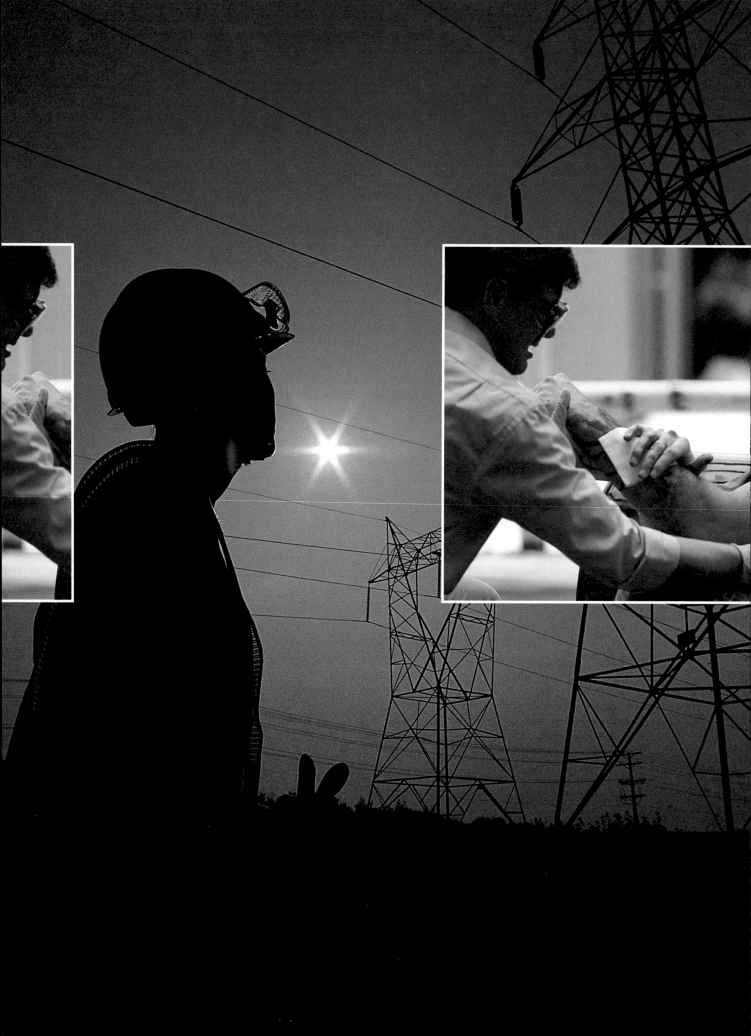

# Part Five

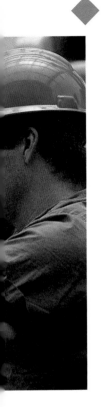

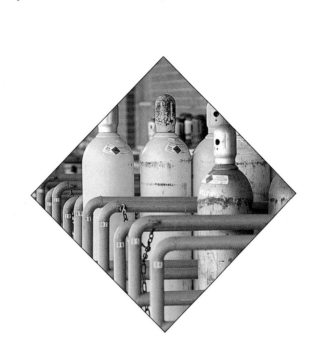

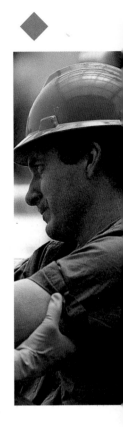

# Medical Emergencies

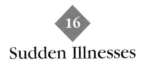

**16**

Sudden Illnesses

**17**

Poisoning

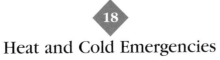

**18**

Heat and Cold Emergencies

## ◆ INTRODUCTION

*You are summoned to assist with an emergency. As you arrive, you notice an elderly woman lying motionless on her side on the floor. An elderly man is kneeling helplessly next to her. Bystanders are gathering, but no one is helping her. There is an empty medicine container without a label on the floor nearby. You notice her body is limp. Saliva is dribbling from her mouth. Her face seems distorted; her mouth droops to one side. She does not respond when you speak to her and tap her on the shoulder. You bend over her and observe that she is breathing rapidly. Her skin is cool and she is sweating heavily.*

*You ask the man what happened and how long she has been like this. He says he is not sure. He came out of his office and found her lying face down on the floor. Then he rolled her over. You summon more advanced medical personnel. You ask the man and the bystanders if anyone knows whether the woman has any medical problems, is taking any medications, or is allergic to anything. The man looks confused and replies "no" to each question.*

*Thoughts race through your mind. What could her problem be? Heart problems? Poisoning? An allergic reaction? A stroke? A diabetic problem? A head injury from a fall? Did she have a seizure? Did the man tell everything he knew about the situation?*

*You know that the EMTs will arrive in about 8 minutes. You try to remain calm. You ask bystanders for a blanket to help warm the woman's cool body. You make certain her airway is clear. You administer oxygen. You decide not to move her but examine her carefully for any clues as to what the problem could be. You want to help the woman more but because you do not know what the problem is, you are unsure about how to proceed. You feel somewhat helpless. What more should you do?*

## The Dilemma of Medical Emergencies

The dilemma in the preceding scenario is not rare. You could someday face a similar situation involving an unclear medical emergency. Unlike easily identifiable problems, such as external bleeding, medical emergencies are rarely as clear. Therefore, you may feel more uncertain about providing care.

When you face an emergency you do not understand, it is normal to feel helpless or indecisive. Yet, like everyone, you still want to help to the best of your ability. Take comfort from the fact that giving initial care, even for medical emergencies you do not understand, does not require extensive knowledge. You do not have to "diagnose" or choose among possible problems to be able to provide appropriate care. By following the emergency action principles and the guidelines for care in previous chapters, you can provide appropriate care until more advanced medical personnel arrive. Knowing this, you can approach an unclear medical emergency with confidence.

The elderly woman could have been experiencing a stroke, a diabetic emergency, or some other medical emergency, but you could not have known this. None of the bystanders knew the nature of her problem, and she was not wearing a medical alert bracelet. Did it matter that you could not diagnose exactly what her condition was? Not at all. You correctly focused on the following basics of care:

- *Do no further harm.* It was right not to reposition the woman since she was lying on her side. She was not conscious, and there was no immediate threat requiring that she be moved.
- *Monitor the ABCs.* Keeping her positioned on one side kept her airway clear by letting fluid drain from the mouth so that it would not obstruct the airway. You could easily determine that she was breathing by watching and listening to her inhale and

exhale. Since she was breathing, you knew she had a pulse. She did not have any severe external bleeding.

◆ *Summon more advanced medical personnel.* This ensured a rapid response for a person who needed more advanced attention. By sending a bystander to make the call, you were able to continue to provide care.

◆ *Do a secondary survey to check for any additional injuries.* When you surveyed the woman's body looking for any clues to her condition or additional problems, you did not find any. Therefore, you did not need to give further care.

◆ *Minimize shock.* Maintaining normal body temperature with a blanket, keeping her positioned on the floor, and administering oxygen helped minimize shock.

In this instance, everything that needed to be done was done. What if other information had been available, such as a medical alert bracelet indicating the woman was a diabetic? Would that have helped you care for this person? No, even if you had known she was a diabetic, it would not have affected the care you provided. Since she was not conscious, your care would have been the same. Almost all the care you will give a casualty having a medical emergency is as simple as following these basics of care, whether the casualty is conscious or unconscious.

## The Onset of Medical Emergencies

Medical emergencies can develop very rapidly (acute conditions) or develop gradually and persist for a long time (chronic conditions). They can result from illness or disease. They include chronic problems caused by diseases, such as heart and lung disease. They can involve hormone imbalances, such as diabetes. They can involve sudden unexplained conditions, such as fainting. Medical emergencies also can involve illnesses, such as epilepsy, in which an occasional seizure occurs, or allergies, in which exposure to a certain substance causes a severe reaction. Overexposure to heat or cold also can cause serious illness.

In the previous unit, you learned that injury is the leading cause of death and disability for people between the ages of 1 and 44. In this unit, you will learn about medical conditions that also can cause death and disability in the 1-to-44 age group and that are also a major problem for those over age 45.

# Sudden Illnesses

# 16

## ◆ Key Terms ◆

**Diabetic (di ah BET ik):** A person with the condition called diabetes mellitus, which causes the body to produce insufficient insulin.

**Diabetic emergency:** A situation in which a person becomes ill because of an imbalance of insulin.

**Epilepsy (EP I lep se:** A chronic condition characterised by seizures that vary in type and duration; can usually be controlled by medication.

**Fainting:** A loss of consciousness resulting from a temporary reduction of blood flow to the brain.

**Hyperglycaemia (hi per gli SE me ah):** A condition in which too much sugar is in the bloodstream.

**Hypoglycaemia (hi po gli SE me ah):** A condition in which too little sugar is in the bloodstream.

**Insulin (IN su lin):** A hormone that enables the body to use sugar for energy; frequently used to treat diabetes.

**Seizure (SE zhur):** A disorder in the brain's electrical activity, marked by loss of consciousness and often uncontrollable muscle movement.

**Stroke:** A disruption of blood flow to a part of the brain that causes permanent damage; also called a cerebrovascular accident (CVA).

**Transient (TRANZ e ent) ischemic (is KE mik) attack:** A temporary disruption of blood flow to the brain; sometimes called a mini-stroke or TIA.

## ◆ For Review ◆

Before reading this chapter, you should review the guidelines for when to summon more advanced medical personnel (Chapters 1, 2, and 5) and be familiar with the body systems (Chapter 3).

## ◆ INTRODUCTION

Certain illnesses can occur suddenly. Sometimes there are no warning signs and symptoms to alert you or the casualty that something is about to happen. At other times, the casualty may feel ill or state that he or she feels that something is wrong.

Sudden illnesses may have a variety of signs and symptoms. They may cause changes in a person's level of consciousness. A casualty may complain of feeling lightheaded, dizzy, or weak. He or she may feel nauseated or may vomit. Breathing, pulse, and skin characteristics may change. If a casualty looks and feels ill, there is a problem.

Several conditions, such as diabetes, stroke, epilepsy, poisoning, and shock, can cause a change in consciousness. In an emergency, you may not know what caused the change, but the cause is not important. You do not need to know the exact cause to provide appropriate care for the casualty. In this chapter, you will learn that knowing and following the emergency action principles and basic principles of care are all you need to care for a casualty of sudden illness.

Faced with an unknown illness, you should summon more advanced medical personnel. Sometimes, as with simple fainting, the illness can pass quickly. At other times, the problem may not be resolved quickly and easily. The condition may get worse. Therefore, it is better to err on the side of caution and summon more advanced medical personnel.

This chapter provides information about some sudden illnesses you may encounter.

These include fainting, diabetic emergencies, seizure, and stroke. Even though each of these sudden illnesses occurs for a different reason, many of the same signs and symptoms are present. The care for these illnesses follows the same general guidelines:

- Prevent further harm.
- Monitor the vital signs.
- Summon more advanced medical personnel.
- Help the casualty rest comfortably.
- Maintain normal body temperature.
- Provide reassurance.
- Administer oxygen if available.

## ◆ SPECIFIC SUDDEN ILLNESSES

### Fainting

One of the most common sudden illnesses is fainting. *Fainting* is a partial or complete loss of consciousness. It is caused by a temporary reduction of blood flow to the brain, such as occurs when blood collects in the legs and lower body. When the brain is suddenly deprived of its normal blood flow, it momentarily shuts down and the casualty faints.

Fainting can be triggered by an emotional shock, such as the sight of blood. It may be caused by pain, by specific medical conditions such as heart disease, by standing for a long time, or by overexertion. Some people, such as pregnant women or the elderly, are more likely to faint when suddenly changing positions, for example, when moving from lying to standing up. Anytime changes inside the body momentarily reduce the blood flow to the brain, fainting may occur.

### Signs and Symptoms of Fainting

Fainting may occur with or without warning. Often, the casualty may initially feel lightheaded or dizzy. Because fainting is one form of shock, he or she may show signs of shock, such as pale, cool, moist skin. The casualty may feel nauseated and complain of numbness or tingling in the fingers and toes. The casualty's breathing and/or pulse may become faster.

## Care for Fainting

Fainting often resolves itself. When the casualty moves from an upright position to a horizontal position, normal circulation to the brain often resumes. The casualty usually regains consciousness within a minute.

Fainting itself does not usually harm the casualty, but injury may occur from falling. If you suspect head or spinal injury, take the necessary precautions when providing care. If you can reach a casualty starting to collapse, lower him or her to the ground or other flat surface and position on the back. Loosen any restrictive clothing, such as a tie or collar. Check the ABCs. Do not give the casualty anything to eat or drink. This can increase the chance of vomiting. Do not splash water on the casualty's face. This does little to stimulate the casualty, and the casualty could aspirate the water. Administer oxygen if it is available.

Usually a casualty who has fainted recovers quickly with no lasting effects. However, since you will not be able to determine whether the fainting is linked to a more serious condition, more advanced medical personnel should be summoned.

## Diabetic Emergencies

To function normally, body cells need sugar as a source of energy. Through the digestive process, the body breaks down food into sugars, which are absorbed into the bloodstream. However, sugar cannot pass freely from the blood into the body cells; it needs an escort. *Insulin,* a hormone produced in the pancreas, takes sugar into the cells. Without a proper balance of sugar and insulin, the cells will starve and the body will not function properly (Fig. 16-1).

The condition in which the body does not produce enough insulin is called **diabetes mellitus,** or more commonly, sugar diabetes. A person with this condition is a *diabetic.*

There are two major types of diabetes. Type I, insulin-dependent diabetes, occurs when the body produces little or no insulin. Since this type of diabetes tends to begin in childhood, it is often called juvenile diabetes. Most insulin-dependent diabetics have to inject insulin into their bodies daily.

Type II, noninsulin-dependent diabetes, occurs when the body produces insulin but not in a quantity sufficient for the body's needs. This condition is called maturity-onset diabetes and usually occurs in older adults.

Anyone with diabetes must carefully monitor his or her diet and exercise. Insulin-dependent diabetics must also regulate their use of insulin (Fig. 16-2). When a diabetic fails to control these factors, either of two problems can occur—too much or too little sugar in the body.

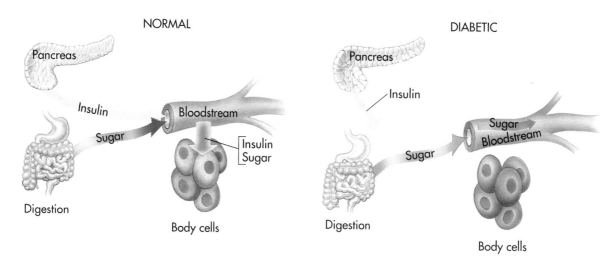

**Figure 16-1** The hormone insulin is needed to take sugar from the blood into the body cells.

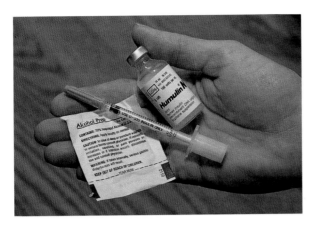

**Figure 16-2**   Insulin-dependent diabetics inject insulin to regulate the amount in the body.

This imbalance causes illness, which can become a *diabetic emergency.*

When the insulin level in the body is too low, the sugar level in the blood is high. This condition is called *hyperglycaemia* (Fig. 16-3, *A*). Sugar is present in the blood but cannot be transported from the blood into the cells without insulin. When this occurs, body cells become starved for sugar. The body attempts to meet its need for energy by using other stored food and energy sources, such as fats. However, converting fat to energy produces waste products and increases the acidity level in the blood, causing a condition called acidosis. As this occurs, the casualty becomes ill. If it continues, the hyperglycaemic condition deteriorates into its most serious form, **diabetic coma.**

On the other hand, when the insulin level in the body is too high, the casualty has a low sugar level. This condition is known as *hypoglycaemia* (Fig. 16-3, *B*). The sugar level can become too low if the diabetic—

♦ Takes too much insulin.
♦ Fails to eat adequately.
♦ Overexercises and burns off sugar faster than normal.
♦ Experiences great emotional stress.

In this situation, the small amount of sugar is used up rapidly and there is not enough for the brain to function properly. This results in an acute condition called **insulin reaction,** which can be life threatening.

## Signs and Symptoms of Diabetic Emergencies

The signs and symptoms of hyperglycaemia and hypoglycaemia differ somewhat, but the major signs and symptoms are similar. These include—

♦ Changes in the level of consciousness, including dizziness, drowsiness, and confusion.
♦ Rapid breathing.

**DIABETIC EMERGENCIES**

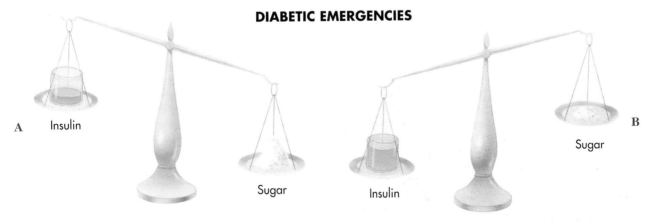

**DIABETIC COMA (HYPERGLYCEMIA)**    **INSULIN REACTION (HYPOGLYCEMIA)**

**Figure 16-3   A,** Hyperglycemia occurs when there is insufficient insulin in the body, causing a high level of sugar in the blood. **B,** Hypoglycemia occurs when the insulin level in the body is high, causing a low level of sugar in the blood.

- Rapid pulse.
- Feeling and looking ill.

It is not important for you to differentiate between insulin reaction and diabetic coma. The basic care for both conditions is the same.

### Care for Diabetic Emergencies

First, do a primary survey and care for any life-threatening conditions. If the casualty is conscious, do a secondary survey, looking for anything visibly wrong. Ask if he or she is a diabetic, and look for a medical alert tag. If the casualty is a known diabetic and exhibits the signs and symptoms previously stated, then suspect a diabetic emergency.

If the conscious casualty can take food or fluids, give him or her sugar (Fig. 16-4). Most candy, fruit juices, and nondiet soft drinks have enough sugar to be effective. Common table sugar, either dry or dissolved in a glass of water, can restore the blood sugar level to normal. Commercially available sugar sources also work well. Sometimes, diabetics will be able to tell you what is wrong and will ask for something with sugar in it. If the casualty's problem is low sugar (hypoglycaemia), the sugar you give will help quickly. If the casualty already has too much sugar (hyperglycaemia), the excess sugar will do no further harm.

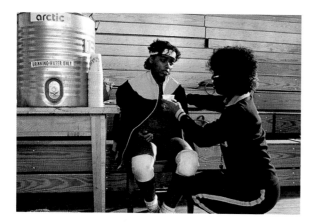

**Figure 16-4** If a casualty of a diabetic emergency is conscious, give him or her food or fluids containing sugar.

Do not try to assist the casualty by administering insulin. Unless the casualty is fully conscious, do not give anything by mouth. Instead, monitor the ABCs, maintain normal body temperature, summon more advanced medical personnel, and administer oxygen if available. If the casualty is conscious but does not feel better within approximately 5 minutes after taking sugar, summon more advanced medical personnel. Oxygen should be administered if available.

## Seizures

When the normal functions of the brain are disrupted by injury, disease, fever, or infection, the electrical activity of the brain becomes irregular. This irregularity can cause a loss of body control known as a *seizure.*

Seizures may be caused by an acute or a chronic condition. The chronic condition is known as *epilepsy,* which is usually controlled with medication. Still, some epileptics have seizures from time to time. Others, who go a long time without a seizure, may think the condition has gone away and stop taking their medication. They may then have a seizure again.

### Signs and Symptoms of Seizure

Before a seizure occurs, the casualty may experience an **aura.** An aura is an unusual sensation or feeling, such as a visual hallucination; a strange sound, taste, or smell; or an urgent need to get to safety. If the casualty recognizes the aura, he or she may have time to tell bystanders and sit down before the seizure occurs.

Seizures range from mild blackouts that others may mistake for daydreaming to uncontrolled muscular contractions (convulsions) lasting several minutes. Infants and young children are at risk for seizures brought on by high fever. These are called febrile (heat-induced) seizures. When a casualty has a seizure, breathing may become irregular and even stop temporarily.

## Care for Seizure

Although it may be frightening to see someone having a seizure, you can easily care for the casualty. Remember that he or she cannot control any muscular contractions that may occur. Do not try to stop the seizure. Do not attempt to restrain the casualty. This can cause musculoskeletal injuries.

Your objectives for care are to protect the casualty from injury and manage the airway. First, move away nearby objects, such as furniture, that might cause injury. Protect the casualty's head by placing a thin cushion, such as folded clothing, beneath it. If there is fluid, such as saliva or vomitus, in the casualty's mouth, position him or her on one side so that the fluid can drain from the mouth.

Do not try to place anything between the casualty's teeth. People having seizures rarely bite their tongues or cheeks with enough force to cause any significant bleeding. However, some blood may be present, so positioning the casualty on his or her side will help any blood drain out of the mouth.

In most instances, the seizure will be over by the time you arrive to help. The casualty will be drowsy and disoriented. Do a secondary survey, checking to see if he or she was injured during the seizure. Offer comfort and reassurance. The casualty will be tired and want to rest. If the seizure occurred in public, the casualty may be embarrassed and self-conscious. Ask bystanders not to crowd around the casualty. Stay with the casualty until he or she is fully conscious and aware of the surroundings.

If the casualty is known to have periodic seizures, you do not necessarily need to summon more advanced medical personnel immediately. The casualty usually will recover from a seizure in a few minutes. However, more advanced medical personnel should be called if—

- The seizure lasts more than a few minutes.
- The casualty has repeated seizures.
- The casualty appears to be injured.
- You are uncertain about the cause of the seizure.
- The casualty is pregnant.
- The casualty is a known diabetic.

- The casualty is an infant or child.
- The seizure takes place in water.
- The casualty fails to regain consciousness after the seizure.

## Stroke

A *stroke,* also called a cerebrovascular accident (CVA), is a disruption of blood flow to a part of the brain, serious enough to damage brain tissue (Fig. 16-5).

Most commonly, a stroke is caused by a blood clot, called a **thrombus** or **embolism,** that forms or lodges in the arteries that supply blood to the brain. Another common cause is bleeding from a ruptured artery in the brain. A head injury,

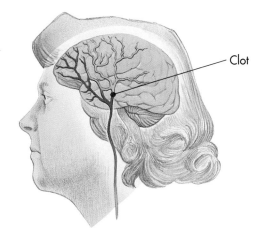

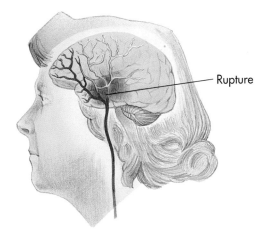

**Figure 16-5**  A stroke can be caused by a blood clot or bleeding from a ruptured artery in the brain.

high blood pressure, a weak area in an artery wall **(aneurysm),** or fat deposits lining an artery (atherosclerosis) may cause a stroke. Less commonly, a tumour or swelling from a head injury may cause a stroke by compressing an artery.

A *transient ischemic attack (TIA)* is a temporary episode that is like a stroke. TIAs are sometimes called "mini-strokes." Like a stroke, a TIA is caused by reduced blood flow to part of the brain. Unlike a stroke, the signs and symptoms of a TIA disappear within a few minutes or hours, although the casualty is not out of danger. Someone who experiences a TIA has nearly a 10 times greater chance of having a stroke in the future.

## Preventing Stroke

The risk factors for stroke and TIA are similar to those for heart disease. Some risk factors are beyond your control, such as age, gender or a family history of stroke, TIA, diabetes, or heart disease.

You can, however, control other risk factors. One of the most important is **hypertension,** or high blood pressure. Hypertension increases your risk of stroke approximately seven times. High blood pressure puts pressure on arteries and makes them more likely to burst. Even mild hypertension can increase your risk of stroke. You can often control high blood pressure by losing weight, changing your diet, exercising routinely, and managing stress. If those measures are not sufficient, your physician may prescribe medication.

Cigarette smoking is another major risk factor for stroke. Smoking is also linked to heart disease and cancer. It increases blood pressure and makes blood more likely to clot. If you do not smoke, do not start. If you do smoke, seek help to try to stop. No matter how difficult or painful quitting may be, it is well worth it. The benefits of not smoking start as soon as you stop.

Diets that are high in saturated fats and cholesterol increase your chance of stroke by increasing the possibility of fatty materials building up on

## The Brain Makes a Comeback

Neuroscientists have been mystified for years by the capricious effects of stroke. For many stroke survivors, talking becomes a tangle of words, a word like "piddlypop" spilling out in place of "hello." One man spoke normally unless he was asked to name fruits and vegetables. Each stroke survivor seemed to have a unique, perplexing set of problems, and doctors found recovery equally unpredictable.

But research into brain function after a stroke has shed new light on the way the brain works. Many strokes are caused when blood flow to the brain is cut off by a blood clot or haemorrhage. The oxygen-deprived brain cells rupture and die. Neuroscientists once believed that the cells died from lack of oxygen. However, their conclusion did not explain why stroke survivors sometimes get worse over several hours.

The oxygen-deprived brain cells actually start an avalanche of death when they rupture. The ruptured cells release huge quantities of the amino acid glutamate that gushes into surviving brain cells and destroys them. Normally, small amounts of glutamate act as transmitters between the cells, but large amounts are extremely damaging.

Researchers believe that if they could inhibit the reaction of glutamate within the cell, they could stop the avalanche. Researchers are developing several drugs to try to block the amino acid avalanche after a stroke. Oddly enough, they have found that drugs similar to phencyclidine, a potent animal tranquilizer and street drug known as PCP, have proven the most effective. Like PCP, the drugs cause temporary hallucinations. But doctors say the promising results outweigh the side effects.

Strokes still present many mysteries, but with more than 2 million people surviving strokes in North America, doctors are hopeful that the drugs will eventually eliminate the long-term effects.

the walls of your blood vessels. Keep your intake of these foods at a moderate level.

Regular exercise reduces your chances of stroke by increasing blood circulation, which develops more channels for blood flow. These additional channels provide alternate routes for blood if the primary channels become blocked.

### Signs and Symptoms of Stroke

As with other sudden illnesses, the primary signs and symptoms of stroke or TIA are looking or feeling ill, changes in consciousness, or abnormal behaviour. Others include sudden weakness and numbness of the face, arm, or leg. Usually, this occurs only on one side of the body. The casualty may have difficulty talking or understanding speech. Vision may be blurred or dimmed; the pupils of the eyes may be of unequal size. The casualty may experience a sudden severe headache, dizziness, confusion, changes in mood, or ringing in the ears. The casualty may become unconscious or lose bowel or bladder control.

### Care for Stroke

If the casualty is unconscious, make sure he or she has an open airway and care for any life-threatening conditions that may occur. If there is fluid or vomitus in the casualty's mouth, position him or her on their unaffected side to allow any fluids to drain out. You may have to use a finger sweep to remove some of the material from the mouth. Summon more advanced medical personnel, stay with the casualty, and monitor his or her ABCs.

If the casualty is conscious, do a secondary survey. A stroke can make the casualty fearful and anxious. Offer comfort and reassurance. Often he or she does not understand what has happened. Have the casualty rest in a comfortable position. Do not give him or her anything to eat or drink. If the casualty is drooling or having difficulty swallowing, place him or her on their unaffected side to help drain any fluids or vomitus from the mouth. Summon more advanced medical personnel, stay with the casualty, monitor his or her ABCs, and administer oxygen if available.

### ◆ SUMMARY

Sudden illness can strike anyone at anytime. The signs and symptoms for each of the sudden illnesses described in this chapter are very similar. Recognizing their *general* signs and symptoms, such as changes in the level of consciousness, sweating, confusion, weakness, and the appearance of illness, will indicate to you the necessary initial care you should provide. Usually you will not know the cause of the illness. Diabetic emergencies, seizures, fainting, and stroke are all sudden illnesses, each with an individual, specific cause. Fortunately, you can provide proper care without knowing the cause. Following the emergency action principles and the general guidelines of care for any emergency will help prevent the condition from becoming worse. When providing care for sudden illnesses, you should—

- ◆ Do no further harm.
- ◆ Monitor the vital signs.
- ◆ Summon more advanced medical personnel.
- ◆ Help the casualty rest comfortably.
- ◆ Maintain normal body temperature.
- ◆ Provide reassurance.
- ◆ Administer oxygen if available.

**YOU ▼ ARE THE RESPONDER**

*It is a hot afternoon and the swimming pool is crowded. You notice a child acting strangely in the shallow end of the pool. He appears to stagger and then suddenly falls face down in the water. He is seizing. His arms and legs flail wildly about. You rush into the water, support his body, and keep his head above water. The seizure soon stops. His rigid body goes limp as you move him toward the side of the pool where another lifeguard is waiting to remove him from the water. What care will you give?*

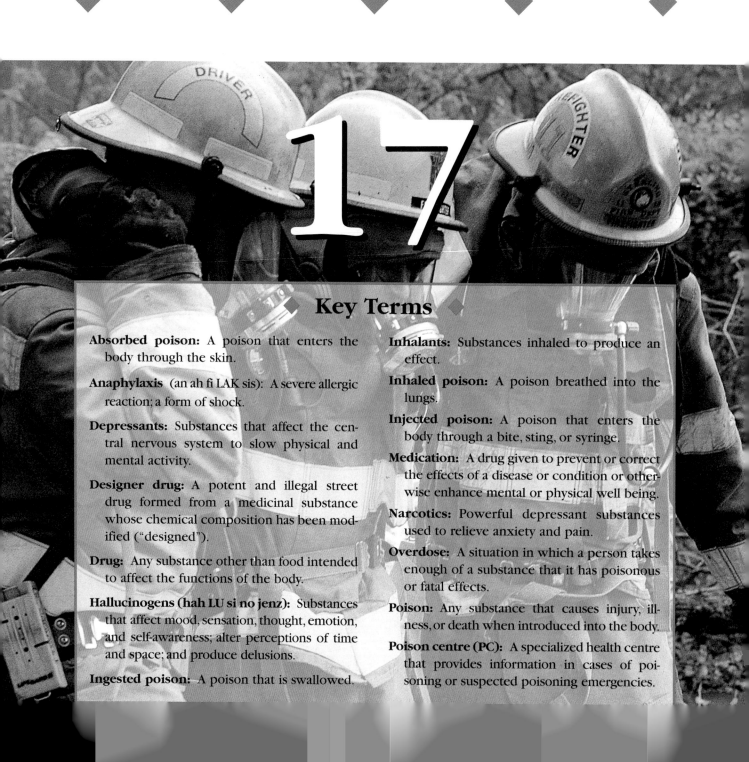

# Poisoning

## 17

### ◆ Key Terms ◆

**Absorbed poison:** A poison that enters the body through the skin.

**Anaphylaxis** (an ah fi LAK sis): A severe allergic reaction; a form of shock.

**Depressants:** Substances that affect the central nervous system to slow physical and mental activity.

**Designer drug:** A potent and illegal street drug formed from a medicinal substance whose chemical composition has been modified ("designed").

**Drug:** Any substance other than food intended to affect the functions of the body.

**Hallucinogens (hah LU si no jenz):** Substances that affect mood, sensation, thought, emotion, and self-awareness; alter perceptions of time and space; and produce delusions.

**Ingested poison:** A poison that is swallowed.

**Inhalants:** Substances inhaled to produce an effect.

**Inhaled poison:** A poison breathed into the lungs.

**Injected poison:** A poison that enters the body through a bite, sting, or syringe.

**Medication:** A drug given to prevent or correct the effects of a disease or condition or otherwise enhance mental or physical well being.

**Narcotics:** Powerful depressant substances used to relieve anxiety and pain.

**Overdose:** A situation in which a person takes enough of a substance that it has poisonous or fatal effects.

**Poison:** Any substance that causes injury, illness, or death when introduced into the body.

**Poison centre (PC):** A specialized health centre that provides information in cases of poisoning or suspected poisoning emergencies.

## ◆ Key Terms ◆

**Stimulants:** Substances that affect the central nervous system to speed up physical and mental activity.

**Substance abuse:** The deliberate, persistent, excessive use of a substance without regard to health concerns or accepted medical practices.

**Substance misuse:** The use of a substance for unintended purposes or for intended purposes but in improper amounts or doses.

## ◆ For Review ◆

Before reading this chapter, you should review the information on breathing emergencies (Chapter 4) and sudden illnesses (Chapter 16).

## ◆ INTRODUCTION

Chapter 16 described sudden illnesses caused by conditions inside the body. Poisoning can also be a sudden illness, but unlike sudden illnesses, such as fainting and stroke, poisoning results when an external substance enters the body. The substance may be a chemical, or it may be a germ or virus that enters the body through a bite or sting. In this chapter, you will learn how to recognise and care for poisoning.

Poisoning is the third-most common cause of accidental death in Canada, with over 500 deaths by poisoning every year. Most poisonings occur in the home, and most are unintentional.

## ◆ HOW POISONS ENTER THE BODY

A *poison* is any substance that causes injury or illness when introduced into the body. Some poisons can cause death. Poisons include solids, liquids, and fumes (gases and vapours). A poison can enter the body in four ways: ingestion, inhalation, absorption, and injection (Fig. 17-1).

To ingest means to swallow. *Ingested poisons* include foods, such as certain mushrooms and shellfish; substances, such as alcohol; medications, such as aspirin; and household and garden items, such as cleaning products, pesticides, and plants. Many substances not poisonous in small amounts are poisonous in larger amounts.

Poisoning by inhalation occurs when a person breathes in toxic fumes. *Inhaled poisons* include—

- Gases, such as carbon monoxide, from an engine or other combustion.
- Gases, such as carbon dioxide, that can occur naturally from decomposition.
- Gases, such as nitrous oxide, used for medical procedures.
- Gases, such as chlorine, found in commercial swimming facilities.
- Fumes from household products, such as glues and paints.
- Fumes from drugs, such as marijuana.

An *absorbed poison* enters the body after coming in contact with the skin or other **membranes** (thin sheets of tissue that cover a structure or line a cavity, such as the mouth or nose). Absorbed poisons come from plants, such as poison ivy, poison oak, and poison sumac, and from fertilizers and pesticides used in lawn and plant care. They can also come from drugs, such as cocaine, that can be absorbed through the mucous membranes in the mouth and nose.

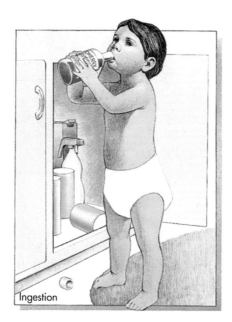

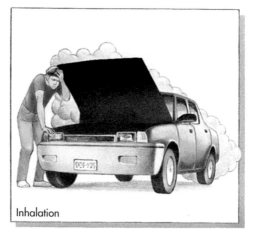

Inhalation

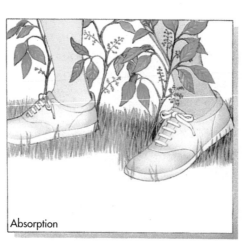

Absorption

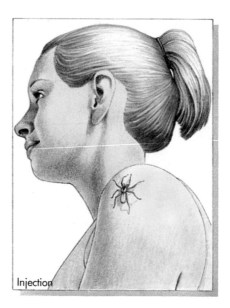

Injection

**Figure 17-1** A poison can enter the body in four ways: ingestion, inhalation, absorption, and injection.

***Injected poisons*** enter the body through bites or stings of insects, spiders, ticks, animals, and snakes or as drugs or medications injected with a hypodermic syringe.

## ◆ POISONING PREVENTION

The best approach to poisoning emergencies is to prevent them from occurring in the first place. This is a simple principle, but often people do not take enough precautions.

By following these general guidelines, people will be able to prevent most poisoning emergencies:

- Keep all medications and dangerous products well out of the reach of children.
- Use childproof safety caps on medication containers and other potentially dangerous products.
- Keep products in their original containers with the labels in place.
- Use poison symbols to identify dangerous substances.

◆ Dispose of outdated products.
◆ Use potentially dangerous chemicals only in well-ventilated areas.
◆ When working with a poisonous substance, wear clothing that can prevent contact with the substance.

# ◆ SIGNS AND SYMPTOMS OF POISONING

The most important thing is to recognize that *a poisoning may have occurred.* As with other serious emergencies, such as severe chest pain or head and spinal injury, evaluate the scene, the condition of the casualty, and any information given by the casualty or bystanders. If you then have even a slight suspicion that the casualty has been poisoned, seek more advanced medical assistance immediately.

As you approach the casualty, survey the scene. Be aware of any unusual odours, flames, smoke, open or spilled containers, an open medicine cabinet, an overturned or damaged plant, or other signs of possible poisoning.

When you reach the casualty, do a primary survey. If the casualty has no life-threatening conditions, do a secondary survey. The casualty of poisoning generally displays signs and symptoms common to other sudden illnesses. These include nausea, vomiting, diarrhea, chest or abdominal pain, breathing difficulty, sweating, altered level of consciousness, and seizures.

Other signs of poisoning are burn injuries around the mouth or on the skin. You may also suspect a poisoning based on any information you have from or about the casualty. Look also for any **drug paraphernalia,** such as pipes, paper for rolling, syringes, or containers.

If you suspect a poisoning, try to get answers to the following questions:

◆ What type of poison was taken?
◆ How much was taken?
◆ When was it taken?

This information will help you provide the most appropriate initial care and provide more advanced medical personnel with valuable information that may affect additional care.

# ◆ POISON CENTRES

A poisoning emergency can sometimes pose a unique problem for those trying to provide appropriate care. The severity of the poisoning depends on the type and amount of the substance, how it entered the body, and the casualty's size, weight, and age. Some poisons act fast and have characteristic signs and symptoms. Others act slowly and cannot be easily identified. Sometimes you will be able to identify the specific poison, sometimes not.

To help responders on all levels deal with poisonings, poison centres exist throughout Canada. Medical professionals in these centres have access to information about virtually all poisonous substances. They can tell you how to counteract the poison. You should know your closest poison centre number and keep it posted in your first aid kit.

If the casualty is unconscious, summon more advanced medical personnel immediately. The dispatcher can link you with the poison centre. The dispatcher may also monitor your discussion with the poison centre and provide additional information to the responding ambulance crew (Fig. 17-2). In some instances, this eliminates the need for a second call and saves time.

# ◆ CARE FOR POISONING

Follow these general principles for any poisoning emergency:

◆ Survey the scene to make sure it is safe to approach and gather clues about what happened.
◆ Remove the casualty from the source of the poison.
◆ Do a primary survey to assess the casualty's airway, breathing, and circulation.

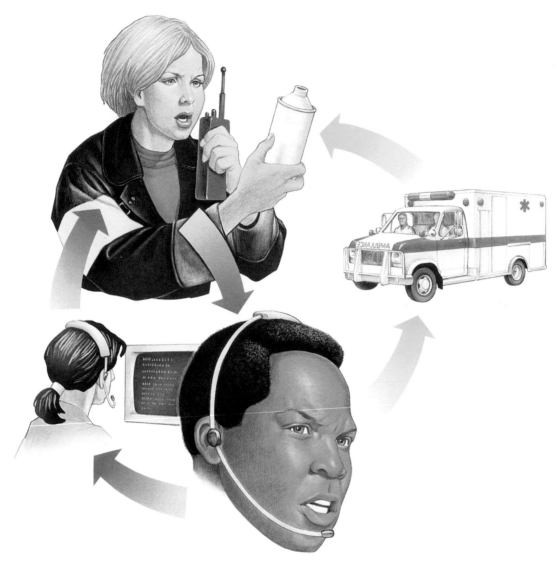

**Figure 17-2** A dispatcher can link you with the poison centre, monitor your discussion, and provide additional information to the responding ambulance crew.

- Care for any life-threatening conditions.
- If the casualty is conscious, do a secondary survey to gather additional information. Look for containers, pills, etc.
- Contact the poison centre or summon more advanced medical personnel.
- Follow the directions of the poison centre.
- Do not give the casualty anything by mouth unless advised by medical professionals. If the poison is unknown and the casualty vomits, save some of the vomitus, which may be analysed later to identify the poison.

## Ingested Poisons

Besides following these general principles for any poisoning, you may also need to provide additional care for specific types of poisons. Usually, if the casualty has ingested the poison in the last hour, the stomach should be emptied. The poison centre may instruct you to induce vomiting.

If the poison centre advises you to induce vomiting with **syrup of ipecac,** follow their directions and use the dose they direct. Vomiting usually occurs within 20 minutes.

There are some instances when vomiting *should not* be induced. These include when the casualty—

◆ Is unconscious.
◆ Is having a seizure.
◆ Is pregnant.
◆ Has ingested a corrosive substance (an acid or alkali) or a petroleum product (such as kerosene or gasoline).
◆ Is known to have heart disease.

Since vomiting removes only about half of the poison, the poison centre may ask you to neutralize the amount that remains with **activated charcoal**. Activated charcoal is available in both liquid and powder forms. Follow the direction from the poison centre. Both syrup of ipecac and activated charcoal may be part of your first aid supplies (Fig. 17-3).

You can dilute some ingested poisons by giving the casualty water to drink. Examples of such poisons are corrosive chemicals, like acids or alkalies, that damage or destroy tissues. Vomiting these corrosives could burn the esophagus, throat, and mouth. Diluting the corrosive substance decreases the potential for damaging tissues.

Diluting poisons taken in tablet or capsule form is usually not a good idea. The increased fluid could dissolve them more rapidly in the stomach, speeding the body's absorption of the poison. As always, follow the advice of the poison centre or other medical professionals.

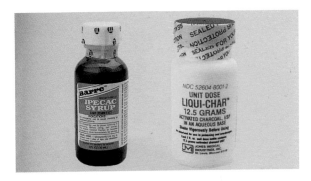

**Figure 17-3** Syrup of ipecac and activated charcoal.

skin colour that indicates a lack of oxygen may signal carbon monoxide poisoning. For years, people were taught that carbon monoxide poisoning was indicated by a cherry-red colour of the skin and lips. This, however, is a poor *initial indicator* of carbon monoxide poisoning. The red colour occurs later, usually after death.

All casualties of inhaled poison need to be removed from the poison as soon as possible. First and foremost, however, remember the emergency action principles. Survey the scene to determine if it is safe for you to help. If you can remove the casualty from the source of the poison without endangering your life, then do so. You can help a conscious casualty by just getting him or her to fresh air and then summoning more advanced medical personnel. Remove an unconscious casualty from the environment, and maintain an open airway. If the person is not breathing, begin rescue breathing. Administer oxygen, if available, to anyone suffering from having inhaled poison.

## Inhaled Poisons

Toxic fumes come from a variety of sources. They may have an odour or be odour free. Carbon dioxide ($CO_2$), for example, is an inhaled poison given off by decomposing organic matter, some wells, and sewers. It is also found in the fumes from certain industrial and home spray chemicals.

A more common inhaled poison is carbon monoxide (CO). It is present in car exhaust and can be produced by defective cooking equipment, fires, and charcoal grills. A pale or bluish

## Absorbed Poisons

People often contact poisonous substances that can be absorbed into the body. Thousands of people each year suffer from contact with poison ivy, poison oak, and poison sumac (Fig. 17-4). Other common poisons absorbed through the skin include dry and wet chemicals, such as those found in insecticides and toxic industrial chemicals, which may also burn the surface of the skin.

To care for poison contact, immediately wash the affected area with water. Rinse the area with

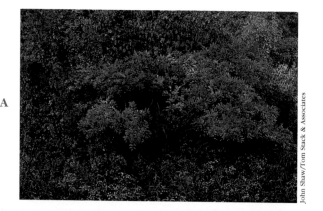

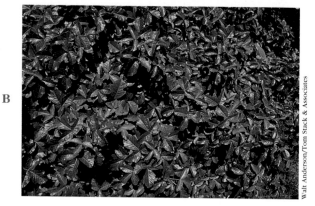

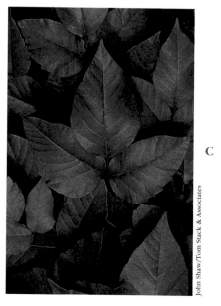

**Figure 17-4** Annually, millions of people suffer from contact with poisonous plants whose poisons are absorbed into the body: **A,** poison sumac; **B,** poison oak; **C,** poison ivy.

cool water and pat dry. Keep the area clean and dry. Instruct casualty to see a doctor if the condition gets worse. If poisons, such as dry or wet chemicals, contact the skin, flush the affected area continuously with large amounts of water (Fig. 17-5). Summon more advanced medical personnel immediately. Continue to flush the area until they arrive.

If running water is not available, brush off dry chemicals, such as lime. Take care not to get any in your eyes or the eyes of the casualty or any bystanders. Dry chemicals are activated by contact with water, but if continuous running water is available, it will flush the chemical from the skin before activating it. Running water reduces the threat to you and quickly and easily removes the substance from the casualty.

## Injected Poisons

Insect and animal stings and bites are among the most common sources of injected poisons. This text cannot consider all possible types of stings and bites that could result in poisoning.

The following sections describe the care for common stings and bites of insects, spiders, ticks, marine life, snakes, and warm-blooded animals.

### Insects

Although insect stings are painful, they are rarely fatal. Fewer than 100 reported deaths occur each year. Some people, however, have a

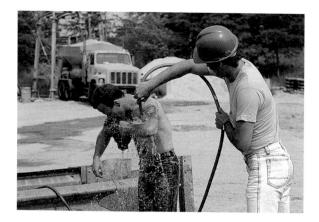

**Figure 17-5** Whenever chemical poisons come in contact with the skin, flush the affected area continuously with large amounts of water.

severe allergic reaction to an insect sting, resulting in the life-threatening condition ana- phylaxis discussed in Chapter 6 and in more detail later in this chapter.

To care for an insect sting, first examine the sting site to see if the stinger is in the skin. If it is, remove it to prevent any further poisoning. Scrape the stinger away from the skin with your fingernail or a plastic card, such as a credit card. Often the venom sac will still be attached to the stinger. Do not remove the stinger with tweezers, since putting pressure on the venom sac can cause further poisoning.

Next, wash the site with soap and water. Cover it to keep it clean. Apply ice or a cold pack to the area to reduce the pain and swelling. Observe the casualty periodically for signs and symptoms of an allergic reaction.

## Spiders and Scorpions

Few spiders in North America have venom that causes death. But the bites of the black widow and brown recluse spiders can be fatal. You can identify them by the unique designs on their bodies (Fig. 17-6). The black widow spider is black with a reddish hourglass shape on its underbody. The brown recluse spider is light brown with a darker brown, violin-shaped marking on the top of its body.

Both spiders prefer dark, out-of-the-way places where they are seldom disturbed. Bites usually occur on the hands and arms of people reaching into places such as wood, rock, and brush piles or rummaging in dark storage areas. Often, the casualty will not know that he or she has been bitten until signs or symptoms develop.

If the spider is identified as either a black widow or brown recluse, the casualty should get immediate care at a medical facility. The wound will be cleansed and medication pro- vided to reduce the pain and inflammation. An antivenin, a substance used to counteract or reduce the poisonous effects of snake or other venom, is available for black widow bites.

Scorpions live in dry regions of the south- western United States and Mexico (Fig. 17-7). Like spiders, only a few species of scorpions are fatally

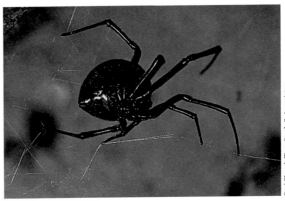

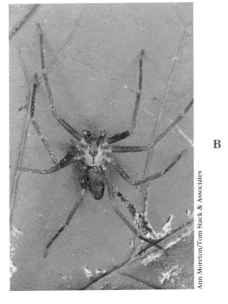

**Figure 17-6  A,** The black widow spider, and **B,** the brown recluse spider have characteristic markings.

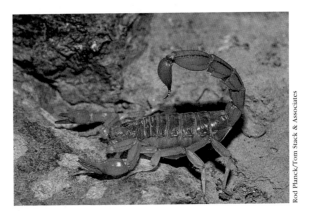

**Figure 17-7**  The bites of only a few species of scorpions can be fatal.

poisonous. They live under rocks, logs, and the bark of certain trees and are most active at night.

Signs and symptoms of spider bites and scorpion stings include—

- Nausea and vomiting.
- Difficulty breathing or swallowing.
- Sweating and salivating profusely.
- Irregular heart rhythms that can lead to cardiac arrest.
- Severe pain in the sting or bite area.
- Swelling on or around the site.
- A mark indicating a possible bite or sting.

To care for a scorpion sting, wash the wound and apply a cold pack to the site. A casualty who has these signs and symptoms needs to go to a medical facility.

## Marine Life

Sting rays, sea anemones, certain fish, jellyfish, and some other marine animals can give painful stings that may cause serious problems, such as allergic reaction, paralysis, and cardiac and respiratory difficulties (Fig. 17-8). Always remove the person who has been stung from the water as soon as possible. Summon more advanced medical personnel if the casualty—

- Has a history of allergic reactions to marine life stings.
- Is stung on the face or neck.
- Develops severe problems, such as difficulty breathing.

If the sting is from a jellyfish, sea anemone, or man-of-war, soak the injured part in vinegar.

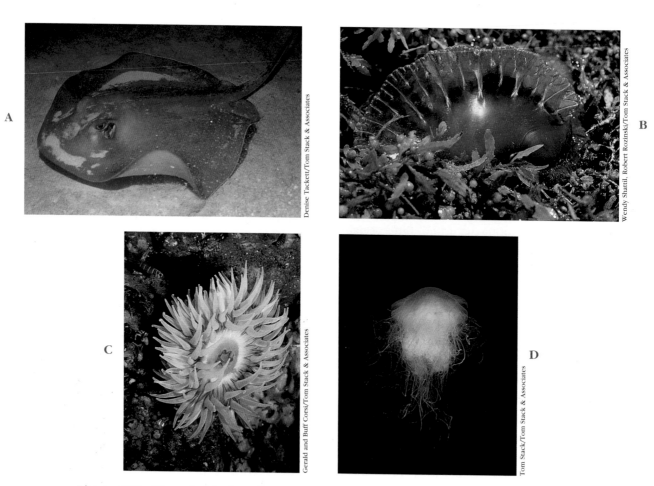

**Figure 17-8**   The painful sting of some marine animals can cause serious problems: **A,** sting ray; **B,** man-of-war; **C,** sea anemone; **D,** jellyfish.

Vinegar often works best to deactivate the toxin. Rubbing alcohol or baking soda may also be used. Do not rub the wound or apply fresh water or ammonia since this will increase pain. Meat tenderizer is no longer recommended.

If the sting is from a stingray, sea urchin, or spiny fish, flush the wound with sterile saline or water. Tap or ocean water also may be used. Immobilize the injured part, usually the foot, and soak the affected area in nonscalding hot water (as hot as the casualty can stand) for about 30 minutes or until the pain subsides. Then carefully clean the wound and apply a bandage. Remind the casualty to watch for signs of infection and check with a health-care provider to determine if a tetanus shot is needed.

## Snakes

Few areas of medicine have provoked more controversy about care for an injury that claims so few lives. Snakebite care issues, such as whether to use a tourniquet, cut the wound, apply ice, apply suction, use electric shock, or capture the snake, have been discussed at length over the years. All this controversy is rather amazing, since few people die of snakebites. Furthermore, just because a snake bites does not mean that venom is injected. Rattlesnakes account for most snakebites and nearly all deaths from snakebites. Figure 17-9 shows the four kinds of poisonous snakes found in North America. Most deaths occur because the casualty has an allergic reaction or a weakened body system or because significant time passes before the casualty receives medical care.

Elaborate care is usually unnecessary because, in most cases, the casualty can reach advanced medical care within 30 minutes.

Follow these guidelines to provide initial care for someone bitten by a snake:

◆ Wash the wound.
◆ Immobilize the affected part.
◆ Keep the affected area lower than the heart if possible.
◆ Summon more advanced medical personnel.

When a casualty cannot get advanced medical care within 30 minutes, you may apply a **constricting band.** This is a band placed around an arm or leg to slow the flow of venom throughout the body. You may also use a commercial kit to suction the wound. You should follow your local protocols regarding extended care for a casualty of snakebite.

Regardless of what you may have otherwise heard or read—

◆ *Do not* apply ice. Recent studies show that cooling the bite can cause as much harm as good.
◆ *Do not* cut the wound. Cutting the wound can further injure the casualty and has not been shown to remove any significant amount of venom.
◆ *Do not* apply a tourniquet. A tourniquet severely restricts blood flow to the extremity, which could result in the loss of the extremity.
◆ *Do not* use electric shock. This technique has not been conclusively shown to affect the poison and can be dangerous.

## Animals

The bite of a domestic or wild animal carries the risk of infection, as well as soft tissue injury. The most serious possible result is **rabies,** a disease transmitted through the saliva of diseased animals, such as skunks, bats, raccoons, cats, dogs, cattle, and foxes.

Animals with rabies may act in unusual ways. For example, nocturnal animals, such as raccoons, may be active in the daytime. A wild animal that usually tries to avoid humans may not run away when you approach. Rabid animals may salivate, appear partially paralysed, or act irritable, aggressive, or strangely quiet. Do not pet or feed wild animals, and do not touch the body of a dead wild animal.

If not treated, rabies is fatal. Anyone bitten by an animal suspected of having rabies must get medical attention. To prevent rabies from developing, the casualty receives a series of injections to build up immunity. In the past, caring for

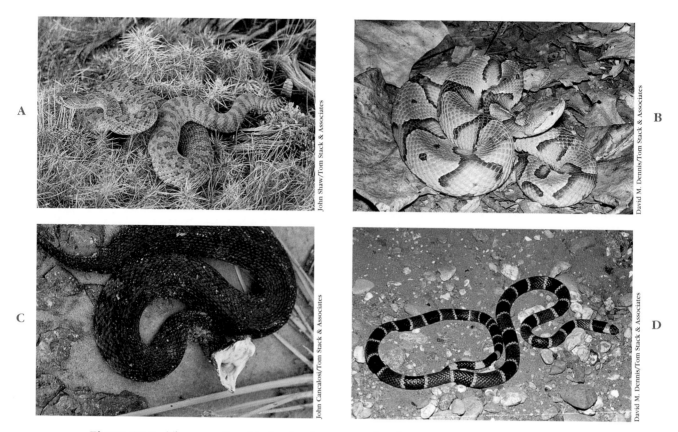

**Figure 17-9** There are four kinds of poisonous snakes found in North America: **A,** rattlesnake; **B,** copperhead; **C,** water moccasin; **D,** coral snake.

rabies meant a lengthy series of painful injections that had many unpleasant side effects. The vaccines used now require fewer injections and have less severe side effects.

If someone is bitten by an animal, try to get him or her away from the animal without endangering yourself. If possible, try to get a good description of the animal and the area in which it was last seen. Do not try to restrain or capture the animal. If the wound is minor, wash it with soap and water and then control any bleeding. If the wound is bleeding seriously, control the bleeding first. Do not clean the wound. The wound will be properly cleaned at a medical facility. Summon more advanced medical personnel for any wounds with serious bleeding. The dispatcher will be able to notify the proper authorities, such as animal control. Any person who has been bitten by an animal must see his or her physician. Local laws

or protocols may require you to report the bite to the proper authorities.

**Ticks**

Ticks can carry and transmit disease to humans. In the past, Rocky Mountain spotted fever was widely publicized as a tick disease. It is still occurring today, but more recently, attention has been focused on a new disease transmitted by ticks.

This disease, known as **Lyme disease** or Lyme borreliosis, is an illness that people get from the bite of an infected tick. Lyme disease is affecting a growing number of people, and people in areas where Lyme disease occurs should take appropriate precautions to protect against it.

Not all ticks carry Lyme disease. Lyme disease is spread primarily by a type of tick that commonly attaches itself to field mice and deer. It is sometimes called a deer tick. This tick is found around beaches and in wooded and grassy areas. Like all ticks, it attaches itself to *any* warm-blooded animal that brushes by it, including humans.

Deer ticks are very tiny and difficult to see. They are much smaller than the common dog tick or wood tick. They can be as small as a poppy seed or the head of a pin (Fig. 17-10). Even in the adult stage, they are only as large as a grape seed. A deer tick can attach to you without your knowledge. Many people who develop Lyme disease cannot recall having been bitten.

A person can get Lyme disease from the bite of an infected tick at any time of the year, but this occurs most often in summer, when ticks are most active and people spend more time outdoors.

The first sign of infection may appear a few days or a few weeks after a tick bite. Typically, a rash starts as a small red area at the site of the bite. It may spread up to 12 to 17 centimetres (5 to 7 inches) across (Fig. 17-11). In fair-skinned people, the centre is lighter in colour, and the outer edges are red and raised, sometimes giving the rash a bull's-eye appearance. In dark-skinned people, the area may look black and blue, like a bruise.

Signs and symptoms of Lyme disease include fever, headache, weakness, and joint and muscle pain similar to the pain of "flu." These signals may develop slowly and may not occur at the same time as a rash. In fact, a person can have Lyme disease without developing a rash.

Lyme disease can get worse if not treated. In its advanced stages it may cause arthritis, numbness, memory loss, problems in seeing or hearing, high fever, and stiff neck. Some of these symptoms could indicate brain or nervous system problems. An irregular or rapid heartbeat could indicate heart problems.

If you find a tick, remove it by pulling steadily and firmly. Grasp the tick with fine-tipped tweezers, as close to the skin as possible, and pull *slowly* (Fig. 17-12). If you do not have tweezers, use a glove, plastic wrap, a piece of paper, or a leaf to protect your fingers. If you use your bare fingers, wash your hands immediately. Do not try to burn a tick off with a hot match or a burning cigarette. Do not use other home remedies, like coating the tick with Vaseline or nail polish or pricking it with a pin.

If you are unable to remove the tick or if its mouth parts stay in the skin, the casualty should obtain medical care, such as from a family physician. Once the tick is removed, wash the area immediately with soap and water. If an antiseptic or antibiotic ointment is available, apply it to prevent wound infection. The casualty should be told to observe the site periodically thereafter. If a rash or flu-like symptoms develop, he or she should seek medical help. A physician will usually use antibiotics to treat Lyme disease. Antibiotics work best and most

Bernard Funival/Fran Heyl Associates

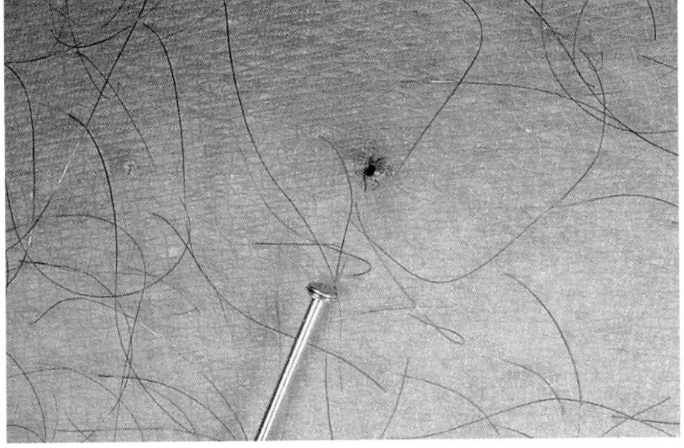

**Figure 17-10** A deer tick can be as small as the head of a pin.

Michael Weissmann, M.D./Fran Heyl Associates

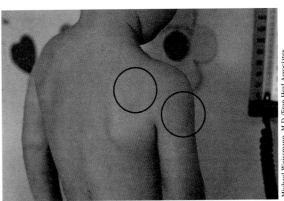

**Figure 17-11** A person with Lyme disease may develop a rash.

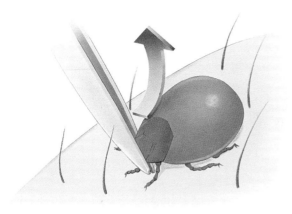

**Figure 17-12** Remove a tick by pulling steadily and firmly with fine-tipped tweezers.

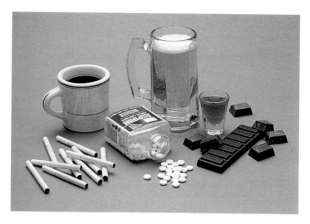

**Figure 17-13** Substance abuse and misuse involve improper use of a broad range of medical and nonmedical substances.

quickly when taken *early*. Treatment is slower and less effective in advanced stages.

### ◆ SUBSTANCE MISUSE AND ABUSE

Alcohol and over-the-counter medications, such as aspirin, sleeping pills, and certain stimulants, are among the most often misused or abused substances. The misuse or abuse of a substance results in the poisoning of the body.

*Substance misuse* is the use of a substance for unintended purposes or for appropriate purposes but in improper amounts or doses. *Substance abuse* is the deliberate, persistent, and excessive use of a substance without regard to health concerns or accepted medical practices. Many substances that are abused or misused are not illegal. Other substances are legal when prescribed by a physician. Some are illegal only for those under age. Figure 17-13 shows some commonly misused and abused substances.

A *drug* is any substance other than food taken to affect body functions. A drug used to prevent or treat a disease or otherwise enhance mental or physical well being is a *medication*.

An *overdose* occurs if someone takes enough of a substance that it has toxic (poisonous) or fatal effects. An overdose may occur if the casualty takes more than is needed for medical purposes. One may occur unintentionally when a casualty takes too much medication at one time. An elderly casualty, for example, may not remember that he or she has already taken the medication and may take another dose (Fig. 17-14). Or a person with failing eyesight may mistake one medication for another.

An overdose may also be intentional, such as in suicidal attempts. Sometimes the suicide casualty takes a sufficient quantity of a substance to cause certain death. Other times, to gain attention or help, the casualty takes enough of a substance to need medical attention but not enough to cause death.

The term **withdrawal** describes the condition produced when someone stops using or abusing a drug to which he or she is addicted. Withdrawal may occur because of someone's deliberate decision to stop or because he or she is unable to obtain the specific drug. Withdrawal from certain substances, such as alcohol, can cause severe mental and physical discomfort and can become a serious medical condition.

### Commonly Misused and Abused Substances

Substances are categorized according to their effects on the body. The basic categories are

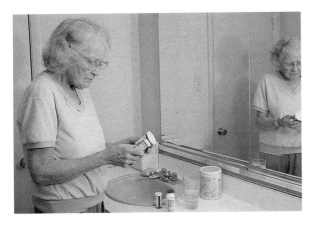

**Figure 17-14**  Misuse of a medication can occur unintentionally for an elderly person or a person with failing eyesight.

stimulants, depressants, and hallucinogens. The category to which a substance belongs depends mostly on the effects it has on the central nervous system. Some substances depress the nervous system, whereas others speed up its activity. Some are not easily categorized because they have various effects. Figure 17-15 shows a variety of misused and abused substances.

## Stimulants

*Stimulants* affect the central nervous system to speed up physical and mental activity. They have limited medical value. They produce temporary feelings of alertness, improve task performance, and prevent sleepiness. They are sometimes used for weight reduction because they suppress appetite.

Many stimulants are ingested as pills, but some can be absorbed or inhaled. Amphetamine, dextroamphetamine, and methamphetamine are stimulants. Their street (slang) names include uppers, bennies, black beauties, speed, crystal, meth, and crank. One of the most recent and dangerous new stimulants is called ice. This is a smokable form of methamphetamine that is extremely addictive.

Cocaine is one of the most publicized and powerful stimulants. Cocaine can be taken into the body in different ways. The most common is sniffing it in powder form, known as snorting. In this method, the drug is absorbed into the blood through the capillaries in the nose. A purer and more potent form of cocaine is crack. Crack is smoked. The vapours that are inhaled into the lungs reach the brain within 10 seconds, causing immediate effects. Crack poses a serious threat because it is highly addictive.

The most common stimulants are legal. Leading the list is caffeine, present in coffee, tea, many kinds of sodas, chocolate, diet pills, and pills used to combat fatigue. Next is nicotine, found in tobacco products. Other stimulants used for medical purposes are inhaled to treat asthma.

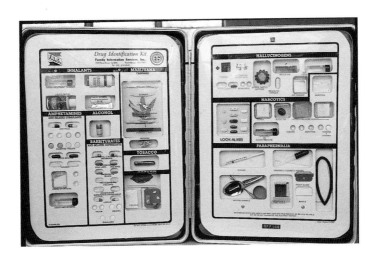

**Figure 17-15**  Misused and abused substances.

# Hallucinogens

*Hallucinogens* at present have no medical uses. They cause changes in mood, sensation, thought, emotion, and self-awareness. They alter perception of time and space and produce delusions.

Among the most widely abused are LSD (lysergic acid diethylamide), commonly called acid; psilocybin, called mushrooms; PCP (phencyclidine), also known as angel dust; and mescaline, otherwise referred to as peyote, buttons, or mesc. These substances are usually ingested, but PCP is also often inhaled.

Hallucinogens often have physical effects similar to stimulants but are classified differently because of the other effects they produce. Hallucinogens sometimes cause what is called "a bad trip." They can cause intense fear, panic, paranoid delusions, vivid hallucinations, profound depression, tension, and anxiety. The casualty may be irrational and feel threatened by any attempt others make to help.

# Depressants

*Depressants* affect the central nervous system to slow down physical and mental activity. Unlike stimulants and hallucinogens, which have limited or no medical value, depressants are commonly used for medical purposes. Common depressants are barbiturates, benzodiazepines, narcotics, alcohol, and inhalants. Most depressants are ingested or injected. Their street names include downers, rainbows, barbs, goofballs, yellow jackets, purple hearts, nemmies, tooies, or reds.

All depressants alter consciousness to some degree. They relieve anxiety, promote sleep, depress respiration, relieve pain, relax muscles, and impair coordination and judgment. Like other substances, the larger the dose or the stronger the substance, the greater its effects.

Alcohol is the most widely used and abused depressant in Canada. In small amounts, its effects are fairly mild. In higher doses, its effects can be toxic. Alcohol is like other depressants in its effects and the risks for overdose. Frequent drinkers may become dependent on the effects of alcohol and increasingly tolerant of them.

Alcohol taken in large amounts or frequently has many unhealthy consequences. The digestive system may be irritated. Alcohol can cause the esophagus to rupture or can injure the stomach lining, causing the casualty to vomit blood. Casualties who have drunk large amounts of alcohol in a short time can experience effects of alcohol use. This type of consumption is life threatening. Chronic drinking can affect the brain and cause a lack of coordination, memory loss, and apathy. Other problems include liver disease, such as **cirrhosis.** In addition, many psychological, family, social, and work problems are related to chronic drinking.

*Narcotics* have effects similar to those of other depressants. They are powerful and are used to relieve anxiety and pain. All narcotics are illegal without a prescription, and some are not prescribed at all. The most common natural narcotics are morphine and codeine. Most other narcotics, including heroin, are synthetic.

Substances inhaled to produce an intoxicating effect are called *inhalants.* Inhalants also have a depressing effect on the central nervous system. In addition, inhalant use can damage the heart, lungs, brain, and liver. Solvents, such as acetone, toluene, butane, gasoline, kerosene, lighter fluid, paints, nail polish and remover, and aerosol sprays, have been inhaled for their effects. The effects are similar to those of alcohol. The user at first appears to be drunk.

# Designer Drugs

Designer drugs are substances that do not fit neatly into any of the three categories mentioned previously. In the early 1980s, the spread of designer drugs was a frightening possibility. Today, it is a reality. Like designer clothes, designer drugs are produced to appeal to a wide audience.

*Designer drugs* are variations of medically prescribed substances, such as narcotics and amphetamines. Through simple and inexpensive methods, the molecular structure of substances produced for medicinal purposes can be modified by street chemists into extremely potent and dangerous street drugs; hence the name designer drug. One designer drug, a form of the commonly used surgical anaesthetic fentanyl, can be made 2000 to 6000 times stronger than its original form.

When the chemical makeup of a drug is altered, as with designer drugs, the user can experience a variety of unpredictable and dangerous effects. In many cases, the chemist has no knowledge of what the effects of the new designer drug could be.

One of the more commonly used designer drugs is "ecstasy" (MDMA). Although ecstasy is structurally related to stimulants and hallucinogens, its effects are somewhat different from either. Ecstasy can evoke a euphoric high that makes it popular among young adults.

The signs and symptoms of ecstasy use range from the stimulant-like effects of high blood pressure, rapid heartbeat, profuse sweating, and agitation to the hallucinogenic-like effects of paranoia, visual distortion, and erratic mood swings.

## Signs and Symptoms of Substance Misuse or Abuse

Like other poisons, the general signs and symptoms of substance misuse and abuse are similar to those of other medical emergencies. The misuse or abuse of stimulants can have many unhealthy effects on the body. These can include moist or flushed skin, sweating, chills, nausea, vomiting, fever, headache, dizziness, rapid pulse, rapid breathing, high blood pressure, and chest pain. In some instances, it can cause respiratory distress, disrupt normal heart rhythms, or cause death. The casualty may appear very excited, restless, talkative, irritable, combative or may suddenly lose consciousness.

Specific signs and symptoms of hallucinogen abuse may include sudden mood changes and a flushed face. The casualty may claim to see or hear something not present. He or she may be anxious and frightened.

Specific signs and symptoms of depressant misuse or abuse may include drowsiness, confusion, slurred speech, slow heart and breathing rates, and poor coordination. An alcohol abuser may smell of alcohol. A casualty who has consumed a great deal of alcohol in a short time may be unconscious or hard to arouse. The casualty may vomit violently. A casualty suffering alcohol withdrawal, a potentially dangerous condition, can be confused and restless. He or she may also be trembling and experiencing hallucinations.

You may be able to find clues that suggest the nature of the problem. Often these clues will come from the casualty, bystanders, or the scene itself. Look for containers, drug paraphernalia, and signs and symptoms of other medical problems. Try to get information from the casualty or from any bystanders or family members. Since many of these physical signs and symptoms of substance abuse mimic other conditions, you may not be able to determine that a casualty has overdosed on a substance.

To provide care for the casualty, you need only recognize abnormalities in breathing; pulse; skin colour, temperature, and moisture; and behaviour that may indicate a condition requiring professional help.

## Care for Substance Misuse or Abuse

As with other medical emergencies, you do not have to diagnose substance misuse or abuse to provide care. Your initial care for substance misuse or abuse does not require that you know the specific substance taken. Since substance abuse or misuse is a form of poisoning, care follows the same general steps. Follow these general steps as you would for any poisoning:

- Survey the scene to be sure it is safe to help the casualty.
- Do a primary survey and care for any life-threatening conditions.
- Contact the poison centre or summon more advanced medical personnel.
- Question the casualty or bystanders during your secondary survey to try to find out what substance was taken, how much was taken, and when it was taken.

- Try to keep the casualty calm by minimizing movement, loud noises, etc.
- If the casualty is unconscious, maintain an open airway.
- Maintain normal body temperature.
- If the casualty vomits or has vomited, place the casualty on one side and clear any matter out of the mouth. (Save a sample of the vomitus, if possible.)
- Withdraw from the area if the casualty becomes violent or threatening.
- If you suspect that someone has used a designer drug, tell the responding advanced medical personnel. This is important because a casualty who has overdosed on a designer drug frequently does not respond to usual medical treatment.

## ♦ ANAPHYLAXIS

Severe allergic reactions to poisons are rare. But when one occurs, it is truly a life-threatening medical emergency. This reaction is called anaphylaxis and was discussed in Chapter 6. *Anaphylaxis* is a form of shock. It can be caused by an insect bite or sting or by contact with drugs, medications, foods, and chemicals. Anaphylaxis can result from any of the kinds of poisoning described in this chapter.

## Signs and Symptoms of Anaphylaxis

Anaphylaxis usually occurs suddenly, within seconds or minutes after contact with the substance. The skin or area of the body that came in contact with the substance usually swells and turns red (Fig. 17-16). Other signs and symptoms include hives, itching, rash, weakness, nausea, vomiting, dizziness, and breathing difficulty that includes coughing and wheezing. This breathing difficulty can progress to an obstructed airway as the tongue and throat swell. Death from anaphylaxis usually occurs because the casualty's breathing is severely impaired.

## Care for Anaphylaxis

If an unusual inflammation or rash is noticeable immediately after contact with a possible source, it could be an allergic reaction. Assess the casualty's airway and breathing. If the casualty has any breathing difficulty or complains that his or her throat is closing, summon more advanced medical personnel immediately. Help the casualty into the most comfortable position for breathing. Administer oxygen if available. Monitor the ABCs and try to keep the casualty calm.

People who know they are extremely allergic to certain substances usually try to avoid them, although this is sometimes impos-

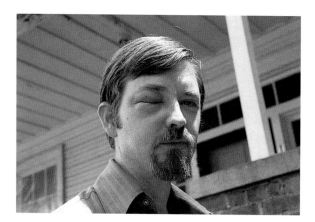

**Figure 17-16** In anaphylaxis, the skin usually swells and turns red.

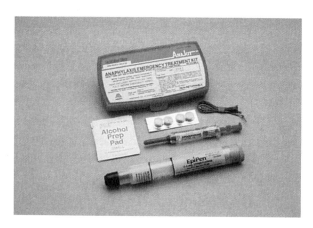

**Figure 17-17** The contents of an anaphylaxis kit.

sible. These people may carry an anaphylaxis kit in case they have a severe allergic reaction. Such kits are available by prescription only (Fig. 17-17). The kit contains a single dose of the drug epinephrine that can be injected into the body to counteract the anaphylactic reaction. If you are allergic to a substance, contact your doctor to discuss whether you need such a kit.

## ◆ SUMMARY

Poisonings can occur in four ways: ingestion, inhalation, absorption, and injection. Substance abuse and misuse are types of poisoning that can occur in any of these ways. Substance abuse and misuse can produce a variety of signs and symptoms, most of which are common to other types of poisoning. You do not need to be able to determine the cause of a poisoning to provide appropriate initial care. If you see any of the signs and symptoms of sudden illness, follow the emergency action principles and the basics of care for any sudden illness.

For suspected poisonings, contact your local or regional poison centre or summon more advanced medical personnel. Beyond following the general guidelines for giving care for a suspected poisoning, medical professionals may advise you to provide some specific care, such as inducing vomiting. The best way to avoid poisoning is to take steps to prevent it.

### YOU ▼ ARE THE RESPONDER

*You are on your way to work when you see a station wagon on the highway go out of control, narrowly miss hitting other cars, bounce off a guard rail, and come to a stop, fortunately on the shoulder. You stop, go over to the car, and find the driver coughing and wheezing, and clutching his throat. You notice a red, swollen mark on his left arm, and you see a hornet buzzing on the windshield. What do you do?*

# Heat and Cold Emergencies

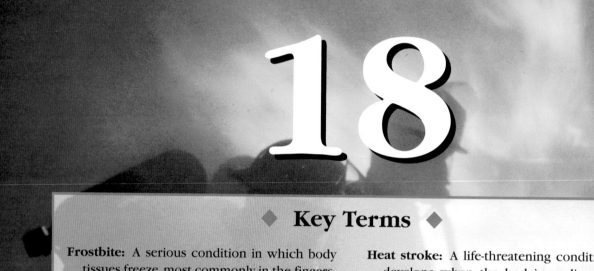

# 18

### ◆ Key Terms ◆

**Frostbite:** A serious condition in which body tissues freeze, most commonly in the fingers, toes, ears, and nose.

**Heat cramps:** Painful spasms of skeletal muscles following exercise or work in warm or moderate temperatures; usually involve the calf and abdominal muscles.

**Heat exhaustion:** A form of shock, often resulting from strenuous work or exercise in a hot environment.

**Heat stroke:** A life-threatening condition that develops when the body's cooling mechanisms are overwhelmed and body systems begin to fail.

**Hypothermia:** A life-threatening condition in which the body's warming mechanisms fail to maintain normal body temperature and the entire body cools.

## ◆ For Review ◆

Before reading this chapter, you should have a basic understanding of the functions of the circulatory and integumentary systems (Chapter 3). You should also know the signs and symptoms of shock (Chapter 10) and of sudden illness (Chapter 16).

## ◆ INTRODUCTION

*The race leader has only another 10 minutes or so to the finish line. You are part of the mobile aid team that has been following the lead pack throughout the gruelling race. At the end of the first two legs of the triathlon, you noticed that the leader had a remarkable time. He looked fresh and ready for the final leg. You knew he had trained hard for this race. But now you observe that he looks exhausted. Urged forward by the cheering crowd, the leader appears to summon up his last energies to push ahead, but instead, his legs begin to falter. He looks ill and you suddenly see him shiver, even though it is a hot day. Others begin to pass him. You hear him say he is dizzy and nauseated.*

*He states he does not remember falling. He barely remembers voices shouting for help and indistinguishable people moving him to a nearby tub of cool water. He says things are now coming into focus. The sounds around him are becoming clearer. He says he hears a siren very near. He asks if someone needs help. Suddenly, he is overwhelmed by the realization that he is the one in trouble. He is on his way to the hospital in an ambulance. His moment of glory ended—just short of the finish line. He has fallen casualty to the heat—a condition to which not even champions are immune.*

The human body is equipped to withstand extremes of temperature. Usually, its mechanisms for regulating body temperature work very well. However, when the body is overwhelmed by extremes of heat and cold, illness occurs.

Extreme temperatures can occur anywhere, both indoors and outdoors, but a person can develop a heat- or cold-related illness even if temperatures are not extreme. The effects of humidity, wind, clothing, living and working environment, physical activity, age, and an individual's health are all factors in heat- and cold-related illnesses.

Illnesses caused by exposure to temperature extremes are progressive and can become life threatening. Once the signs and symptoms of a heat- or cold-related illness begin to appear, a casualty's condition can rapidly deteriorate and lead to death. If the casualty shows any of the signs and symptoms of sudden illness, notice the weather conditions and decide if they suggest the possibility of a heat- or cold-related illness. If so, give the appropriate care. Immediate care can prevent the illness from becoming life threatening. In this chapter, you will learn how extremes of heat and cold affect the body, how to recognize temperature-related emergencies, and how to provide care.

## ◆ HOW BODY TEMPERATURE IS CONTROLLED

Body temperature must remain constant for the body to work efficiently. Normal body temperature is 37 degrees Celsius (98.6 degrees F). Body heat is generated primarily through the conversion of food to energy. Heat is also produced by muscle contractions, as in exercise or shivering.

Heat always moves from warm areas to cooler ones. Since the body is usually warmer than the surrounding air, it tends to lose heat to the air. The body maintains its temperature by constantly balancing heat loss with heat production (Fig. 18-1). The heat produced in routine activities is usually enough to balance normal heat loss.

When body heat increases, the body removes heat through the skin. Blood vessels near the

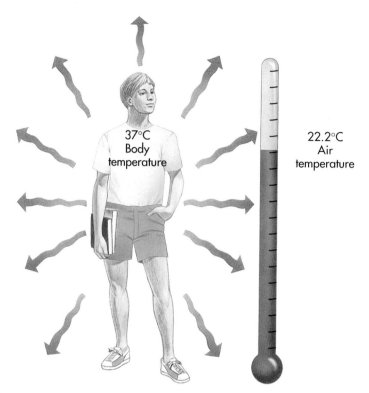

**Figure 18-1**  Since the body is usually warmer than the surrounding air, it tends to lose heat to the air.

skin dilate (widen) to bring more warm blood to the surface. Heat then escapes and the body cools (Fig. 18-2, *A*).

The body is also cooled by the evaporation of sweat. When the air temperature is very warm, dilation of blood vessels is a less effective means of removing heat. Therefore, sweating increases. But when humidity is high, sweat does not evaporate as quickly. It stays on the skin longer and has little or no cooling effect.

When the body reacts to cold, blood vessels near the skin constrict (narrow), which moves warm blood to the centre of the body. Thus less heat escapes through the skin, and the body stays warm (Fig. 18-2, *B*). When constriction of blood vessels fails to keep the body warm, shivering results. Shivering produces heat through muscle action.

Three external factors affect how well the body maintains its temperature: air temperature, humidity, and wind. Humidity and wind

multiply the effects of heat or cold. Extreme heat or cold accompanied by high humidity hampers the body's ability to effectively maintain normal body temperature (Fig. 18-3). A cold temperature combined with a strong wind rapidly cools exposed body parts. The combination of temperature and wind speed form the "wind chill factor."

Other factors, such as the clothing you wear, how often you take breaks from exposure to extreme temperature, how much and how often you drink water, and how intense your activity is, also affect how well your body manages temperature extremes. These are all factors you can control to prevent heat or cold emergencies.

## Preventing Heat or Cold Emergencies

Generally, emergencies caused by overexposure to extreme temperatures are preventable.

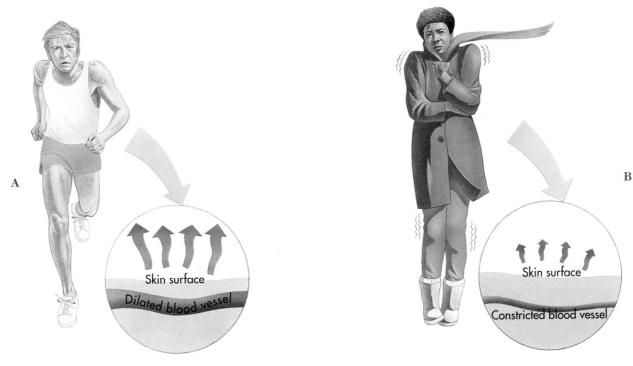

**Figure 18-2  A,** Your body removes heat by dilating the blood vessels near the skin's surface. **B,** The body conserves heat by constricting the blood vessels near the skin.

To prevent heat or cold emergencies from happening to you or anyone you know, follow these guidelines:

- Avoid being outdoors in the hottest or coldest part of the day.
- Change your activity level according to the temperature.
- Take frequent breaks.
- Dress appropriately for the environment.
- Drink large amounts of fluids.

The easiest way to prevent emergencies caused by temperature extremes is to avoid being outside during the time of day temperatures are most intense. For instance, if you plan to work outdoors in hot weather, plan your activity for the early morning and evening hours when the sun is not as strong. Likewise, if you must be outdoors on cold days, plan your activities for the warmest part of the day.

However, not everyone can avoid extremes of temperature. Often work or other situations require exposure to extreme conditions. But you can take additional precautions, such as changing your activity level and taking frequent breaks. For instance, in very hot conditions, exercise only for brief periods, then rest in a cool, shaded area. Frequent breaks allow your body to readjust to normal body temperature, enabling it to better withstand brief periods of exposure to temperature extremes (Fig. 18-4). Avoid heavy exercise during the hottest or coldest part of the day. Extremes of temperature promote fatigue, which hampers the body's ability to adjust to them.

Always wear clothing appropriate to the environmental conditions and your activity level. When possible, wear light-coloured cotton clothing in the heat. Cotton absorbs perspiration and lets air circulate through the material. This lets heat escape and perspiration evaporate, cooling the body. Light-coloured clothing reflects the sun's rays.

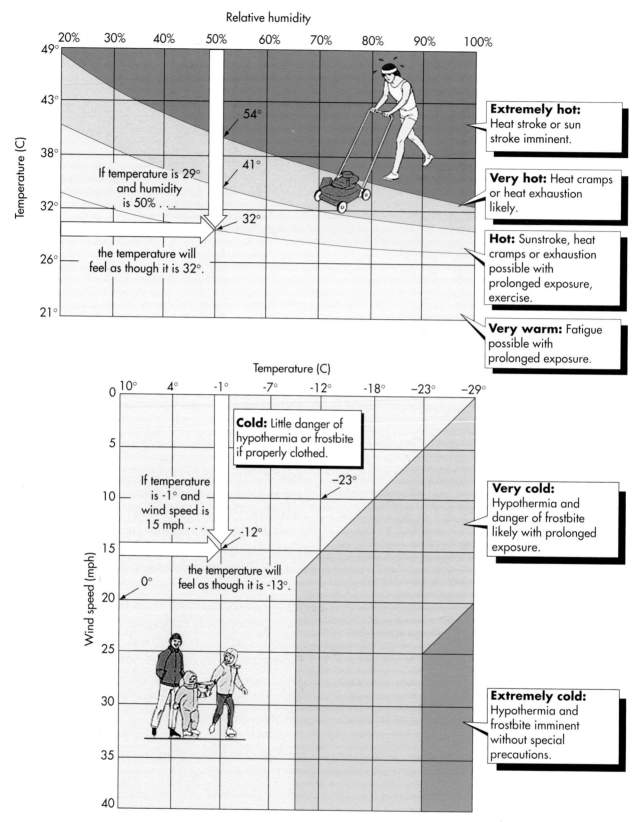

**Figure 18-3** Temperature, humidity, and wind are the three main environmental factors affecting body temperature.

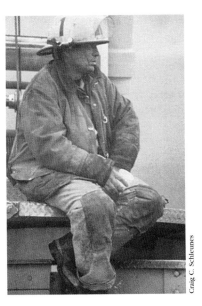

**Figure 18-4**  Taking frequent breaks when working in very hot conditions will allow your body to readjust to normal body temperature.

When you are in the cold, wear layers of clothing made of tightly woven fibres, such as wool that trap warm air against your body. Wear a head covering in both heat and cold. A hat protects the head from the sun's rays in the summer and prevents heat from escaping in the winter. Also protect other areas of the body, such as the fingers, toes, ears, and nose, from cold exposure by wearing protective coverings.

Whether in heat or cold, always drink enough fluids. Drinking plenty of fluids is the most important thing you can do to prevent heat or cold related illnesses. Plan for fluids when you take a break. Just as you would drink cool fluids in the summer, drink warm fluids in the winter. Cool and warm fluids help the body maintain a normal temperature. If cold or hot drinks are not available, drink plenty of plain water. Do not drink beverages containing caffeine or alcohol. Caffeine and alcohol hinder the body's temperature-regulating mechanism.

# ◆ PEOPLE AT RISK FOR HEAT OR COLD RELATED ILLNESSES

People at risk for heat or cold related illnesses include—

- ◆ Those who work or exercise strenuously outdoors or in unheated or poorly cooled indoor areas.
- ◆ Elderly people.
- ◆ Young children.
- ◆ Those with health problems.
- ◆ Those who have had a heat or cold related illness in the past.
- ◆ Those who have respiratory or cardiovascular disease or other conditions that cause poor circulation.
- ◆ Those who take medications (diuretics) to eliminate water from the body.

Usually, people seek relief from an extreme temperature before they begin to feel ill. However, some people do not or cannot easily escape these extremes (Fig. 18-5). Athletes and those who work outdoors or in hot, humid indoor conditions often keep working even after they develop the first signs or symptoms of illness, which they may not even recognize.

Heat and cold related illnesses occur more frequently in the elderly, especially those living in poorly ventilated and insulated buildings or in

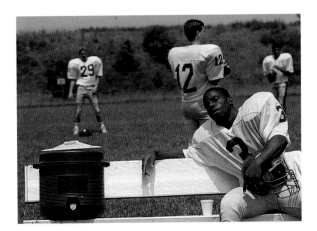

**Figure 18-5**  In certain situations it is difficult to escape temperature extremes.

buildings with poor heating or cooling systems. Young children and people with health problems are also at risk because their bodies do not respond as effectively to temperature extremes.

# ◆ HEAT EMERGENCIES

Heat cramps, heat exhaustion, and heat stroke are conditions caused by overexposure to heat. Heat cramps are the least severe but are often the first indicator of a problem. Heat exhaustion and heat stroke are more serious conditions. Heat exhaustion and heat stroke are heat related illnesses.

## Heat Cramps

*Heat cramps* are painful spasms of skeletal muscles. The exact cause is not known, although it is believed to be a combination of fluid and salt loss caused by heavy sweating. Heat cramps develop fairly rapidly and usually occur after heavy exercise or work outdoors in warm or even moderate temperatures. Heat cramps are characterized by severe muscle contractions, usually in the legs and the abdomen, but can occur in any voluntary muscle. Body temperature is usually normal, and the skin is moist. However, heat cramps may also indicate that a casualty is in the early stages of a more severe heat related emergency.

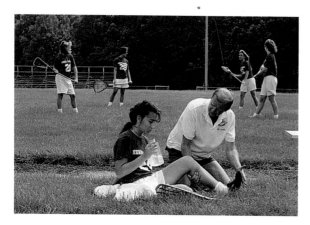

**Figure 18-6** Resting, lightly stretching the affected muscle, and drinking fluid will help the body recover from heat cramps.

To care for heat cramps, have the casualty rest comfortably in a cool place. Provide cool water or a commercial sports drink. Usually, rest and fluids are all the body needs to recover. Lightly stretch the muscle and gently massage the area (Fig. 18-6). The casualty should *not* take salt tablets or salt water. Ingesting high concentrations of salt, whether in tablet or liquid form, can increase the onset of heat related illness.

Once the cramps stop and there are no other signs or symptoms of illness, the casualty can usually resume activity. Caution the casualty to be aware of signs and symptoms of developing heat related illness. Tell the casualty to continue to drink plenty of fluids during and after activity.

## Heat Related Illnesses

### Heat Exhaustion

*Heat exhaustion* is the early stage and the most common form of heat related illness. It typically occurs after long periods of strenuous exercise or work in a hot environment. Although heat exhaustion is commonly associated with athletes, it also affects fire fighters, construction workers, factory workers, and others who work and wear heavy clothing in a hot, humid environment. Heat exhaustion is an early indication that the body's temperature-regulating mechanism is becoming overwhelmed. It is not always preceded by heat cramps. Over time, the casualty loses fluid through sweating, which decreases blood volume. Blood flow to the skin increases, reducing blood flow to the vital organs. Because the circulatory system is affected, the casualty goes into mild shock.

The signs and symptoms of heat exhaustion include—

◆ Normal or below normal body temperature.
◆ Cool, moist, pale skin. (Skin may be red in the early stage, immediately following exertion.)
◆ Headache.
◆ Nausea.
◆ Dizziness and weakness.
◆ Exhaustion.

In its early stage, heat exhaustion can usually be reversed with prompt care. Often the casualty feels better when he or she rests in a cool place and drinks cool water. If heat exhaustion is allowed to progress, the casualty's condition will worsen. Body temperature will continue to climb. A casualty may vomit and begin to show changes in his or her level of consciousness. Without prompt care, heat exhaustion can quickly advance to a more serious stage of heat related illness—heat stroke.

## Heat Stroke

*Heat stroke* is the least common and most severe heat related illness. It most often occurs when casualties ignore the signs and symptoms of heat exhaustion. Heat stroke develops when the body systems are overwhelmed by heat and begin to stop functioning. Sweating stops because body fluid levels are low. When sweating stops, the body cannot cool itself effectively, and body temperature rapidly rises. It soon reaches a level at which the brain and other vital organs, such as the heart and kidneys, begin to fail. If the body is not cooled, convulsions, coma, and death will result. Heat stroke is a *serious* medical emergency. You must recognize the signs and symptoms of this later stage of heat related illness and provide care immediately.

The signs of heat stroke include—

- High body temperature (often as high as 41 degrees Celsius or 106 degrees F).
- Red, hot, dry skin.
- Progressive loss of consciousness.
- Rapid, weak pulse.
- Rapid, shallow breathing.

Someone having a heat stroke may at first have a strong, rapid pulse, as the heart works hard to rid the body of heat by dilating blood vessels and sending more blood to the skin. As consciousness deteriorates, the circulatory system begins to fail and the pulse becomes weak and irregular. Without prompt care, the casualty will die.

## Care for Heat Related Illness

When signs or symptoms of sudden illness develop and you suspect the illness is caused by overexposure to heat, follow these general care steps immediately:

- Cool the body.
- Give fluids.
- Minimize shock.

When you recognize heat related illness in its early stages, you can usually reverse it. Remove the casualty from the hot environment and give him or her cool water to drink. Moving the casualty out of the sun or away from the heat allows the body's own temperature-regulating mechanism to recover, cooling the body more quickly.

Remove any tight or heavy clothing. Cool the body by any means available (Fig. 18-7). This can be done by applying cool, wet cloths, such as towels or sheets, to the skin. You can also fan the casualty to help increase evaporation. If you only have ice or cold packs, place them on areas such as the casualty's wrists and ankles, in each armpit, and on the neck to cool the large blood vessels. *Do not* apply rubbing (isopropyl) alcohol. Alcohol closes the skin's pores and prevents heat loss.

If the casualty is conscious, have him or her drink cool water slowly. This will help replenish the vital fluids lost through sweating. The casualty is likely to be nauseated, and water is less

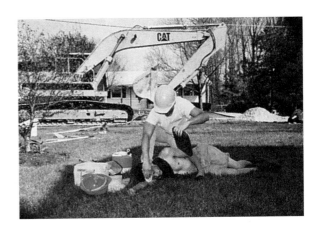

**Figure 18-7**  Cool the body of a person who has a heat related illness.

likely than other fluids to cause vomiting. It also is more quickly absorbed into the body from the stomach. Do not let the casualty drink too quickly. Give one-half glass (120 ml or 4 ounces) about every 15 minutes. Let the casualty rest in a comfortable position, and watch carefully for changes in his or her condition. Caution a casualty of heat related illness not to resume normal activities the same day.

Refusing water, vomiting, and changing level of consciousness are signs that the casualty's condition is worsening. Summon more advanced medical personnel immediately, if you have not already done so. If the casualty vomits, stop giving fluids and position the casualty on one side. Make sure the airway is clear. Monitor vital signs. Keep the casualty lying down and continue to cool the body. A casualty having a heat stroke may experience respiratory or cardiac arrest. Be prepared to do rescue breathing or CPR.

# ◆ COLD EMERGENCIES

Frostbite and hypothermia are two types of cold emergencies. Frostbite occurs in body parts exposed to the cold. *Hypothermia* is a general body cooling that develops when the body can no longer generate sufficient heat to maintain normal body temperature.

## Frostbite

*Frostbite* is the freezing of body tissues. It usually occurs in exposed areas of the body, depending on the air temperature, length of exposure, and the wind. Frostbite can affect superficial or deep tissues. In superficial frostbite, the skin is frozen but the tissues below are not. In deep frostbite, also called freezing, both the skin and underlying tissues are frozen. Both types of frostbite are serious. The water in and between the body's cells freezes and swells. The ice crystals and swelling damage or destroy the cells. Frostbite can cause the loss of fingers, hands, arms, toes, feet, and legs.

The signs and symptoms of frostbite include—

* Lack of feeling in the affected area.
* Skin that appears waxy.
* Skin that is cold to the touch.
* Skin that is discoloured (flushed, white, yellow, blue).

## Care for Frostbite

When caring for frostbite, handle the area gently. Never rub an affected area. Rubbing causes further damage because of the sharp ice crystals in the skin.

Warm the area gently by soaking the affected part in water no warmer than 38 to 40 degrees Celsius (100 degrees F to 105 degrees F). Use a thermometer to check the water, if possible. If not, test the water temperature yourself. If the temperature is uncomfortable to your touch, the water is too warm. Do not let the affected body part touch the bottom or sides of the container (Fig. 18-8, *A*). Keep the frostbitten part in the water until it appears red and feels warm. Bandage the area with a dry, sterile dressing. If fingers or toes are frostbitten, place cotton or gauze between them (Fig. 18-8, *B*). Avoid breaking any blisters. Seek professional medical attention as soon as possible.

Do not thaw the area if transport may be delayed or if there is a possibility of the area refreezing.

## Hypothermia

In hypothermia, the entire body cools when its warming mechanisms fail. The casualty will die if not given care. In hypothermia, body temperature drops below 35 degrees C (95 degrees F). Hypothermia progresses from mild to severe stages (Table 18-1). As the body temperature cools, the heart begins to beat erratically and eventually stops. Death then occurs.

The signs and symptoms of hypothermia include—

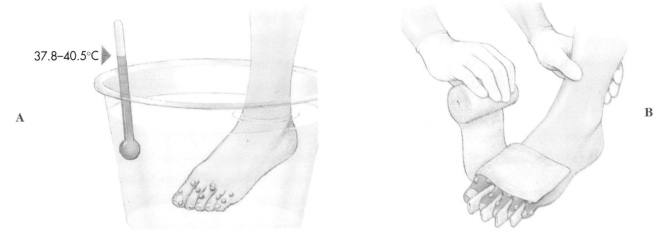

37.8–40.5°C

A

B

**Figure 18-8  A,** Warm the frostbitten area gently by soaking the area in water. Do not allow the frostbitten area to touch the container. **B,** After rewarming, bandage the area with dry, sterile dressing. If fingers or toes are frostbitten, place gauze between them.

**Table 18-1    Progression of Clinical Signs and Symptoms of Hypothermia**

| Class | Core Temperature | | Signs and Symptoms |
|---|---|---|---|
| | **°C** | **°F** | |
| Mild | 36° | 96.8° | Increased metabolic rate, maximum shivering, thermogenesis |
| | 34° | 93.2° | Impaired judgment, slurred speech |
| Moderate | 30° | 86.0° | Respiratory depression, myocardial irritability, bradycardia, atrial fibrillation, Osborne waves |
| Severe | <30° | <86.0° | Basal metabolic rate that is 50% of normal, loss of deep tendon reflexes, fixed and dilated pupils, spontaneous ventricular fibrillation |

- Shivering (may be absent in later stages).
- Slow, irregular pulse.
- Numbness.
- Glassy stare.
- Apathy and decreasing levels of consciousness.

The air temperature does not have to be below freezing for people to develop hypothermia. Elderly people in poorly heated homes, particularly people who receive poor nutrition and who get little exercise, can develop hypothermia at higher temperatures. The homeless and the ill are also at risk. Certain substances, such as alcohol and barbiturates, can also interfere with the body's normal response to cold, causing hypothermia to occur more easily. Medical conditions, such as infection, insulin reaction, stroke, and brain tumour, also make a person more susceptible. Anyone remaining in cold water or wet clothing for a prolonged time may also easily develop hypothermia.

## Care for Hypothermia

To care for hypothermia, do a primary survey and care for any life-threatening conditions. Summon more advanced medical personnel. Remove any wet clothing and dry the casualty.

Warm the body gradually by wrapping the casualty in blankets or putting on dry clothing and moving him or her to a warm environment. Hot water bottles, heating pads (if the casualty is dry), or other heat sources can aid in rewarming the body. Keep a barrier, such as a blanket, towel, or clothing, between the heat source and the casualty to avoid burning him or her. If the casualty is alert, give warm liquids to drink (Fig. 18-9). *Do not* warm the casualty too quickly, by immersing in warm water, for instance. Rapid rewarming can cause dangerous heart rhythms. Be extremely gentle in handling the casualty.

In cases of severe hypothermia, shivering will cease and the casualty may be unconscious. Breathing may have slowed or stopped. The pulse may be slow and irregular. The body may feel stiff as the muscles become rigid. Rescue breathing should be started immediately if the casualty is not breathing. Be prepared to start CPR. Before starting CPR, check the casualty's signs of circulation and pulse for up to 45 seconds. If you cannot detect a pulse or signs of circulation, begin CPR. Summon more advanced medical personnel.

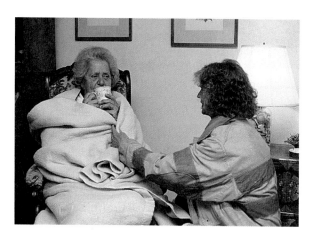

**Figure 18-9** If the hypothermia casualty is alert, give something warm to drink and rewarm the body gradually.

## ◆ SUMMARY

Overexposure to extreme heat and cold may cause a person to become ill. The likelihood of illness also depends on factors such as physical activity, clothing, wind, humidity, working and living conditions, and a person's age and physical condition.

Heat cramps are an early indication that the body's normal temperature-regulating mechanism is not working efficiently. They may signal that the casualty is in the early stage of a heat related illness. For heat related illnesses, it is important to stop physical activity, cool the body, and summon more advanced medical personnel.

Frostbite and hypothermia are serious cold related conditions, and the casualty of either needs professional medical care. Hypothermia can be life threatening. For both hypothermia and frostbite, it is important to warm the casualty. For hypothermia, warm the entire body. For frostbite, warm the affected area.

### ▼ YOU ◆ ARE THE RESPONDER

*On a winter day, you are summoned to check on an elderly woman who has not answered her phone or a neighbour's repeated attempts to get her to come to her door. You go to the house with the neighbour and knock. No one answers. The door is heavy, closed, but not locked. You enter and realize immediately that inside it is no warmer than outside. A woman bundled in a blanket is huddled close to a space heater. You speak to her and ask how she is. She appears disoriented and responds weakly. She is shivering uncontrollably. What care would you give this woman? Why?*

◆ **NOTES:**

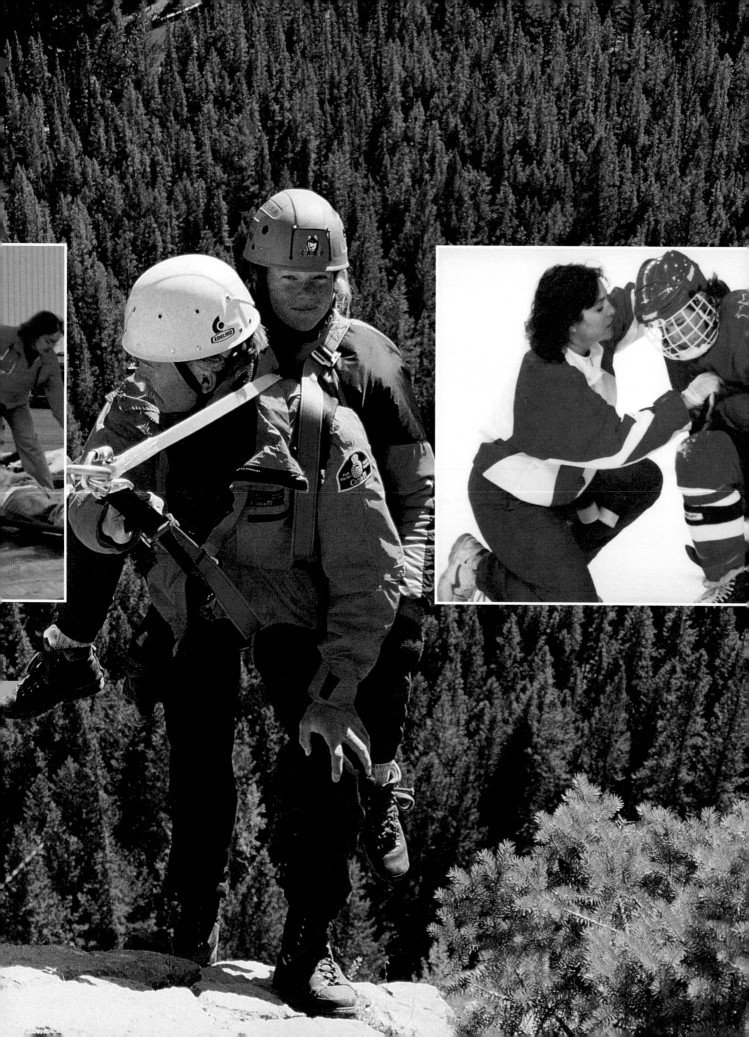

# Part Six

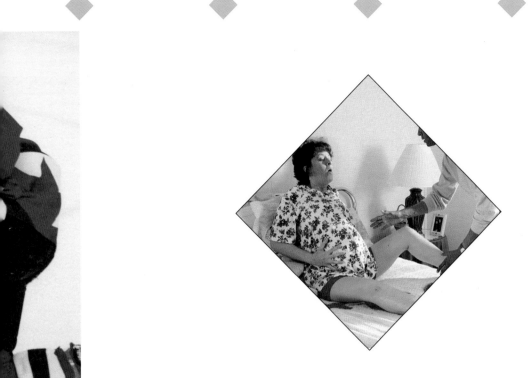

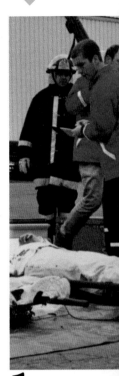

# Special Populations and Situations

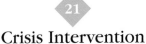

# Special Populations

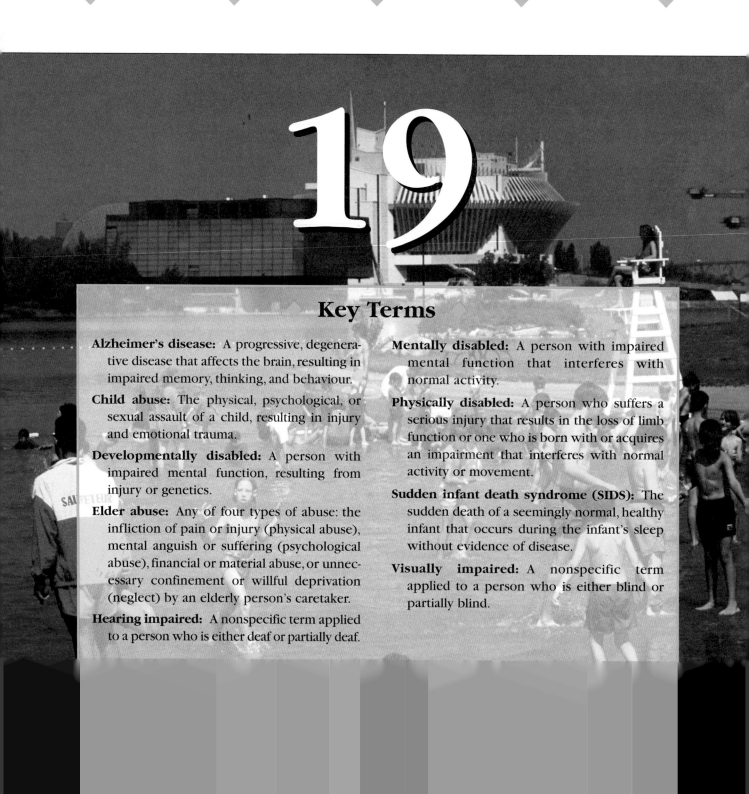

## Key Terms

**Alzheimer's disease:** A progressive, degenerative disease that affects the brain, resulting in impaired memory, thinking, and behaviour.

**Child abuse:** The physical, psychological, or sexual assault of a child, resulting in injury and emotional trauma.

**Developmentally disabled:** A person with impaired mental function, resulting from injury or genetics.

**Elder abuse:** Any of four types of abuse: the infliction of pain or injury (physical abuse), mental anguish or suffering (psychological abuse), financial or material abuse, or unnecessary confinement or willful deprivation (neglect) by an elderly person's caretaker.

**Hearing impaired:** A nonspecific term applied to a person who is either deaf or partially deaf.

**Mentally disabled:** A person with impaired mental function that interferes with normal activity.

**Physically disabled:** A person who suffers a serious injury that results in the loss of limb function or one who is born with or acquires an impairment that interferes with normal activity or movement.

**Sudden infant death syndrome (SIDS):** The sudden death of a seemingly normal, healthy infant that occurs during the infant's sleep without evidence of disease.

**Visually impaired:** A nonspecific term applied to a person who is either blind or partially blind.

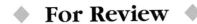

## ◆ For Review ◆

Before reading this chapter, you should have a basic understanding of how to conduct primary and secondary surveys (Chapter 5).

---

## ◆ INTRODUCTION

*You are summoned to assist an elderly man who states he is feeling ill. As you question him, you notice that he does not appear to be listening to you. In fact, the answers he gives are not consistent with your questions. Is some condition causing him to be disoriented? Is he fully conscious? Is this the way he normally behaves? Are you missing something?*

*A seven-year-old has been involved in a bike incident. She was thrown over the handlebars, landing on her head. As you approach, you notice her sitting quietly on her mother's lap. She clings to her mother and appears lethargic. Is she having a problem associated with head injury? Is this a reaction to a stranger, or is this normal behaviour for her?*

As a first responder, you are likely to encounter individuals who fit the title of "Special Populations." What makes these people special are their needs and considerations. This chapter focuses on three special populations: children, the elderly, and the mentally and physically disabled. By being able to understand the special needs of a particular person, you will be better able to communicate with him or her. As a result, you will be able to provide more effective care.

## ◆ THE PEDIATRIC CASUALTY

Nearly 10 percent of all emergency responses involve children. As a result, at some time you will probably be summoned to assist an ill or injured child. If you are, you must keep several considerations in mind. The most important is that children are not simply small adults. They have unique needs and require special care. They do not readily accept strangers. This can make it difficult to accurately assess a child's condition. Young children can be especially difficult to assess, since they often will not be able to tell you what is wrong.

It is often difficult for adults to imagine how a young child with a serious illness or injury feels. The fears that a child experiences are real. One of a child's primary emotions is fear. A child is afraid of the unknown. He or she is afraid of being ill or hurt, of being touched by strangers, and of being separated from his or her parents. Being aware of the fears of a child and knowing how to cope with them will enable you to provide more effective care.

### Assessing the Child

When assessing a child, follow the same steps as for an adult. That is, you do the primary survey first. Any problems that threaten the child's airway, breathing, and circulation must be taken care of as soon as they are found. Once you have completed the primary survey, you can begin the secondary survey.

During the secondary survey, you will interview the casualty and any bystanders, such as the child's parent or adult guardian. How you interact with the child and the parent or guardian is very important. You must establish a good rapport. This means reducing anxiety and panic in both child and parent or guardian. There are a few basic guidelines that will help you assess an injured or ill child.

◆ **Observe the child before touching him or her.** Information can be obtained before actually touching the child. Look for signs that indicate changes in the level of consciousness, any breathing difficulty, and any apparent injuries or conditions. All may change as soon as you touch the child because he or she may become anxious or upset.

- **Communicate clearly with the parent or guardian and the child.** If the family is excited or agitated, the child is likely to be so too. When you can calm the family, the child will often calm down as well. Explain what you wish to do. Get at eye level with the child (Fig. 19-1). Talk slowly and use simple words when speaking with the child. Ask questions that can be easily answered.
- **Remain calm.** Caring for children, especially those who are seriously ill or injured, can be very stressful. Calmness on your part will show confidence and help keep the child and parent or guardian calm.
- **Do not separate the child from loved ones unless necessary.** This is especially true for younger children (under age 7 or 8). Often a parent or guardian will be holding a crying child. In this case, you can assess the child's condition while the parent or guardian continues to hold the child (Fig. 19-2).
- **Gain trust through your actions.** Explain to the child and parent or guardian what you are going to do before you do it. Be sure to use terms and language appropriate for the child's age.

In doing the secondary survey, it is often easier to do the head-to-toe examination before you check vital signs. Furthermore, the head-to-toe examination is often better performed in reverse order, as a toe-to-head examination, on a conscious child. The child is more likely to accept you first touching the feet and progressing to the head. You should still look and feel for the same things.

As you may recall, children up to 1 year of age are commonly referred to as **infants.** Young infants, those less than 6 months old, are relatively easy to examine. Your presence will not generally bother children of this age group. Older infants, however, will often exhibit "stranger anxiety." They are uncomfortable around strangers and may cry and cling to a parent or guardian.

Children 1 and 2 years of age are called **toddlers.** These children are frequently uncooperative. As a result, they are often best examined in the parent's or guardian's lap. A toddler will be concerned that he or she will be separated from the parent or guardian. Reassurance that this will not happen will often comfort a concerned child of this age.

Children aged 3, 4, and 5 are generally referred to as **preschoolers.** Children in this age group are usually easy to examine if approached properly. Use their natural curiosity. Allow them to inspect equipment or supplies, such as oxygen tubing or bandages. This can allay many fears and distract them during your assessment.

**School-aged** children are those between 6 and 12 years of age. They are usually cooperative and can be a good source of information regarding what happened. You should be readily

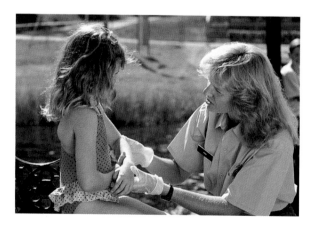

**Figure 19-1** You must communicate clearly with a child casualty.

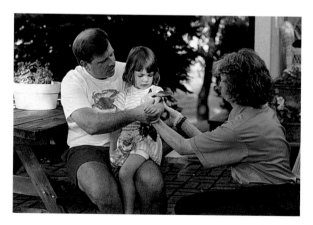

**Figure 19-2** Allow a parent to hold the child while you do the head-to-toe examination.

able to converse with them. Children in this age group are becoming conscious of their bodies and do not like exposure. Respect the child's modesty.

**Adolescents** are between 13 and 18 years of age. They are typically more adult than child. Direct questions to them instead of to parents or guardians. However, allow input from a parent or guardian. Occasionally, in the presence of a parent or guardian, it may not be possible to get an accurate history. Adolescents do not like having their bodies exposed and often respond better to a caregiver of the same gender. Respect the adolescent's modesty.

When checking a child's vital signs, such as breathing and pulse, during the secondary survey, do not be alarmed at finding faster rates. A child's resting pulse and breathing are normally faster than that of an adult. A normal resting heart rate for an adult ranges from 60 to 100 beats per minute. Infants and toddlers, on the other hand, have normal resting heart rates from approximately 100 to 160 beats per minute. As the child ages, his or her resting heart rate will become slower. By the time the child reaches adolescence, his or her resting heart rate will be approximately the same as an adult's.

This is also true for a child's breathing rate. In response to a heart that is beating faster, the child also breathes faster. Average resting breathing rates for preadolescent children are 20 to 40 breaths per minute.

## Special Problems

### Injury

Injury remains the number one cause of death for children in Canada. Many of these deaths result from motor vehicle crashes. The greatest dangers to a child involved in a vehicle incident that results in serious injury are airway obstruction and bleeding. Because a child's head is usually large in proportion to the rest of the body, the head is often injured.

To avoid some of the needless deaths of children associated with motor vehicles, laws requiring safety seats and seat belts have been imposed. As a result, more lives will be saved but also more injured children will need to be cared for while in car seats (Fig. 19-3). A car seat does not normally pose any problem when you are trying to assess a child. A child involved in a motor vehicle crash and found in a car seat should be left in the car seat if the device has not been damaged. If the child is to be transported to a medical facility for evaluation, he or she can be easily secured in the car seat.

### High Fever

A high fever in a child indicates some type of infection. Because a young child's temperature-regulating mechanism has not fully developed, even a minor infection can result in a rather high fever. This is often defined as a temperature above 39 degrees Celsius (103 degrees F). Prolonged or excessively high fever can result in seizures known as febrile seizures. Summon more advanced medical personnel. Your initial care for a child with high fever is to gently cool the child. This includes removing excessive clothing or blankets and sponging lukewarm water on the child.

### Respiratory Distress

Infections of the respiratory system are more common in children than adults. These can range from minor infections, such as the

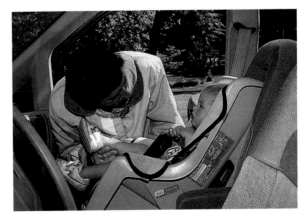

**Figure 19-3** A child involved in a motor vehicle crash and found in a car seat should be left in the car seat if the device has not been damaged.

common cold, to life-threatening infections that block the airway. Signs and symptoms of respiratory distress in children include—

- Unusually fast or slow breathing.
- Noisy breathing.
- Skin discolouration.
- Retraction of the spaces between the ribs during breathing.
- Diminished level of consciousness.

A common childhood illness that causes respiratory distress is croup. Croup is a viral infection that causes swelling of the tissues below the vocal cords. Besides the basic signs and symptoms of respiratory distress and a cough that sounds like the bark of a seal, croup is often preceded by 1 or 2 days of illness, sometimes with a fever. Croup occurs more often in the winter months, and the signs and symptoms of croup are often more evident in the evening. It generally is not life threatening. The child will often improve when exposed to cool air, such as the air outdoors or cool steam from a vaporizer.

Another childhood problem is epiglottitis, a bacterial infection that causes a severe inflammation of the epiglottis. You may recall that the epiglottis is a flap of tissue above the vocal cords that protects the airway during swallowing. When it becomes infected, it can swell to a point at which the airway is completely obstructed. The child with epiglottitis will appear quite ill and have a high fever. He or she will often be sitting up and straining to breathe. The child will be very frightened. Saliva will often be drooling from his or her mouth. This is because swelling of the epiglottis prevents the child from swallowing.

You will not need to distinguish between croup and epiglottitis, since the care you provide will be the same for either situation. To care for a child in respiratory distress, allow him or her to remain in the most comfortable position for breathing and administer oxygen. Do not attempt to place any object in the child's mouth or examine the mouth. Summon more advanced medical personnel immediately. This is extremely important because the child needs immediate transport to a medical facility.

## Child Abuse

Child abuse is unfortunately an all too common occurrence in our society. *Child abuse* commonly refers to the physical, psychological, or sexual assault of a child, resulting in injuries and emotional trauma. Children of all ages are victimized. You should suspect child abuse if a child's injuries are not consistent with the explanation you are given by the child or parent or guardian as to what happened.

The child abuser can come from any geographic, ethnic, religious, occupational, or socioeconomic background. The abuser is most often a parent or an adult guardian. The signs of child abuse include—

- Obvious fractures in a child less than 2 years of age.
- Injuries in various stages of healing, especially bruises and burns.
- More injuries than are usually seen in a child of the same age.
- An injury that does not fit the description of what caused the injury.

When caring for a child who may have been abused, always care for the child's injuries first. An abused child may be frightened, hysterical, or withdrawn. He or she may be unwilling to talk about the incident in an attempt to protect the abuser. As you provide care for any injuries, attempt to talk with the child. Do not make any accusations. Instead, explain your concerns to responding law enforcement or EMS personnel. Accurately complete an incident report, noting in detail anything you were told and any injuries you noted when you first examined the child.

## Sudden Infant Death Syndrome (SIDS)

*Sudden infant death syndrome (SIDS)* is defined as the sudden death of a seemingly healthy infant that occurs during the infant's sleep and without evidence of disease. Usually, a thorough medical examination fails to reveal a cause of death. SIDS is sometimes mistaken for child abuse because of the unexplained death of an otherwise normal child and the bruiselike blotches on the casualty's body. However, SIDS is not related to child abuse. It is not caused by vomiting and aspiration of stomach contents. It is also not believed to be hereditary but does tend to recur in families. What causes SIDS is not yet clear. You will not be able to "diagnose" SIDS. When the infant is found, he or she will be in cardiac arrest. You should care for the infant as you would other cardiac arrest casualties.

## ◆ THE ELDERLY CASUALTY

The elderly are generally considered those over 65 years of age. These individuals are quickly becoming the fastest growing population group in Canada. A major reason for this occurrence is an increase in life expectancy because of advances in health care. Since 1900, there has been a 53 percent increase in life expectancy. For example, in 1900, the average life expectancy was 49 years. Today, the average life expectancy exceeds 75 years.

There are many changes that occur with age. Overall, there is a general decline in body function, with some changes beginning as early as age 30. One of the first body systems affected by age is the respiratory system. The capacity of the respiratory system begins to decrease around age 30. By the time we reach age 65, our respiratory system may be only half as effective as it was in our youth. The heart also suffers the effects of aging. The amount of blood pumped by the heart with each beat decreases, and the heart rate slows. The blood vessels harden, causing increased work for the heart. The number of functioning brain cells also decreases with age. Hearing and vision usually decline, often causing some degree of sight and hearing loss. Reflexes become slower, and arthritis may affect joints, causing movement to become painful.

As a result of slower reflexes, failing eyesight and hearing, arthritis, and problems, such as numbness, related to the blood vessels, the elderly are at increased risk of injury from falls. Falls frequently result in fractures because the bones become weaker and more brittle with age.

An elderly person is also at increased risk of serious head injuries. This is primarily because of the difference in proportion between the brain and the skull. As we age, the size of the brain decreases, which results in increased space between the surface of the brain and the inside of the skull. This allows more movement of the brain within the skull, which can increase the likelihood of serious head injury. Occasionally, an elderly casualty may not develop the symptoms of a head injury until days after a fall. Therefore, you should always suspect a head injury as a possible cause of unusual behaviour in an elderly casualty, especially if there is a history of a fall or blow to the head.

The elderly are also prone to nervous system disorders. The most common in the elderly is stroke, discussed in Chapter 16. In addition, the elderly are at increased risk of altered thinking patterns and confusion. Some deterioration in mental function caused by aging is normal. The most common of these is ***Alzheimer's disease,*** a progressive, degenerative disease that affects the brain. It results in impaired memory, thinking, and behaviour.

If you are providing care for a confused elderly casualty, try to determine whether the confusion is the result of injury or a preexisting condition. Get at the casualty's eye level so he or she can see and hear you more clearly (Fig. 19-4). Sometimes confusion is actually the result of decreased vision or hearing.

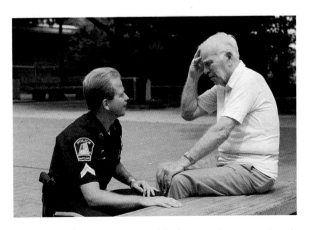

**Figure 19-4** Speak to an elderly casualty at eye level.

Your care for the elderly casualty requires you to keep in mind the special problems and concerns of the elderly and to communicate appropriately. Often, an elderly casualty's problem will seem insignificant to him or her. However, he or she may not recognize the signs or symptoms of a serious condition. For example, an elderly person may complain of weakness. On further questioning, you may learn that she has been having fainting episodes with periods of numbness and tingling in one side of the body. Some elderly casualties may purposely minimize their symptoms from fear of losing their independence or of being placed in a nursing home or similar institution. If the casualty takes medications, you should gather them and see that they are with the casualty if he or she is being taken to a medical facility.

## Elder Abuse

Elder abuse is a growing problem in our society. **Elder abuse** involves any of four types of abuse: the infliction of pain or injury (physical abuse), mental anguish or suffering (psychological abuse), financial or material abuse, or unnecessary confinement or willful deprivation (neglect) by an elderly person's caretaker. Typically the abuser is a relative and lives with the abused elder.

The signs and symptoms of elder abuse generally include any unexplained injury or any physical situation in which the elderly person seems to be being neglected. Provincial laws may require the reporting of such abuse if suspected. Follow your local protocol.

## ◆ THE PHYSICALLY OR MENTALLY DISABLED CASUALTY

Other special populations include those with physical or mental disabilities. The terms *physical disability* and *mental disability* mean different things to different people. What comes to mind when you hear these words? A person who uses a wheelchair? An amputee? Someone said to be mentally retarded?

Though these are examples of physical or mental disabilities, the individuals facing these challenges are not without a future. A person who suffers a serious injury that results in the loss of a limb, or who is born lacking a limb, is often referred to as *physically disabled.* So is someone who suffers the paralysing effects of a stroke.

A *mentally disabled* person has an impairment of mental function that interferes with normal activity. Anyone at any age can find himself or herself challenged by a physical or mental impairment that interferes to some degree with normal activities. Some of the more common types of mental or physical disabilities that you will encounter include persons who are visually impaired, hearing impaired, and physically and developmentally disabled.

## Visually Impaired

People who are unable to see adequately or at all are often called blind or partially blind. These people are also said to be *visually impaired.* Blindness can occur from many causes. Some persons are born blind. Others are born with the ability to see, then subsequently lose it through injury or illness. Visual impairment is not necessarily a problem in the eyes. It can occur because of problems in the visual centres of the brain.

Persons who are visually impaired have usually adapted well to their condition and are not embarrassed by it. It should be no more difficult to communicate with this casualty than with one who can see. It is not necessary to speak loudly or in overly simple terms. In fact, your assessment of the visually impaired casualty should be little different from one of a casualty who is not impaired. The casualty may not be able to tell you certain things about how an injury occurred but can generally give you a good description based on his or her interpretation of sounds and touch.

If you are called to assist a casualty who is visually impaired, explain to him or her what is going on and what you are doing. This will help alleviate anxiety. It will also allow the casualty to orient himself or herself to the environment and then provide you with information regarding his or her care. If you must move a blind casualty who can walk, stand beside the casualty and have the casualty hold on to your arm (Fig. 19-5). Walk at a normal pace and alert him or her to any hazards, such as stairs, during the move. If the casualty has a seeing eye dog, try to keep them together. These dogs are usually not aggressive.

## Hearing Impaired

Persons who are unable to hear or who experience any other type of hearing disability are termed ***hearing impaired*** and are often referred to as deaf or partially deaf. Deafness can occur as a result of injury or illness affecting the ear, the nerves leading from the ear to the brain, or the brain itself. As with blindness, deafness can be present at birth or can develop later because of injury or illness. Some rescuers become anxious when called to treat a hearing-impaired casualty. This anxiety is unfounded. Casualties with a hearing impairment should be cared for in basically the same manner as the hearing. You may only have to modify your assessment somewhat so that you can obtain necessary information.

You may not even be aware initially that a casualty is deaf. Often, the casualty will tell you. Others may point at their ear and shake their head, "No." A child may carry a card stating that he or she is deaf. You may see a hearing aid in a casualty's ear. The biggest obstacle you must overcome in caring for the hearing impaired is how to best communicate (Fig. 19-6). If you know how to use sign language, then you may communicate in this manner. Often the casualty will be able to read lips. If the casualty's illness or injury does not distract from the ability to read your lips, then communicate in this manner. Position yourself where the casualty can see you. You must look at the casualty when you speak and speak slowly. Do not modify the way you form words. If the casualty cannot read lips and communication through sign is impossible, you can write messages on paper and have the casualty respond. This system is slow, but effective. Some hearing-impaired people have a machine called a Telecommunications Device for the Deaf (TDD), which is generally used for telephone communication. You can use this device to type messages and questions to the casualty, and the casualty can type replies to you.

Hearing-impaired casualties are usually not embarrassed by their condition. They have adapted to it by learning to lip read, sign, or both. Most deaf casualties can also speak. One casualty's speech will be quite clear, whereas another's will be more difficult to understand. If you do not understand what the casualty is saying, ask him or her to repeat. Do not pretend that you understand.

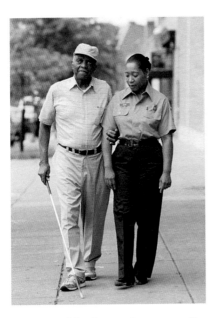

**Figure 19-5**  If a blind casualty can walk, stand beside the casualty and have him or her hold your arm.

## Physically Disabled

The term ***physically disabled*** also refers to a person who is unable to move normally. The

A
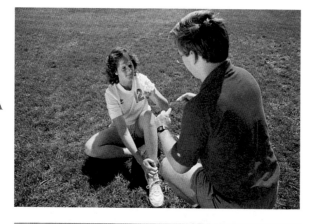

B
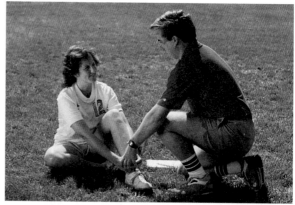

C
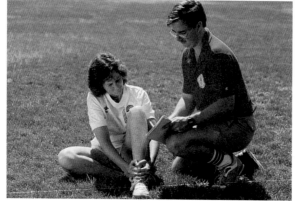

D
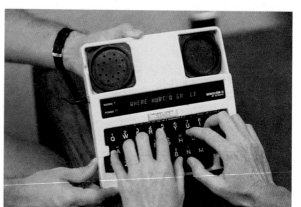

**Figure 19-6**  Communicate with a hearing-impaired casualty in the best way possible: **A,** signing; **B,** lip reading; **C,** writing; **D,** TDD.

impairments causing a disability can be diverse. Physical impairments are generally the result of problems with the muscles or bones or the nerves controlling them. Causes include stroke, cerebral palsy, multiple sclerosis, muscular dystrophy, polio, and brain and spinal cord injuries. Some physically disabled persons have adapted well to their situation and others have not. Care for the person who is physically disabled with respect and compassion. You will often need to be very patient. Many persons have adapted to life without assistance, so be careful not to make assumptions about a person's ability.

The physically disabled person who is injured poses unique problems because it may be difficult to determine which problems are new and which are preexisting conditions. If this situation occurs, care for any detected problems as if they are new, and you can hardly go wrong.

## Developmentally Disabled

Impairment of mental function occurs with greater frequency than you might expect. A person who is mentally challenged is often labelled *developmentally disabled.* As with physical impairments, mental impairments also can be diverse. Some types of mental impairment, such as Down's syndrome, are genetic. Others result from injuries or infections that occur during pregnancy, after birth, or later in life. Some occur for reasons never determined.

Often, you will be able to determine easily whether a casualty is developmentally disabled. However, in some situations, you will not be able to determine this. Always approach the casualty as you would any other person in his or her age group. When you speak, try to determine the casualty's level of understanding. If the casualty is confused, rephrase your statement or question in simpler terms. Listen carefully to what the casualty is saying. Casualties who are developmentally disabled often lead very orderly lives. A sudden illness or injury can interrupt this order and cause a great deal of anxiety and fear. You should expect this and offer reassurance. Take time to explain to the casualty who you are and what you are going to do. Try to gain the casualty's trust. If a parent or guardian is present, ask him or her to assist you in providing care.

◆ **SUMMARY**

As a first responder, you will likely be called to assist a wide variety of special populations. When dealing with children, remember that they are not small adults. They must be approached gently and in a manner appropriate for their age. You need to recognize and try to alleviate their fears. Your assessment will be modified slightly because of the special needs of the child. Certain illnesses, such as croup and epiglottitis, can cause respiratory distress that should be cared for promptly. When caring for

the child, do not forget the parent or guardian. They can make your job easier, so allow them to remain with the ill or injured child and to assist in care when appropriate.

Besides the pediatric casualty, you are likely to encounter an elderly person or a person with a physical or mental disability. Remember to care for these individuals based on individual need. You should recognize their limitations and work around them. As with the pediatric casualty, proper communication will be the most important thing for you to establish.

### YOU ARE THE RESPONDER

*A six-year-old has been struck in the face by a swing seat pushed by a playmate. The incident occurred at a playground adjacent to a ball field where you are located. A distraught older girl is carrying the bleeding child toward you. The child is screaming and is bleeding from a laceration to the forehead and upper lip. Blood is draining into the child's mouth. Describe how you would care for this child.*

# Childbirth

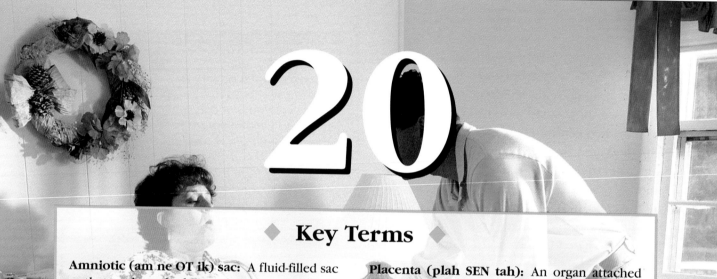

## ♦ Key Terms ♦

**Amniotic (am ne OT ik) sac:** A fluid-filled sac that encloses, bathes, and protects the developing baby; commonly called the bag of waters.

**Birth canal:** The passageway from the uterus to the vaginal opening through which a baby passes during birth.

**Breech birth:** The delivery of a baby feet or buttocks first.

**Cervix:** The upper part of the birth canal.

**Contraction:** The rhythmic tightening of muscles in the uterus during labour.

**Crowning:** The time in labour when the baby's head is at the opening of the vagina.

**Labour:** The birth process; beginning with the contraction of the uterus and dilation of the cervix and ending with the stabilization and recovery of the mother.

**Placenta (plah SEN tah):** An organ attached to the uterus and unborn child through which nutrients are delivered to the baby; expelled after the baby is delivered.

**Prolapsed cord:** A complication of childbirth in which a loop of umbilical cord protrudes through the vagina prior to delivery of the baby.

**Umbilical cord:** A flexible structure that attaches the placenta to the unborn child, allowing for the passage of blood, nutrients, and waste.

**Uterus:** A pear-shaped organ in a woman's pelvis in which an embryo forms and develops into a baby.

**Vagina:** The lower part of the birth canal.

**For Review**

Before reading this chapter, you should have a basic understanding of the reproductive system (Chapter 3).

## ◆ INTRODUCTION

*A woman calls 9-1-1 or the local EMS number and asks for an ambulance. She says she thinks her baby is coming fast. The response time of the ambulance to reach her rural home is nearly 25 minutes. A police officer nearby hears the call on her radio and decides to help until ambulance personnel arrive.*

*As the officer approaches the house, she notices the front door is partially opened. She goes in and finds the woman lying on the floor, in obvious pain. She sees bloody fluid on the floor. When she examines the woman, she sees the infant's head at the opening of the birth canal. Childbirth is occurring and will not wait for the ambulance crew to arrive. The police officer prepares to help deliver the baby.*

Someday you may be faced with a similar situation, requiring that you assist with childbirth. If you have never seen or experienced childbirth, your expectations probably consist of what others have told you.

Terms such as exhausting, stressful, exciting, fulfilling, painful, and scary are sometimes used to describe a planned childbirth, one that occurs in the hospital or at home under the supervision of a health-care provider. If you find yourself assisting with the delivery of a baby, however, it is probably not happening in a planned situation. Therefore, your feelings, as well as those of the expectant mother, may be intensified by fear of the unexpected or the possibility that something might go wrong.

Take comfort in knowing that things rarely go wrong. Childbirth is a natural process. Thousands of children all over the world are born each day, without complications, in areas where no medical assistance is available during childbirth.

By following a few simple steps, you can effectively assist in the birth process. This chapter will help you better understand the birth process, how to assist with the delivery of a baby, how to provide care for both the mother and newborn, how to recognize complications, and what complications could require more advanced care.

## ◆ PREGNANCY

**Pregnancy** begins when an egg (ovum) is fertilized by a sperm, forming an **embryo.** The embryo implants itself within the mother's **uterus,** a pear-shaped organ that lies at the top centre of the pelvis. The embryo is surrounded by the **amniotic sac.** This is a fluid-filled sac also called the "bag of waters." The fluid is constantly renewed and helps protect the baby from injury and infection.

As the embryo grows, its organs and body parts develop. After about 8 weeks, the embryo is called a **fetus.** To continue to develop properly, the fetus must receive nutrients. The fetus receives these nutrients from the mother through a specialized organ attached to the uterus called the **placenta.** The placenta is attached to the fetus by a flexible structure called the **umbilical cord.** The fetus will continue to develop for approximately 40 weeks (about 9 months), at which time the birth process will begin (Fig. 20-1).

## ◆ THE BIRTH PROCESS

The birth process begins with the onset of labour. **Labour** is the final phase of pregnancy. It is a process in which many systems work together to bring about birth. Labour begins with a rhythmic contraction of the uterus. As these contractions continue, they dilate the **cervix**—a short tube of muscle at the upper end of the **birth canal,** the passageway from

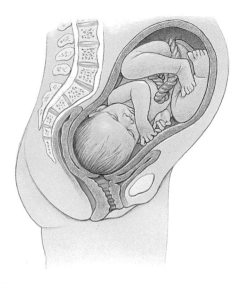

**Figure 20-1** Mother and fetus at 40 weeks.

the uterus to the vaginal opening. When the cervix is sufficiently dilated, it allows the baby to travel from the uterus through the birth canal. The baby passes through the birth canal and emerges from the *vagina,* the lower end of the canal, to the outside world. For first-time mothers, this process normally takes between 12 and 24 hours. Subsequent babies are usually delivered more quickly.

## The Labour Process

The labour process has four distinct stages. The length and intensity of each stage vary.

## Stage One—Preparation

In the first stage, the mother's body prepares for the birth. This stage covers the period of time from the first contraction until the cervix is fully dilated. A *contraction* is a rhythmic tightening of the muscles in the uterus. It is like a wave. It begins gently, rises to a peak of intensity, then drops off and subsides. The muscles then relax, and there is a break before the next contraction starts. As the time for delivery approaches, the contractions become closer together, last longer, and feel stronger. Normally, when contractions are less than 3 minutes apart, childbirth is near.

## Stage Two—Delivery of the Baby

The second stage of labour involves the actual delivery of the baby. It begins once the cervix is completely dilated and ends with the birth of a baby. The baby's head will become visible as it emerges from the vagina. When the top of the head begins to emerge, it is called *crowning* (Fig. 20-2). When crowning occurs, birth is imminent and you must be prepared to receive the baby.

## Stage Three—Delivery of the Placenta

Once the baby's body emerges, the third stage of labour begins. During this stage, the placenta usually separates from the wall of the uterus and exits from the birth canal. This process normally occurs within 20 minutes of the delivery of the baby.

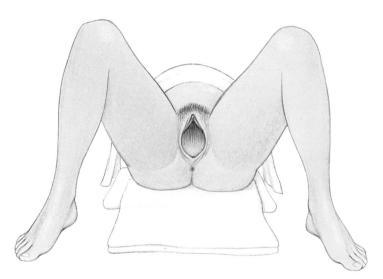

**Figure 20-2** When crowning begins, birth is imminent.

Chapter 20 *Childbirth* ◆ **357**

## Stage Four—Stabilization

The final stage of labour involves the initial recovery and stabilization of the mother after childbirth. Normally, this stage lasts for approximately 1 hour. During this time, the uterus contracts to control bleeding and the mother begins to recover from the physical and emotional stress that occurred during childbirth.

## Assessing Labour

If you are called to assist a pregnant woman, you will want to determine whether she is in labour. If she is in labour, you should determine how far along she is in the birth process and whether she expects any complications. You can determine these factors by asking a few key questions and making some quick observations. Ask the following:

- Is this the first pregnancy? The first stage of labour normally takes longer with first pregnancies than with subsequent ones.
- Has the amniotic sac ruptured? When this happens, fluid flows from the vagina in a sudden gush or a trickle. Some women think they have lost control of their bladder. The breaking of the sac usually signals the beginning of labour. People often describe the rupture of the sac as "the water breaking."
- What are the contractions like? Are they very close together? Are they strong? The length and intensity of the contractions will give you valuable information about the progress of labour. As labour progresses, contractions become stronger, last longer, and are closer together.
- Is there a bloody discharge? This pink or light red, thick discharge from the vagina is the mucous plug that falls from the cervix as it begins to dilate, also signalling the onset of labour.
- Does she have an urge to bear down? If the expectant mother expresses a strong urge to push, this signals that labour is far along.
- Is the baby crowning? If the baby's head is visible, the baby is about to be born.

## ◆ PREPARING FOR DELIVERY

## Preparing Yourself

There comes a time when you realize that you are about to assist with childbirth. Though this is often exciting, it is rarely comforting. Childbirth is messy. It involves a discharge of watery, sometimes bloody, fluid at stages one and two of labour and what appears to be a rather large loss of blood after stage two. Try not to be alarmed at the loss of blood. It is a normal part of the birth process. Only bleeding that cannot be controlled after the baby is born is a problem. Take a deep breath and try to relax. Remember that you are only assisting in the process; the expectant mother is doing all the work.

## Helping the Mother Cope With Labour and Delivery

Explain to the expectant mother that the baby is about to be born. Be calm and reassuring. A woman having her first child often feels fear and apprehension about the pain and the condition of the baby. Labour pain ranges from discomfort similar to menstrual cramps to intense pressure or pain. Many women experience something in between. Factors that can increase pain and discomfort during the first stage of labour include—

- Irregular breathing.
- Tensing up because of fear.
- Not knowing what to expect.
- Feeling alone and unsupported.

You can help the expectant mother cope with the discomfort and pain of labour. Begin by reassuring her that you are there to help. Explain what to expect as labour progresses. Suggest specific physical activities that she can do to relax, such as regulating her breathing. Ask her to breathe in slowly and deeply through the nose and out through the mouth. Ask her to try to focus on one object in the room while regulating her breathing. By staying calm, firm, and confident and offering encouragement, you can help reduce fear and apprehension. This will aid in reducing pain and discomfort.

The use of slow, deep breathing through the mouth during labour can help in several ways:

- Aids muscle relaxation.
- Offers a distraction from the pain of strong contractions as labour progresses.
- Ensures adequate oxygen to both the mother and the baby during labour.

Taking childbirth classes, such as those offered at local hospitals, can help you become more competent in techniques used to help the expectant mother relax.

## ◆ ASSISTING WITH DELIVERY

It is difficult to predict how much time you have before the baby is delivered. However, if the expectant mother says that she feels the need to push or feels as if she has to have a bowel movement, delivery is near.

You should time the expectant mother's contractions from the beginning of one contraction to the beginning of the next. If they are less than 2 minutes apart, prepare to assist with the delivery of the baby.

Assisting with the delivery of the baby is often a simple process. The expectant mother is doing all the work. Your job is to create a clean environment and to help guide the baby from the birth canal, minimizing the possibility of injury to the mother and baby. Begin by positioning the mother. She should be lying on her back, with her head and upper back raised, not lying flat. Her legs should be bent, with the knees drawn up and apart (Fig. 20-3, *A*). Positioning the mother in this way will make her more comfortable.

Next, establish a clean environment for delivery. Since it is unlikely that you will have sterile supplies, use items such as clean sheets, blankets, towels, or even clothes. To make the area around the mother as sanitary as possible,

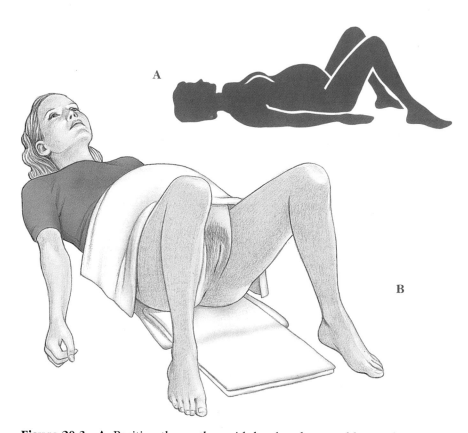

**Figure 20-3**  **A,** Position the mother with her legs bent and knees drawn up and apart.
**B,** Place clean sheets, blankets, towels, or even clothes under the mother.

place these items over the mother's abdomen and under her buttocks and legs (Fig. 20-3, *B*). Keep a clean, warm towel or blanket handy to wrap the newborn. Because you will be coming in contact with the mother's and baby's body fluids, be sure to wear disposable gloves. Wear goggles and a disposable gown, if available, to protect yourself from splashing.

Other items that can be helpful include a bulb syringe to suction secretions from the infant's mouth and nose, gauze or sanitary pads to help absorb secretions and vaginal bleeding, a large plastic bag or towel to hold the placenta after delivery, and oxygen if available.

As crowning occurs, place a hand on the top of the baby's head and apply light pressure (Fig. 20-4). In this way, you allow the head to emerge slowly, not forcefully. This will help prevent tearing of the vagina and injury to the baby. At this point, the expectant mother should stop pushing. Instruct the mother to concentrate on her breathing techniques. Have her "pant like a dog." This technique will help her stop pushing and help prevent a forceful birth.

As the head emerges, the baby will turn to one side (Fig. 20-5). This will enable the shoulders and the rest of the body to pass through the birth canal. Check to see if the umbilical cord is looped around the baby's neck. If it is, gently slip it over the baby's head. If this cannot be done, slip it over the baby's shoulders as they emerge. The baby can slide through the loop.

Guide one shoulder out at a time. Do not pull the baby. As the baby emerges, he or she will be wet and slippery. Use a clean towel to catch the baby. Place the baby on its side, between the mother and you. In this way, you can provide initial care without fear of dropping the newborn. If possible, note the time the baby was born.

Leave the cord in place and do not pull on it. Clamp or tie the cord while waiting for the placenta to be delivered. Use strips of sterile cloth tied tightly at two different locations 10 and 15 centimetres (4 and 6 inches) away from the infant. Do not cut the cord.

## ◆ CARING FOR THE NEWBORN AND MOTHER

### Caring for the Newborn

The first few minutes of the baby's life are a difficult transition from life inside the mother's uterus to life outside. You have two priorities at this point. Your first is to see that the baby's airway is open and clear. Since a newborn baby breathes primarily through the nose, it is important to immediately clear the mouth and nasal

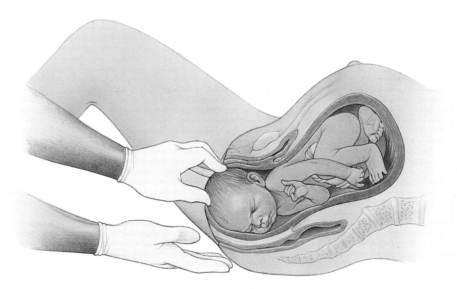

**Figure 20-4** Place your hand on top of the baby's head and apply light pressure.

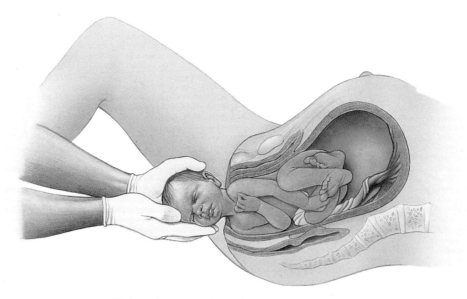

**Figure 20-5**   As the infant emerges, support the head.

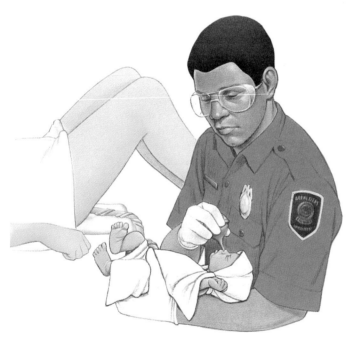

**Figure 20-6**   A bulb syringe can be used to clear a newborn baby's mouth and nose of any secretions.

passages. You can do this by using your finger, a gauze pad, or a bulb syringe (Fig. 20-6).

Most babies begin crying and breathing spontaneously. If the baby has not made any sounds, stimulate the baby to elicit the crying response by flicking your fingers on the soles of the baby's feet. Crying helps clear the baby's airway of fluids and promotes breathing. If the baby does not begin breathing on his or her

own within the first minute after birth, begin rescue breathing. If the baby does not have a pulse, begin CPR. You can review these techniques in Chapters 6 and 7.

If the baby is having difficulty breathing, additional oxygen would be beneficial. If you have oxygen available, you can attach a section of tubing to the flowmeter and deliver oxygen at 4 litres per minute to the newborn. Do this by holding the other end of the tubing near the infant's face (Fig. 20-7).

Your second responsibility is to maintain normal body temperature. Newborns lose heat quickly; therefore, it is important to keep him or her warm. Dry the newborn and wrap him or her in a clean, warm towel or blanket. If possible, record an initial set of vital signs. Most important are breathing, heart rate, and skin colour. You can review vital signs in Chapter 5.

## Caring for the Mother

You can continue to meet the needs of the newborn while caring for the mother. Allow the mother to begin nursing the newborn. This will stimulate the uterus to contract and help slow bleeding. The placenta will still be in the uterus, attached to the baby by the umbilical cord. Contractions of the uterus will usually

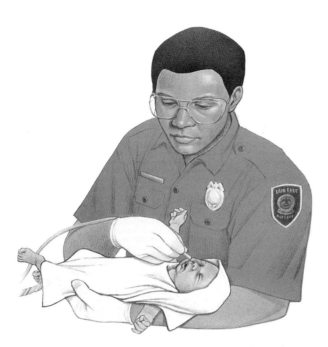

**Figure 20-7** Deliver oxygen to a newborn by holding the end of the oxygen tube near the newborn's face.

expel the placenta within 20 minutes of delivery. Catch the placenta in a clean towel or container. Do not separate the placenta from the newborn or cut the tied umbilical cord. Leave the placenta attached to the newborn and place it in a plastic bag or wrap it in a towel for transport to the hospital.

Expect some additional vaginal bleeding when the placenta is delivered. Using gauze pads or clean towels, gently clean the mother. Place a sanitary pad or towel over the vagina. Do not insert anything inside the vagina. Have the mother place her legs together. Feel for a grapefruit-sized mass in the lower abdomen. This is the uterus. Gently massage the lower portion of the abdomen. Massage will help eliminate any large blood clots within the uterus, cause the uterus to contract, and slow bleeding.

Many new mothers experience shock-like signs or symptoms, such as cool, pale, moist skin, shivering, and slight dizziness, after childbirth. Keep the mother positioned on her back. Administer oxygen if available. Maintain normal body temperature and monitor vital signs.

## ◆ COMPLICATIONS REQUIRING ADVANCED CARE

### Complications During Pregnancy

Complications during pregnancy are rare. One such complication is a spontaneous **miscarriage,** or **abortion.** Since the nature and extent of most complications can only be determined by medical professionals during or after examination, you should not be concerned with trying to "diagnose" a particular problem. Instead, concern yourself with recognizing signs and symptoms that suggest a serious complication during pregnancy. There are two important signs and symptoms you should be concerned with—vaginal bleeding and abdominal pain. Any persistent or profuse vaginal bleeding, or bleeding in which tissue passes through the vagina during pregnancy, is abnormal, as is any abdominal pain.

An expectant mother exhibiting these signs and symptoms needs to receive advanced medical care quickly. While waiting for an ambulance, take steps to minimize shock. These include—

- Helping the woman into the most comfortable position.
- Controlling bleeding.
- Maintaining normal body temperature.
- Administering oxygen if available.

### Complications During Childbirth

The vast majority of all births occur without complication. However, this fact is only reassuring if the one you are assisting with is not complicated. For the few that do have complications, delivery can be stressful and even life threatening for the expectant mother and the baby. All require the help of more advanced medical personnel.

The most common complication of childbirth is persistent vaginal bleeding. Besides seeking more advanced medical care, you should take steps to minimize shock, as explained in earlier chapters. Other childbirth complications include prolapsed cord, breech birth, and multiple births.

## Prolapsed Cord

A ***prolapsed cord*** occurs when a loop of the umbilical cord protrudes from the vagina while the baby is still in the birth canal (Fig. 20-8). If this occurs, it can threaten the baby's life. As the baby moves through the birth canal, the cord will be compressed against the unborn child and the birth canal and blood flow to the baby will stop. Without this blood flow, the baby will die within a few minutes from lack of oxygen. If you notice a prolapsed cord, have the expectant mother assume a knee-chest position (Fig. 20-9). This will help take the pressure off the cord. Administer oxygen to the mother if it is available. Summon more advanced medical personnel if they have not been contacted already.

## Breech Birth

Most babies are born head first. However, on rare occasions, the baby is delivered feet or buttocks first. This condition is commonly called ***breech birth***. If you encounter a breech delivery, support the baby's body as it exits the birth canal while you are waiting for the head to deliver. Do not pull on the baby's body. This will not help to deliver the head.

If, after about 3 minutes, the head has not delivered, you will need to help create an airway for the baby to breathe. Because the weight of the baby's head lodged in the birth canal will reduce or stop blood flow by compressing the cord, the baby will be unable to get any oxygen. Should the baby try to take a spontaneous breath, he or she will also be unable to breathe because the face is pressed against the wall of the birth canal.

To help with a breech delivery, place the index and middle fingers of your gloved hand into the vagina next to the baby's mouth and nose. Spread your fingers to form a "V" (Fig. 20-10). Though this will not lessen the compression on the umbilical cord, it may allow air to enter the baby's mouth and nose. You must maintain this position until the baby's head is delivered. Administer oxygen to the mother if it is available.

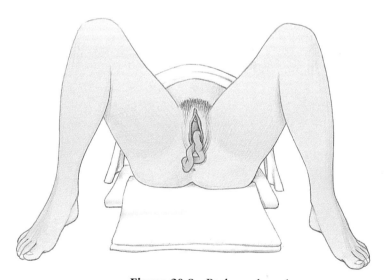

**Figure 20-8**   Prolapsed cord.

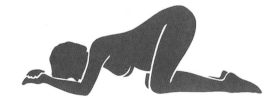

**Figure 20-9**   The knee-chest position will take pressure off the cord.

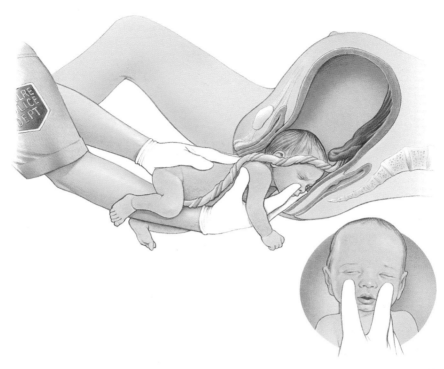

**Figure 20-10**   During a breech birth, position your index and middle fingers to allow air to enter the baby's mouth and nose.

Summon more advanced medical personnel if they have not already been contacted.

### Multiple Births

Although most births involve only a single baby, a few will involve delivery of more than one. If the mother has had proper prenatal care, she will probably be aware that she is going to have more than one baby. Multiple births should be handled in the same manner as single births. The mother will have a separate set of contractions for each child being born. There may also be a separate placenta for each child, though this is not always the case.

### ◆ SUMMARY

Ideally, childbirth should occur in a controlled environment under the guidance of health-care professionals trained in delivery. In this way, the necessary medical care is immediately available for mother and baby should any problem arise. However, there will always be unexpected deliveries occurring outside of the controlled environment that may require your assistance. By knowing how to prepare the expectant mother for delivery, assist in the delivery, and provide proper care for the mother and baby, you will be able to successfully assist in bringing a new child into the world.

### YOU ▼ ARE THE RESPONDER

1. *A 32-year-old woman believes she is in labour. She says that this will be her third child. The amniotic sac ruptured about 1 hour ago. She says she feels a need to move her bowels. Contractions are frequent, about 2 minutes apart. What steps would you take to prepare for delivery of the baby?*
2. *The same woman screams that she feels the need to push. When you examine her, you see the baby's head crowning. What steps would you take to assist in the delivery of the baby?*

# Crisis Intervention

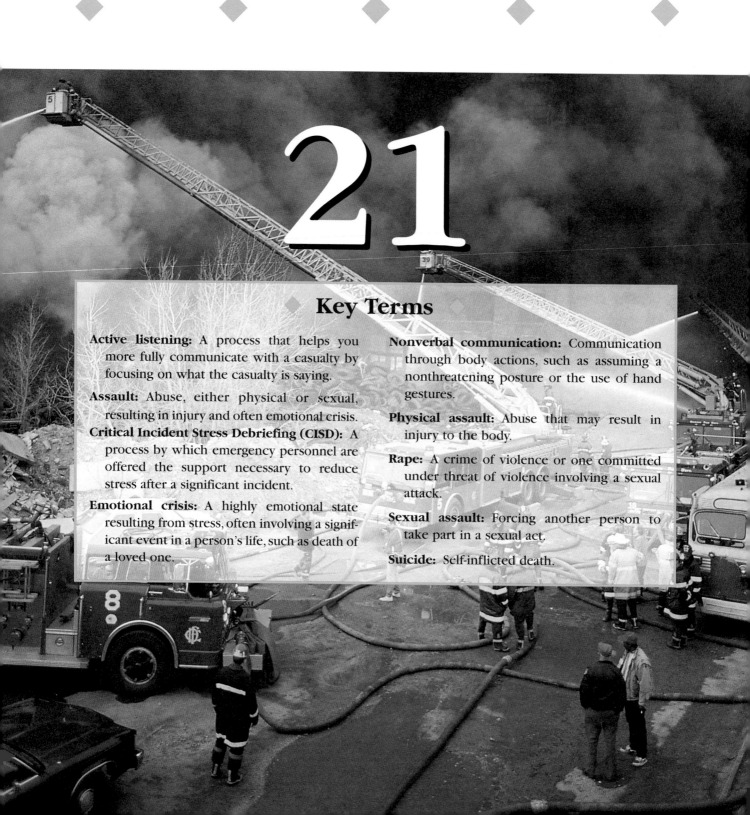

# 21

## ◆ Key Terms ◆

**Active listening:** A process that helps you more fully communicate with a casualty by focusing on what the casualty is saying.

**Assault:** Abuse, either physical or sexual, resulting in injury and often emotional crisis.

**Critical Incident Stress Debriefing (CISD):** A process by which emergency personnel are offered the support necessary to reduce stress after a significant incident.

**Emotional crisis:** A highly emotional state resulting from stress, often involving a significant event in a person's life, such as death of a loved one.

**Nonverbal communication:** Communication through body actions, such as assuming a nonthreatening posture or the use of hand gestures.

**Physical assault:** Abuse that may result in injury to the body.

**Rape:** A crime of violence or one committed under threat of violence involving a sexual attack.

**Sexual assault:** Forcing another person to take part in a sexual act.

**Suicide:** Self-inflicted death.

## ◆ For Review ◆

Before reading this chapter, you should have a basic understanding of your roles and responsibilities as a first responder (Chapter 1) and know the guidelines to follow to ensure your safety at an emergency scene (Chapter 2).

## ◆ INTRODUCTION

In one way or another, a serious injury or sudden illness or death has an emotional impact on everyone involved: casualties, family, friends, bystanders, first responders, and others. The degree of impact varies from person to person. For some, the impact is minimal, the acceptance of injury or illness that results in hospitalization, disability, or even death is handled well. For others, however, even a minor injury can create an extreme *emotional crisis,* a highly emotional state resulting from stress. The way a person responds to an emergency largely depends on his or her emotional makeup and patterns of response. Therefore, the way one person responds to a stressful situation can differ substantially from the response of another person in a similar situation.

Sometimes it is not the fact that injury or illness has occurred that triggers emotional distress, but how it occurred. The nature of an event, such as a sexual assault, can cause great emotional turmoil. A casualty's realization that he or she has been sexually violated can cause extreme stress. Events, such as a *suicide,* self-inflicted death, or attempted suicide, can cause great stress to family and friends of the casualty. They often feel as if they could have done more or should have been able to help.

You may someday encounter a situation involving a casualty who is experiencing an emotional crisis. Besides providing care for any specific injury or illness, you may also need to provide emotional support. In some instances, the casualty will be so distraught that he or she will be entirely dependent on you and your directions. Being able to understand some of what the casualty is feeling can help you cope with the situation.

## ◆ SPECIFIC EMOTIONAL CRISES

Many different situations can result in emotional crisis for the casualty or bystanders. Examples commonly encountered by emergency personnel include attempted suicide, sexual or physical assault, the sudden death of a loved one, or a dying casualty.

### Suicide

*You respond to a call for help from a distraught mother who states her 15-year-old son is having trouble breathing. She says he is in his bedroom crying uncontrollably. She also states that he has been depressed because of the recent death of a close friend and classmate.*

*When you arrive, you approach the bedroom and find the door closed and locked. You speak to the casualty from outside the bedroom. He has stopped crying. You ask him to unlock the door. You can barely make out his shape in the darkened room as he opens the door. He appears to be breathing normally now. He requests that you and his mother leave him alone.*

*You suggest that he come out of the bedroom to talk. He eventually complies and begins to talk about his problems dealing with the recent death of his girlfriend. He says no one understands how he feels. He also says he had thought once about killing himself.*

*Both you and the mother console him. Soon he appears better and states he is OK. You suggest to the mother, in the boy's absence, that she get psychological counselling for him immediately because of his suicide remark. You offer to call a counsellor with a mental health agency. The mother says she has called her minister and he will arrive shortly. She also states that she will seek additional help later today after speaking with her husband who is out of town.*

*You leave the home, feeling as if you have averted an emotional crisis that could have had a serious consequence. You feel you did all that you could and that the mother will get her son the professional help he needs. Unfortunately, you later find out that the boy went drinking several days later with friends and used a handgun to end his life.*

Suicide is more common in Canada than most people realize. Suicide is the second leading cause of death among people aged 15 to 19, accounting for about 25 percent of injury deaths in this age group. Suicide is also common among adults and older adults. Many people who attempt suicide suffer some form of mental or emotional problem or illness. Substance misuse or abuse, primarily of alcohol and barbiturates, plays a major role in attempted suicides.

What motivates a person to suddenly try to commit suicide? It is often a combination of unbearable underlying tensions caused by a major event in a person's life, such as—

- A failing or failed relationship with a spouse, family, or friend.
- Serious illness or death of a close family member or friend.
- Serious, prolonged, or chronic personal illness.
- A long period of failure at work or school.
- A long period of unemployment.
- Failure to achieve sufficient occupational, educational, or financial success.
- Dramatic change in the economy.

## Assault

*Assault* is an all too common occurrence in our society. It can be physical, sexual, or both. It results in injury and often emotional distress to the casualty.

## Sexual Assault

*Sexual assault* occurs when one person takes advantage of another by rape or forces a person to take part in any unnatural sexual act. *Rape* is a crime of violence, or one committed under threat of violence, that involves a sexual attack, either heterosexual or homosexual. Rape is a devastating experience for the casualty. Rape casualties often feel degraded, extremely frightened, and at further risk for attack. Casualties of rape require significant emotional support.

Besides providing emotional support, you must care for any injuries the casualty may have received. When caring for a casualty of sexual assault, do the following:

- Cover the casualty and protect the casualty from unnecessary exposure.
- Clear the area of any bystanders, except those friends or family able to help provide emotional support.
- Do not remove any clothing unless absolutely necessary to provide care for injuries.
- Care for any physical injuries.
- Discourage the casualty from bathing, showering, or douching before a medical examination can be performed.
- Do not disrupt the crime scene by handling items unrelated to the casualty's care.
- Do not question the casualty about the specifics of the assault.
- Summon more advanced medical personnel and law enforcement personnel.

## Physical Assault

*Physical assault* on a child, spouse, or the elderly occurs more frequently than reported. Unfortunately, when you are summoned, the assault has often resulted in more serious injuries. The emergency scene where a physical assault has occurred is not always safe. The attacker may still be present or nearby. If the scene involves domestic violence, it may not be clear what has happened. Substances, such as alcohol, may be involved. Remember that your first concern is always your safety. If you are not trained in law enforcement, do not approach the scene until it is determined to be safe. Wait for additional personnel. As with sexual assault, the scene is a crime scene. Therefore, do not handle items unrelated to the casualty's care. Reassure and comfort the casualty while providing care.

## Death and Dying

You may be summoned to an emergency in which one or more casualties have died or are dying. Though your responses will vary according to the situation, you must recognize that death will have an emotional impact on you, as well as on others involved. Be prepared to handle your feelings and the feelings of others. Remember that reactions to death and dying range from anxiety to acceptance. How well you and others handle the situation will depend on both personal feelings about death and the nature of the incident.

One of the most disturbing situations is that involving sudden death. This could involve a casualty who suffers a sudden illness, becomes unconscious, and later dies. It could also be a casualty involved in what appeared to be a minor motor vehicle collision, who is alert and talkative when you arrive, but who suddenly suffers a cardiac arrest. Especially disturbing to new parents is the sudden unexplained death of an infant in the first few weeks of life. In situations such as these, there is no time to prepare for what has happened. Suddenly a man, woman, or child who had been alive only minutes earlier is now dead.

Sometimes you may be in a situation in which you think someone has been dead for a while and you are unsure whether you should attempt to resuscitate the casualty. The general rule is to always attempt to resuscitate and continue efforts to resuscitate until advanced medical personnel advise you to stop.

To determine that a person is dead, he or she is often placed on a heart monitor and vital signs are assessed. When it is determined that the casualty has no heart rhythm, no pulse, no respiration, and no blood pressure, the casualty is declared dead. In some instances, this will be after prolonged resuscitation attempts. At other times, additional signs, such as decapitation, **rigour mortis, lividity,** and decomposition, may cause resuscitation attempts to be withheld.

Some casualties may have **living wills,** written legal documents saying that they do not wish to be resuscitated or further kept alive by mechanical means. In most instances, the wishes of the casualty expressed in writing should be honoured. However, since provincial and local laws about these situations vary, you should summon more advanced medical personnel immediately.

If you must confront a casualty, family, friends, or bystanders during or after a situation in which death is probable, be cautious about what you say. Avoid making statements about the casualty's condition. You can provide comfort with positive statements such as, "We are doing everything we can."

## ◆ STAGES OF GRIEF

Everyone involved in a sudden, unexpected, and undesired event, such as life-threatening illness or injury or the death of a loved one, experiences grief. The grieving process involves an outpouring of emotions that often follows a common pattern with various stages. These stages are not separate entities and do not necessarily follow one after the other. Instead, they often blend together. These stages include—

- *Anxiety*—A stage characterized by a feeling of worry, uncertainty, and fear. Signs and symptoms include rapid breathing and pulse, increased activity, rapid speech, loud talking or screaming, and agitation.
- *Denial/disbelief*—A stage in which a person refuses to accept the fact that the event, such as the death of a loved one or suffering a debilitating injury, has occurred.

◆ *Anger*—A stage that involves an expression of aggressive verbal or physical behaviour. It is sometimes the result of the frustration of not being able to accept the event or a feeling that not enough was done or is being done to help.

◆ *Bargaining*—A stage that involves an unspoken promise of something in exchange for an extension of life or return to the pre-event condition.

◆ *Guilt/depression*—A stage that involves placing the blame for what happened on yourself, resulting in feelings of guilt or depression. A parent will often feel guilty for the event involving his or her child. A family member may feel guilty for not being of help to another family member who committed suicide.

◆ *Acceptance*—The final stage in which the grieving process ends and the pain and discomfort are eased. The person accepts the event and the outcome. For some people, arriving at the stage of acceptance takes weeks, months, or even years after the event. For others, such as friends or family members who are aware that a casualty's condition is terminal, this stage can occur much more rapidly.

## ◆ CRISIS INTERVENTION

Regardless of the nature of the incident, caring for someone experiencing an emotional crisis involves offering emotional support, as well as care for any specific injury. The most important initial step you can take is to communicate with the casualty in an open manner. Communication can be both verbal and nonverbal.

***Nonverbal communication*** refers to your actions. Sometimes your actions (body language) say more than you intend. You should always be aware of the messages you are sending with your body. General body posture is an important aspect of nonverbal communication. Begin by assuming a nonthreatening posture. This involves getting at eye level with

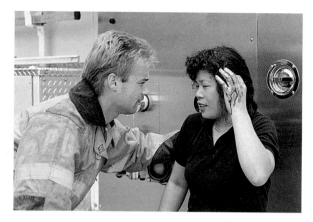

**Figure 21-1** Looking at the casualty at eye level when you talk can be reassuring.

the casualty and looking at the casualty as you talk (Fig. 21-1). Avoid making physical contact. Also, avoid positions such as placing your arms across your chest, your hands on your hips, pointing at the casualty, or leaning over and looking down at the casualty.

As you begin to communicate verbally, remember that communication involves stimulating discussion and listening as much as talking. When you do talk, speak in a calm, reassuring manner. Ask the casualty his or her name, and use it frequently in conversation. One technique used to help you more fully communicate is "active listening." The process of ***active listening*** requires you to listen closely to what the person is saying. It involves four behaviours:

◆ Making every effort to understand fully what the casualty is trying to say.

◆ Repeating back to the casualty, in your own words, what he or she said.

◆ Avoiding criticism, anger, or rejection of the casualty's statements.

◆ Using open-ended questions such as, "You appear to be very sad," or, "What problems are you having?" Generally, avoid questions that can be answered with "yes" or "no."

Casualties of emotional crisis may be withdrawn or hysterical. Some may be entirely dependent on you to help. Avoid being judgmental.

Do not place blame on the casualty. The casualty needs to be cared for gently and with respect. If care is needed for a minor injury, try to get the casualty to help you (Fig. 21-2). By encouraging the casualty to participate, you may help the casualty regain a sense of control that he or she had lost.

Do not be fooled into thinking that you can manage a situation involving emotional crisis yourself. A suicidal person or a rape casualty needs professional counselling. Summon more advanced personnel. This could include law enforcement, EMS, or local mental health or rape crisis centre personnel. While waiting for others to arrive, continue to talk with the casualty. Never leave the casualty alone unless there is a threat to your safety.

# ◆ CRITICAL INCIDENT STRESS DEBRIEFING (CISD)

Researchers have recognized for years that individuals who provide emergency care can experience high levels of stress. Incidents involving multiple casualties, rescues, children, failed resuscitation attempts, and death or serious injury to co-workers tend to cause more stress than others. Critical incident stress can cause a number of signs and symptoms, some of which may appear as long as weeks after the incident:

- ◆ Confusion
- ◆ Lowered attention span
- ◆ Poor concentration
- ◆ Denial
- ◆ Guilt
- ◆ Depression
- ◆ Anger
- ◆ Change in interactions with others
- ◆ Increased or decreased eating
- ◆ Uncharacteristic, excessive humour or silence
- ◆ Unusual behaviour

From the time you begin to establish a rapport with the casualty, you become involved in the casualty's pain and stress. You share to some

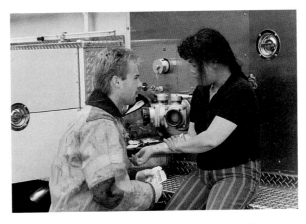

**Figure 21-2** Have the casualty help you when you give care.

degree the thoughts and emotions of the casualty. As a result, the emotional impact of a situation may be too great for you to handle alone. For this reason, you may need counselling to deal with the stress. Such counselling is available through a process called *Critical Incident Stress Debriefing (CISD).* This process brings you together with someone trained to help you express your feelings. Often, this is another person in your line of work.

CISD is not just for those incidents involving death or major disasters. Any incident, such as a dramatic lifesaving rescue, is a potential source of emotional crisis for you. Even though the outcome of such an incident would be completely different from one involving death, the emotions and stress factors would all still be present. For this reason, it is important that the rescuer, rescue teams, and any others closely involved in an incident involving significant stress be debriefed. CISD can also benefit the lay person who performs CPR before you arrive, only to learn that the casualty was pronounced dead soon after arriving at the hospital.

Some people think that participating in CISD is an admission of weakness—quite the contrary. CISD should be, and in many areas is, a routine part of any overwhelming incident, such as an airline disaster. CISD can help in any situation, regardless of how minor you may think the event was. The most important thing you can do to minimize the effects of any emergency is to express your feelings and thoughts after the incident. Check with your local agency to see what resources are available to you.

## ◆ SUMMARY

An emotional crisis often is the result of an unexpected, shocking, and undesired event, such as the sudden loss of a loved one. Although people react differently in different situations, each experiences some or all of the stages associated with grieving. By considering the nature of the incident, you can begin to prepare yourself to deal with its emotional aspects.

Regardless of the nature of the event, however, the care you provide to casualties of any emotional crisis is very similar. Your care involves appropriate verbal and nonverbal communication. It also requires you to under-stand that in some cases death is inevitable. In some situations, you may be overcome by emotion. Remember that self-help involves sharing your feelings with others.

### YOU ARE THE RESPONDER

*You are summoned to a home where a 39-year-old father of three children has attempted suicide by carbon monoxide poisoning. He was found by his oldest child, aged 14, in the car in the garage. You try to resuscitate the casualty until more advanced medical personnel arrive and take over. As they begin to work on him, the casualty's wife comes home. She immediately rushes screaming to her husband. You help restrain her so that the paramedics can continue to try to resuscitate him. You move her away, and the sobbing children run to her. Describe her emotions at this scene. How would you care for this woman and her children?*

◆ **NOTES:**

# Reaching and Moving Casualties

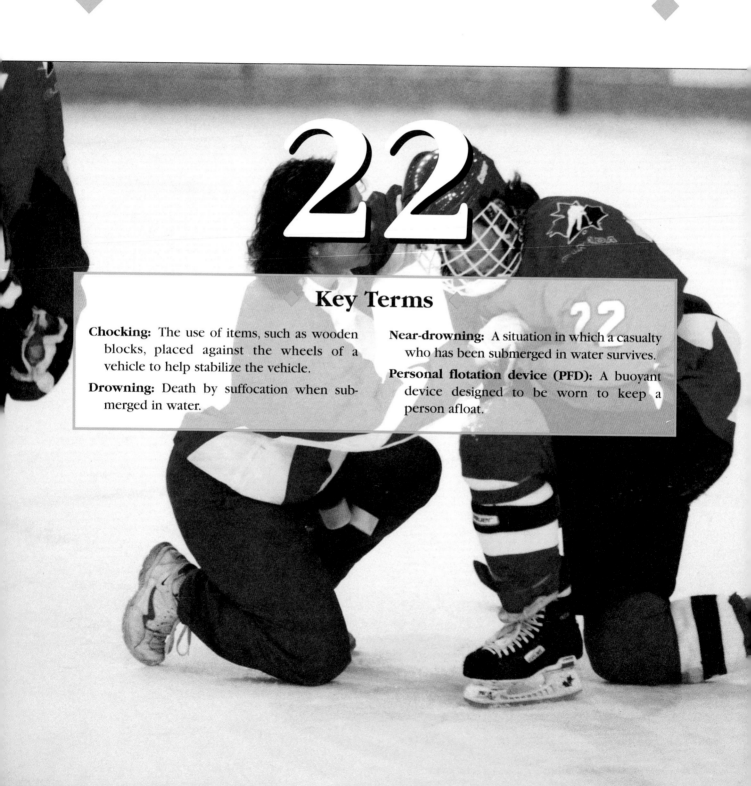

## Key Terms

**Chocking:** The use of items, such as wooden blocks, placed against the wheels of a vehicle to help stabilize the vehicle.

**Drowning:** Death by suffocation when submerged in water.

**Near-drowning:** A situation in which a casualty who has been submerged in water survives.

**Personal flotation device (PFD):** A buoyant device designed to be worn to keep a person afloat.

*debris from a collapsed wall. Your quick decision to act has saved several lives.*

## ◆ For Review ◆

Before reading this chapter, you should have a basic understanding of how to ensure your safety in an emergency situation (Chapter 2).

## ◆ INTRODUCTION

*Your pager goes off just as you are preparing to leave work for the day. At the same time, the fire alarms sound in the building. You are summoned to a recently remodelled adjacent building. As you proceed, you smell something burning. As you near the area, there is a sudden crackling sound followed by an explosion and screams.*

*You arrive to find smoke filling the area. Two people carry an employee through a doorway. Others stagger through and collapse to the ground. Smoke is blowing over them. Flames flicker inside the structure. You hear the sound of sirens, but they are still far off.*

*You make a split-second decision to help. You recruit others and run to the collapsed casualties. Two of them are unconscious. Other employees are still trying to find their way out through the smoke. You recognize the immediate danger to the two unconscious casualties and to the others trying to escape. Time is critical. You need to get everyone to a safer place. With the help of others, you drag casualties away from the building. You return again to help several more casualties who have collapsed nearby and work feverishly to move them. Finally, the smoke becomes too heavy and the flames too hot to continue. You do not know how many may perish in the blaze. You retreat to safety as the fire fighters arrive.*

*The building is nearly fully ablaze as they begin to work. Through the smoke and flames, you see that the doorway where many casualties had collapsed is now covered with burning*

In earlier chapters, you learned how to care for casualties of injury and illness when it is safe to do so. Sometimes, however, you will not have easy access to the casualty. At other times, the casualty may be in a dangerous situation and must be moved before you provide care. In this chapter, you will learn how to quickly and safely reach and move casualties.

## ◆ GAINING ACCESS

One of your primary responsibilities as a first responder is to provide care for an ill or injured casualty. Sometimes, however, providing care is not possible because the casualty is inaccessible. One example is a situation in which someone is able to call 9-1-1 or another local emergency number for help but is unable to unlock the door of the home or office to let in the responders. This is also true in a large number of motor vehicle collisions. Vehicle doors are sometimes locked or crushed, windows may be tightly rolled up, or the vehicle may be unstable. In other instances, fire, water, or other elements may prevent you from reaching the casualty.

In these cases, you must immediately begin to think of how to safely gain access to the casualty before you can begin to provide care. If you cannot reach the casualty, you cannot help him or her. But remember, when attempting to reach a casualty, your safety is the most important consideration. Protect yourself and the casualty by doing only what you are trained to do and by using equipment and clothing appropriate for the situation. Items such as helmets, face shields, goggles, gloves, heavy clothing, blankets, reflective markers or flares, and flashlights will help keep you safe as you attempt to gain access to a trapped casualty. Simple tools, such as a screwdriver, hammer, pocketknife, axe, spare tire, vehicle jack, rope, chains, coat hanger, can also be helpful (see box on next page).

# Motor Vehicles

As with any emergency situation, begin by surveying the scene to see if it is safe. If it is not safe, determine whether you can make it safe so that you can attempt to gain access to the casualty. Well-intentioned first responders and others are injured or killed each year while attempting to help casualties of motor vehicle collisions. Often, these rescuers are struck by oncoming vehicles. Such unfortunate instances can be prevented if you take adequate measures to make the scene safe before trying to gain access and provide care.

## Upright Vehicles

Fortunately, most motor vehicle collisions you encounter will involve upright, stable vehicles. These vehicles are unlikely to move while you attempt to help their occupants. However, there are times when the vehicle will not be stable. Environmental factors can influence the stability of the vehicle. Vehicles on slippery surfaces, such as ice, water, or snow, or on inclined surfaces need to be stabilized. In addition, vehicles positioned where oil has been spilled should also be stabilized.

Stabilizing an upright vehicle is a simple task. Placing blocks or wedges against the wheels of the vehicle will greatly reduce the chance of the vehicle moving. This process is called *chocking* (Fig. 22-1). You can use items such as rocks, logs, wooden blocks, and spare tires. If strong rope or chain is available, these can be attached to the frame of the car and then secured to strong anchor points, such as large trees, guard rails, or another vehicle. Letting the air out of the car's tires also reduces the possibility of movement.

Once you are certain the vehicle is stable, you should attempt to enter it. Begin by checking all of the doors to see if they are unlocked. Though it may seem obvious to check the doors, sometimes in the excitement it is easy to forget this simple, time-saving step. If the doors are locked, the casualties inside might be able to unlock at least one door for you. If the windows are open, you may be able to unlock the door yourself.

Sometimes locked or jammed doors require you to enter the vehicle through a window. If the window is open, or can be rolled down by someone inside the car, this is not a problem. If

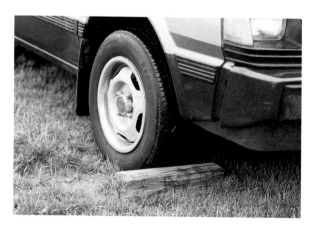

**Figure 22-1** Chocking is used to stabilize a vehicle.

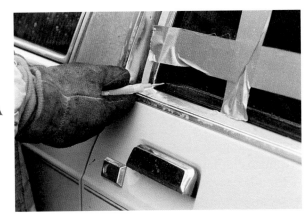
A

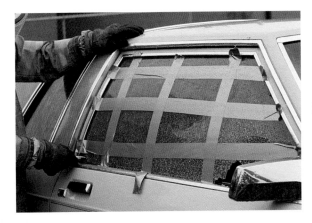
B

**Figure 22-2** **A,** Locate the window farthest from the casualty. Tape it to avoid flying glass. Position the spring-loaded centre punch at a lower corner of the window. **B,** When the punch is pressed against the window, the glass will shatter.

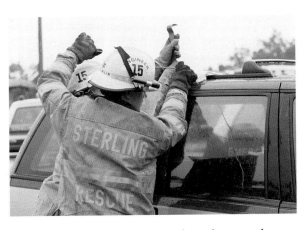

**Figure 22-3** To use a wire and pry bar, pry the door frame with the pry bar and insert the wire. Lift the lock with the wire.

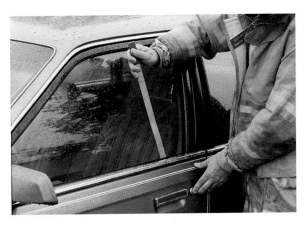

**Figure 22-4** A Slim-Jim can be used to release the locking mechanism in the vehicle door.

the window is rolled up, you can use specific equipment and techniques to get into the car. Figures 22-2, *A* and *B,* 22-3, and 22-4 show three common techniques. Once inside the vehicle, you can further stabilize it by placing the vehicle in "park," turning off the key, and setting the parking brake.

## Overturned Vehicles

It is unusual to find a vehicle overturned or on its side. Consider any vehicle found in either position to be unstable. Though a vehicle on its side or overturned can be stabilized by using

spare tires, jacks, wooden blocks, or other items, it is unlikely that you can adequately stabilize the vehicle. Local fire department and rescue squad personnel specially trained in vehicle stabilization and extrication will respond to the scene when notified.

## Vehicles and Electrical Hazards

When a vehicle is in contact with an electrical wire, you must consider the wire to be energized until you know otherwise. When you arrive on the scene, your first priority is to ensure your safety and that of others in the immediate area. A safety area should be established at a point twice

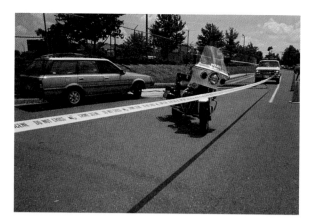

**Figure 22-5** Establish a safety area around a downed electrical wire.

the length of the span of the wire (Fig. 22-5). Attempt to reach and move casualties *only* after the power company has been notified and has removed any electrical current from the downed wire. Do *not* touch any metal fence, metal structure, or body of water in contact with the downed wire. Persons inside the vehicle should be told to remain in the vehicle. You can tell them how to provide care for any injured casualties in the vehicle. Do *not* attempt to deal with electrical hazards unless you are specifically trained to do so.

Once the current has been removed from the wire, you can safely approach the vehicle. Since the vehicle and possibly the casualty(s) were in contact with the current, electrical injury is possible. Signs and symptoms of electrical injury include—

◆ Burns.
◆ Unconsciousness or dazed, confused behaviour.
◆ Respiratory distress or arrest.
◆ Weak, irregular, or absent pulse.

## Hazardous Materials Incidents

When approaching any scene, you should be aware of dangers involving chemicals. Whether a motor vehicle collision or an industrial emergency is involved, you should be able to recognize clues that indicate the presence of hazardous materials. These include—

◆ Signs (placards) on vehicles or storage facilities identifying the presence of hazardous materials.
◆ Spilled liquids or solids.
◆ Unusual odours.
◆ Clouds of vapour.
◆ Leaking containers.

Placards, or signs, are required by law to be placed on any vehicles that contain specific quantities of hazardous materials. In addition, manufacturers and others associated with the production and distribution of these materials are required by law to display the appropriate placard. Placards often clearly identify the danger of the substance. Terms such as "explosive," "flammable," "corrosive," and "radioactive" are frequently used. Universally recognized symbols are also used. Figure 22-6 shows some common labels and placards for identifying hazardous materials.

Unless you have received special training in handling hazardous materials and have the necessary equipment to do so without danger, you should stay well away from the area. Stay out of low areas where vapours and liquids may collect. Stay upwind and uphill of the scene. Be alert for wind changes that could cause vapours to blow toward you. Do not attempt to be a hero. It is not uncommon for responding ambulance crews approaching the scene to recognize a hazardous materials placard and to immediately move to a safe area and summon more advanced help.

Many fire departments have specially trained teams to handle incidents involving hazardous materials. While awaiting help, keep people away from the danger zone. One easy method used to determine the danger zone area is called the rule of thumb. You should position yourself far enough away from the scene so that your thumb, pointing up at arm's length, covers the hazardous area from your view.

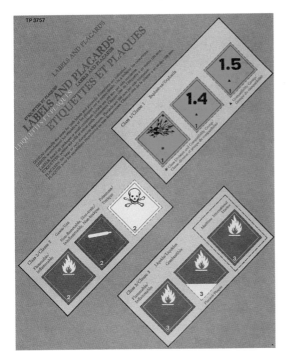
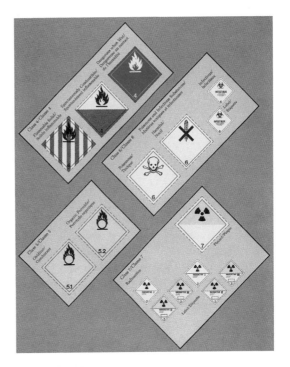
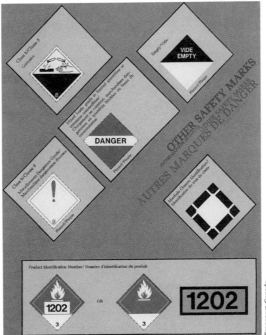

**Figure 22-6** Hazardous materials placards and labels.

Hazardous materials are not found only in industrial sites. They are often transported by rail or truck and may be exposed when a vehicle turns over or is in a collision. Homes contain many hazardous materials, such as natural gas, gasoline, kerosene, and pesticides.

Some hazardous materials, such as natural gas, are flammable and can cause an explosion. Even turning on a light switch or using a telephone or radio may create a spark that sets off an explosion. When you call for help, use a telephone or radio well clear of the scene.

# A Rescue to Remember

**9:30 AM Wednesday.** The emergency call came into the Midland Fire Department from a frantic mother named Reba McClure. Her 18-month-old daughter, who had been playing around an uncapped 8-inch-wide (20 cm) well shaft in the back yard, slipped 22 feet (7 metres) down the dry well.

One of the first police officers to arrive on the scene was Bobbie Jo Hall. She peered into the thin black hole in the earth where Jessica McClure had fallen, but she couldn't see anything. She called out the child's name. Finally, she heard her cry.

Fire fighters, other police, and EMS workers arrived quickly, but neither Hall nor the other rescuers knew much about excavations. However, they knew where to find the help they needed. Soon fire fighters and police were knocking down clotheslines and tearing down fences to move a backhoe into the back yard, but the ditch-digging machine dug 2 or 3 feet (1 metre) and hit rock.

**11:30 AM Wednesday.** The rescuers did not give up hope. Fire Chief James Roberts and Police Chief Richard Czech arrived to take command of the scene and began to develop a plan. One police officer went to get a 50-foot-tall (12 metre) "ratholer," designed to dig holes for pilings, at a nearby road overpass. Another officer had the power company turn off the electricity around the house. The machine was brought in and began digging a hole parallel to the well.

There was no way to determine if Jessica was injured or how long she could survive. Concerned about hypothermia, rescuers set up heaters to blow warm air down the shaft. A microphone lowered into the hole monitored Jessica's breathing. Frightened, Jessica sang songs and cried for her mother, as one hour stretched to six. Digging straight down went fairly smoothly, but when the drillers attempted to connect the tunnel with the well, they again hit solid rock.

**9:00 PM Wednesday.** The work was tortuously slow—an hour's worth of chiselling yielded just a few inches of rock. The drill bits constantly broke off against the limestone. One by one, the volunteers, many of them unemployed oil workers, descended into the black hole and chipped away.

**11:30 AM Thursday.** Fortunately, a Texas businessman arranged to fly a mine rescue expert in from New Mexico. David Lilly was a special investigator for the Mine Safety and Health Administration and had experience with rescue operations. He was quickly put in charge of the dig.

Immediately he changed the angle of the drilling so that the workers would not break the well in directly on Jessica, but 2 feet (2/3 metre) below her. He also switched the type of drill bit to a stronger one made of tungsten carbide. Mud-caked workers continued to drill day and night in the gravelike tunnel.

**4:15 AM Friday.** After nearly 2 days of gruelling effort, workers chipped a small hole into the well. By noon, rescuers thought they could reach Jessica.

Medical authorities warned that Jessica might have spinal injuries, so two paramedics were lowered by harness into the hole to retrieve her. But the tunnel was so small, they could not reach the child.

**3:00 PM Friday.** To make the final cuts, Lilly switched to a high-powered water drill, which was easier to manoeuvre and could cut through the rock more quickly.

**7:25 PM Friday.** Expensive drilling tools helped rescuers reach Jessica, but it was several tubes of K-Y Jelly and forceps that freed her. Smeared with the lubricant, the little girl slipped through the hole on the second rescue attempt. She was strapped to a backboard, attached to a pulley, and lifted to safety. Paramedics rushed the bruised and dehydrated child to the hospital. She had lost 4 of her 21 pounds (1.5 of 8 kg) and 15 percent of her body fluids. Besides saving her life, doctors also tried to save her foot, which had been wedged over her head and lacked circulation during the 58-hour ordeal. After a month in the hospital, Jessica lost a toe and underwent plastic surgery for a sore on her forehead. It took hundreds of people—police, fire fighters, paramedics, construction workers, nurses, and doctors— to rescue the tiny girl. They will never forget the experience.

"I was totally exhausted—totally elated too," said one rescuer. "I said prayers while I was down there, I cussed, I tried it all. I've saved other people's lives before, but there'll never be nothing like this again."

Sources: *Dallas Times Herald, Dallas Morning News, People Weekly,* Midland Police Department Cpl. Jim White.

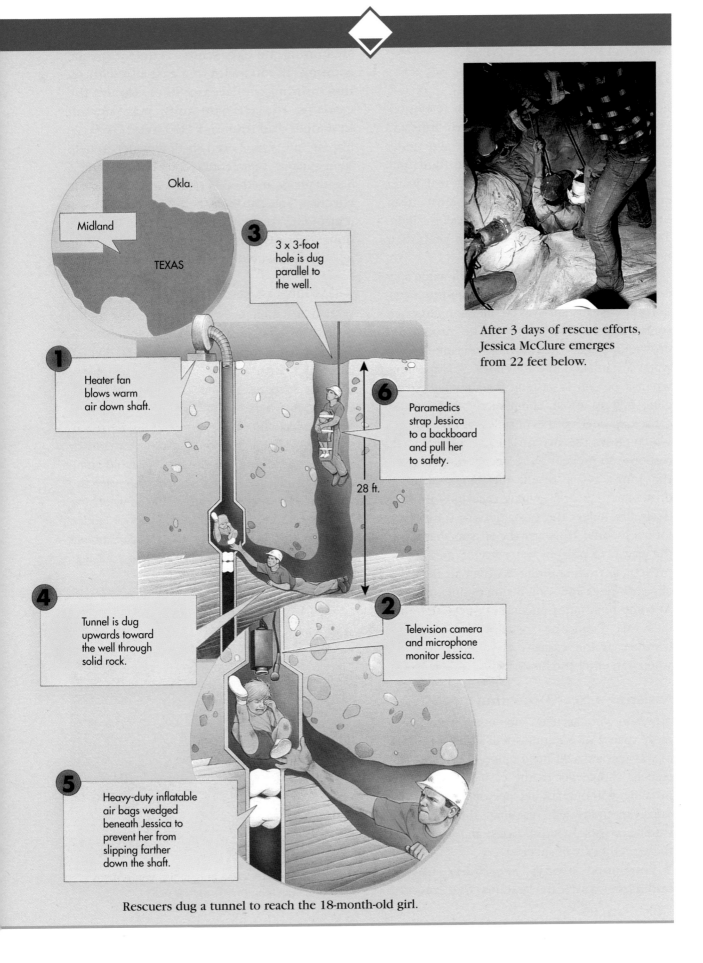

Okla.

Midland

TEXAS

**3** 3 x 3-foot hole is dug parallel to the well.

After 3 days of rescue efforts, Jessica McClure emerges from 22 feet below.

**1** Heater fan blows warm air down shaft.

**6** Paramedics strap Jessica to a backboard and pull her to safety.

28 ft.

**4** Tunnel is dug upwards toward the well through solid rock.

**2** Television camera and microphone monitor Jessica.

**5** Heavy-duty inflatable air bags wedged beneath Jessica to prevent her from slipping farther down the shaft.

Rescuers dug a tunnel to reach the 18-month-old girl.

## ◆ WATER EMERGENCIES

### Drowning

You see it often in movies and on television. People who are drowning wave their arms and shout, "Help, I'm drowning!" They slip under the surface and rise up again. The third time down is supposedly their last. But real water emergencies are not like that. Most near-drowning casualties are unable to call for help. Their energy is spent just trying to keep their head above water.

*Drowning* is death by suffocation when submerged in water. In a *near-drowning* situation, the casualty survives submersion, although sometimes only temporarily. The process of drowning begins whenever small amounts of water are inhaled into the lungs. This happens when a person is gasping for air while struggling to stay afloat. Stimulation by the water causes spasms of the muscles of the larynx, which closes the airway. This is a natural body response to prevent more water from entering the lungs. As a result, the lungs of most drowning or near-drowning casualties are relatively dry unless the casualties are submerged for a long time. However, the spasms that block the airway to prevent water from entering also prevent air from entering. Without air, the casualty suffocates and soon becomes unconscious. At some point after unconsciousness, the muscles relax, and the casualty spontaneously breathes. If the casualty is submerged, more water can enter the lungs.

### Assisting a Near-Drowning Casualty

A person who has been submerged in water for more than 2 or 3 minutes will suffer from lack of oxygen and will need emergency care. The rescuer should get to the casualty as soon as possible without risking personal safety. The safest methods are reaching, throwing, and wading assists. In most cases, at least one of these methods will succeed.

**You must always remember not to endanger yourself. Rescues that require swimming to a casualty require special training. If you swim to a casualty without this training, you are not likely to save the casualty. In fact, you only put yourself in danger and thus risk two lives.** Likewise, leaping into water, even shallow water, to help someone may seem courageous. But choosing a less dramatic method is safer and usually more effective. You can help a casualty only if you remain safe yourself and in control of the situation. The reaching, throwing, and wading methods presented here help you do both.

#### Reaching Assists

With a reaching assist, you reach out to the casualty in the water while remaining in a safe position. First, firmly brace yourself. Extend your reach with any object that will reach the casualty, such as a pole, oar or paddle, tree branch, shirt, belt, or towel (Fig. 22-7).

If you have no objects to extend your reach, try to extend your arm and grasp the casualty or extend your foot to the casualty. To avoid going into the water, lie flat on a pool deck or pier and reach with your arm. If you are in the water, use one hand to get a firm grasp on a pool ladder, overflow trough, piling, or other secure object and extend your free hand or one of your legs to the casualty (Fig. 22-8).

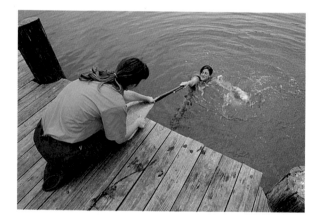

**Figure 22-7** With a reaching assist, you remain safe while reaching out to the casualty.

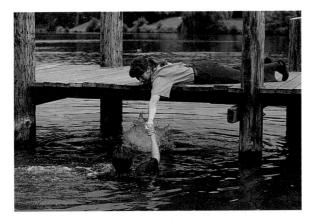

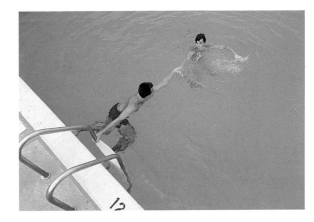

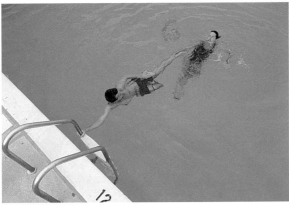

**Figure 22-8** When no object is available to extend to the casualty, try to extend your arm or extend your foot.

### Throwing Assists

With a throwing assist, you throw a heaving line, ring buoy, throw bag, rescue tube, or any other device that the casualty can grab to help stay afloat (Fig. 22-9). If a line is attached, you can pull the person to safety.

When throwing a device, follow these general principles:

- ◆ Get into a safe position where you can keep your balance.
- ◆ Secure the nonthrowing end of the line (Fig. 22-10, *A*).
- ◆ Try to throw the device beyond the casualty (Fig. 22-10, *B*).
- ◆ Throw the device so that the wind or current will bring it back within the casualty's reach.
- ◆ Once the casualty has grasped the device, slowly pull him or her to safety. Lean your body away from the casualty as you pull so that you are less likely to get pulled into the water (Fig. 22-10, *C*).

- ◆ If there is no line on the device, tell the casualty to hold on and kick to safety.

### Wading Assists

If you can enter the water without danger from currents, objects on the bottom, or an unexpected dropoff, wade in and reach to the casualty. If possible, extend your reach using a floatable

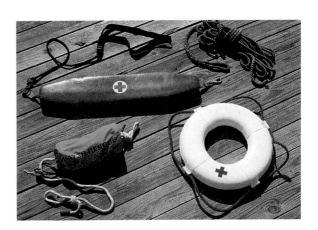

**Figure 22-9** Throwing devices.

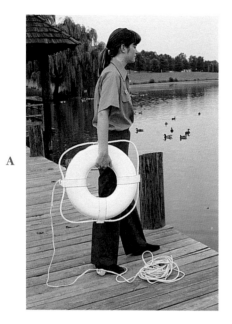

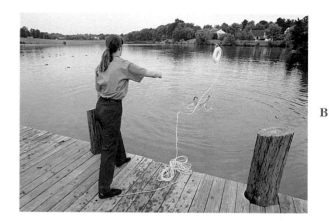

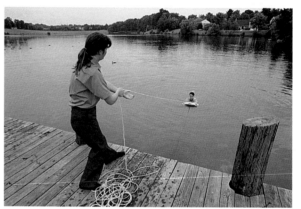

**Figure 22-10 A,** Secure the nonthrowing end of the line before throwing. **B,** Throw the device beyond the casualty. **C,** Lean your body away from the casualty as you slowly pull the casualty in.

item, such as a rescue tube, a ring buoy, a buoyant cushion, a raft, a kickboard, a ***personal flotation device (PFD)*** or a lifejacket. If you do not have a buoyant object, reach out with a tree branch, a pole, or another object (Fig. 22-11).

Whatever object you have, use it for support in the water. Let the casualty grasp the other side of it. You can then pull the casualty to safety, or you can let go of an object that floats and tell the casualty to kick with it toward safety. Keep the safety device between you and the casualty so that a panicky casualty cannot grab you and pull you under.

### After Reaching the Casualty

After reaching the casualty, remove the casualty from the water as quickly as possible. If you sus-pect the casualty may have a head or spinal injury, you must support the casualty's neck and keep it aligned with the body. If it is necessary to turn the casualty on his or her back, the casualty's head, neck, chest, and the rest of the body must be aligned, supported, and turned as a unit. The casualty should be floated on his or her back onto a firm support, such as a backboard or a surfboard, before being moved from the water.

Once the casualty is out of the water, open the airway and check for breathing. Begin ventilation if the casualty is not breathing. If you are unable to get air into the casualty, the airway is probably obstructed. In this case, follow the procedure for an obstructed airway. Once you have been able to get your air in, check for signs of circulation.

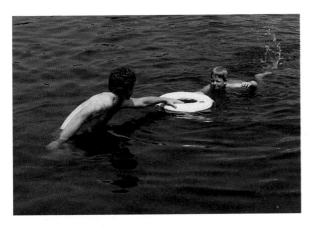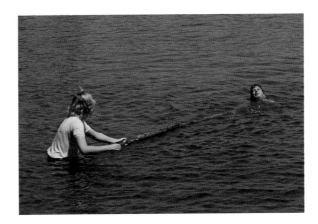

**Figure 22-11** If you can enter the water without endangering yourself, wade out toward the casualty and extend an object for the casualty to grasp.

The pulse may be difficult to detect in a near-drowning casualty and may have to be checked a little longer. If you cannot detect a pulse or signs of circulation, start CPR. Performing chest compressions in the water is not practical. The body needs to be on a hard, firm, horizontal surface for compressions to be effective.

Basic life support should be continued until more advanced medical help is available. Every near-drowning casualty, regardless of how rapid the recovery, should be transported to a medical facility immediately for follow-up care.

You should attempt to resuscitate the casualty even if he or she has been submerged for a prolonged period. People have been successfully resuscitated even after being submerged for longer than 30 minutes. Continue CPR until advanced care can be started.

### Self-Rescue

Besides knowing the skills needed to rescue someone in trouble in the water, you should know what to do to help yourself if you suddenly get into trouble in the water. Whenever you attempt a water rescue in a dangerous water environment, you should wear a PFD.

However, if you unexpectedly fall into the water without a PFD, you may need to remove clothing to swim or float. But some clothing, such as a long-sleeved shirt that buttons, will actually help you float and also help protect you from cold. If your shoes are light enough for you to swim comfortably, leave them on. If they are too heavy, remove them.

Tread water to stay in an upright position while you signal for help or wait for rescue. You may need to tread water while you arrange your clothing to help you float. To tread water, stay vertical and submerge to your chin. Move your hands back and forth and use a kick that you can do effectively and comfortably, using the least amount of energy.

### Ice Rescue

People needlessly die each year as a result of falling through ice. Unfortunately, some of these incidents also involve well-intentioned first responders rushing to aid the casualties. Ice rescues are dangerous. They require special training and equipment.

Ice is not uniformly thick. Just because ice is safe enough to walk on in one area does not

# An Icy Rescue

Rescuers who pulled Michelle Funk from an icy creek near her home thought she was gone. The child's eyes stared dully ahead, her body was chilled and blue, and her heart had stopped beating. The 2½-year-old had been under the icy water for more than an hour. By all basic measurements of life, she was dead.

Years ago, Michelle's family would have prepared for her funeral. Instead, paramedics performed CPR on Michelle's still body as they rushed her to a children's medical centre, where Dr. Robert G. Bolte took over care. Bolte had been reading about a rewarming technique used on adult hypothermia casualties, and he thought it would work on Michelle. Surgeons sometimes intentionally cool a casualty when preparing for surgery and use heart-lung machines to rewarm the casualty's blood after surgery. This cooling helps keep oxygen in the blood longer. Bolte ordered Michelle to the heart-lung machine, which provided oxygen and removed carbon dioxide, in addition to warming the blood. When Michelle's temperature reached 25 degrees Celcius (77 degrees F), the comatose child gasped. Soon her heart was pumping on its own.

Doctors once believed the brain could not survive more than 5 to 7 minutes without oxygen, but miraculous survivals like Michelle's have changed opinions. Ironically, researchers have determined that freezing water actually helps to protect the body from drowning.

In icy water, a person's body temperature begins to drop almost as soon as the body hits the water. The body loses heat in water 32 times faster than it does in the air. Swallowing water accelerates this cooling. As the body's core temperature drops, the metabolic rate drops. Activity in the cells comes to almost a standstill, and they require very little oxygen. Any oxygen left in the blood is diverted from other parts of the body to the brain and heart.

This state of suspended animation allows humans to survive underwater four to five times as long as doctors once believed was possible. Nearly 20 cases of miraculous survivals have been documented in medical journals, although unsuccessful cases are rarely described. Most cases involve children who were 15 minutes or longer

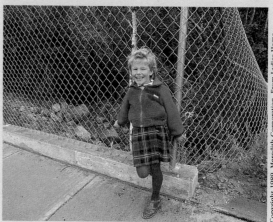

in water temperatures of 5 degrees Celcius (41 degrees F) or less. Children survive better because their bodies cool faster than adult's bodies.

Researchers once theorized that the physiological responses were caused by a "mammalian dive reflex" similar to a response found in whales and seals. They believed the same dive mechanism that allowed whales and seals to stay underwater for long periods of time was triggered in drowning humans. But experiments have failed to support the idea. Many researchers now say the best explanation for the slowdown is simply the body's response to extreme cold.

After being attached to the heart-lung machine for nearly an hour, Michelle was moved into an intensive care unit. She stayed in a coma for more than a week. She was blind for a short period, and doctors weren't sure she would recover. But slowly she began to respond. First she smiled when her parents came into the room, and soon she was talking like a 2½-year-old again. After she left the hospital, she suffered a tremor from nerve damage. But Michelle was one of the lucky ones— eventually she regained her sight, full balance, and coordination.

Although breakthroughs have saved many lives, parents still must be vigilant around their children when near water. Most near-drowning casualties are not as lucky as Michelle. One of every three survivors suffers neurological damage. There is no substitute for close supervision.

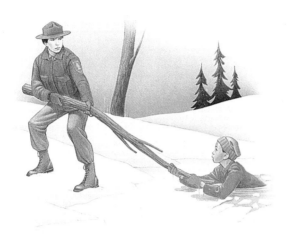

**Figure 22-12** Use an object such as a tree branch to reach a casualty who has fallen through the ice.

mean that it is safe in other areas. While trying to reach the casualty, you could walk on an undetected thin spot and suddenly fall through the ice.

The safest methods of ice rescue are those that do not require you to contact the casualty. Using a reaching device, such as a stick or pole, is your best initial action to reach a casualty who is nearby (Fig. 22-12). If the casualty is farther out on the ice, you should try to throw a line or floatable object to the casualty. If the casualty is beyond your reach or throwing distance, do *not* venture onto the ice yourself. Summon necessary personnel, such as fire and rescue personnel, for assistance.

When attempting any ice rescue, you should always have the following:

- *Adequate personnel*—Never attempt a rescue by yourself. You will often need the assistance of several others to pull the casualty to safety.
- *Proper clothing*—Items such as wet suits or dry suits are required clothing if you are likely to enter the water.
- *Proper equipment*—PFDs for you and the casualty, rope, boat, paddle, and ice pick (screwdriver could substitute) are all necessary items.

- *Appropriate training*—Beyond the basic water rescue skills of reach and throw, rescuers should have the skills needed to operate a rescue boat or ice sled or to move properly over ice toward a casualty. These skills can be obtained through specialized ice rescue courses.

## ◆ MOVING CASUALTIES

Usually when you provide care, you will not face hazards that require moving the casualty immediately. In most cases, you can give care where you find the casualty. Moving a casualty needlessly can lead to further injury. For example, moving a casualty who has a closed fracture of the leg without taking the time to splint it could result in an open fracture if the end of the bone tears the skin. Soft tissue damage, damage to nerves, blood loss, and infection all could result unnecessarily. Needless movement of a casualty with a head or spinal injury could cause paralysis or even death.

There are three general situations requiring you to perform an emergency move:

- *Immediate danger*—Danger to you or the casualty from fire, lack of oxygen, risk of drowning, possible explosion, collapsing structure, or uncontrolled traffic hazards.
- *Gaining access to other casualties*—A person with minor injuries may need to be moved quickly to reach other casualties who may have life-threatening conditions.
- *Providing proper care*—A casualty with a medical emergency, such as a cardiac arrest or heat stroke, may need to be moved to provide proper care. For example, someone in cardiac arrest needs CPR. It should be performed on a firm, flat surface. If the casualty collapses on a bed or in a small bathroom, the surface or space may not be adequate to provide appropriate care. You may have to move the casualty to give the proper care.

Before you act, you must consider the limitations of the situation. Consider the following limitations to ensure moving one or more casualties quickly and safely:

◆ Dangerous conditions at the scene
◆ The size of the casualty
◆ Your own physical ability
◆ Whether others can help you
◆ The casualty's condition

Failing to consider these limitations could result in injury. If you become injured, you may be unable to move the casualty and may risk making the situation worse. In this instance, you will have become part of the problem that arriving personnel with more advanced training will have to deal with. The situation will have become more complicated because now there is one more person to rescue.

To protect yourself and the casualty, follow these guidelines when moving someone:

◆ Only attempt to move a casualty you are sure you can comfortably handle.
◆ Bend your body at the knees and hips.
◆ Lift with your legs, not your back.
◆ Walk carefully, using short steps.
◆ When possible, move forward rather than backward.
◆ Look where you are going.
◆ Support the casualty's head and spine.
◆ Avoid bending or twisting a casualty with possible head or spinal injury.

There are many different ways to move a casualty to safety, but *no one way is best.* As long as you can move a casualty to safety without injuring yourself or causing further injury to the casualty, the move is successful.

Moves used by first responders include assists, carries, and drags. The most common of these are the—

◆ Walking assist.
◆ Pack-strap carry.
◆ Two-person seat carry.

◆ Clothes drag.
◆ Foot drag.

All of these moves can be done by one or two people and without equipment. This is important because with most moves, equipment is not often immediately available and time is critical.

## Walking Assist

The most basic move is the **walking assist.** It is frequently used to help casualties who simply need assistance to walk to safety. Either one or two rescuers can use this method with a conscious casualty. To do a walking assist, place the casualty's arm across your shoulders and hold it in place with one hand. Support the casualty with your other hand around the casualty's waist (Fig. 22-13, *A*). In this way, your body acts as a "crutch," supporting the casualty's weight while you both walk. A second rescuer, if present, can support the casualty in the same way from the other side (Fig. 22-13, *B*).

## Pack-Strap Carry

The pack-strap carry can be used on both conscious and unconscious casualties. To use it on an unconscious casualty requires a second rescuer to help position the casualty on your back. To perform the pack-strap carry, have the casualty stand or have a second rescuer help support the casualty. Position yourself with your back to the casualty, knees bent, so that your shoulders fit into the casualty's armpits. Cross the casualty's arms in front of you and grasp the casualty's wrists (Fig. 22-14, *A*). Lean forward slightly and pull the casualty up onto your back. Stand up and walk to safety (Fig. 22-14, *B*). Depending on the size of your casualty, you may be able to hold both of the casualty's wrists with one hand. This leaves your other hand free to help maintain balance, open doors, and remove obstructions.

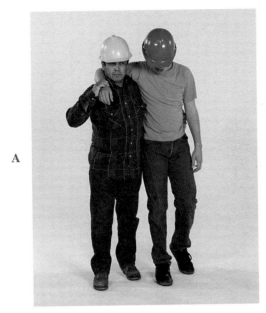

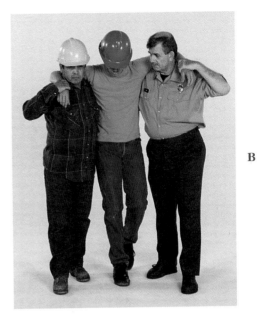

**Figure 22-13  A,** The most basic emergency move is the walking assist. **B,** A second rescuer can support the casualty from the other side.

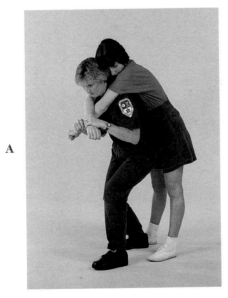

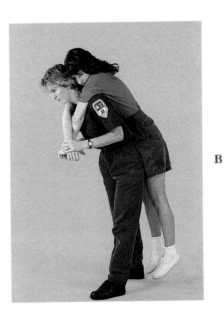

**Figure 22-14  A,** To perform the pack-strap carry, position yourself with your back to the casualty. Cross the casualty's arms in front of you and grasp the casualty's wrists. **B,** Lean forward slightly and pull the casualty onto your back.

## Two-Person Seat Carry

The two-person seat carry is a method for moving a casualty that requires a second rescuer. To perform the two-person seat carry, put one arm under the casualty's thighs and the other across the casualty's back. Interlock your arms with those of a second rescuer under the casualty's legs and across the casualty's back. The casualty is then lifted in the "seat" formed by the rescuers' arms (Fig. 22-15). The move

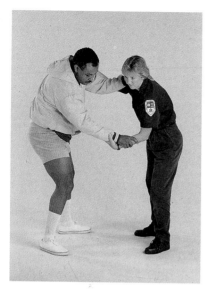
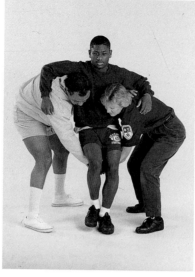
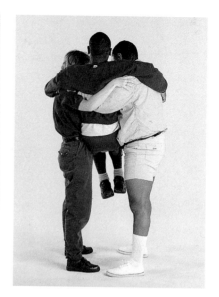

**Figure 22-15**  The two-person seat carry.

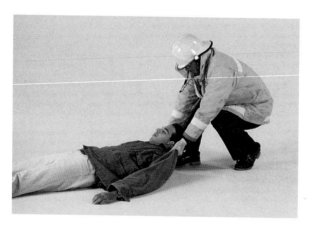

**Figure 22-16**  The clothes drag is most appropriate for moving a person suspected of having a head or spinal injury.

should not be used for a casualty suspected of having serious head or spinal injury.

## Clothes Drag

The clothes drag is an appropriate emergency move for a casualty suspected of having a head or spinal injury. This move helps keep the head and neck stabilized. To do a clothes drag, gather the casualty's clothing behind the casualty's neck. Using the clothing, pull the casualty to safety. During the move, the casualty's head is cradled by both the clothing and the rescuer's hands (Fig. 22-16). This type of emergency move is exhausting and may result in back strain for the rescuer, even when done properly.

## ◆ SUMMARY

Take the time to survey the scene before attempting to gain access to or move the casualty. This is especially true in incidents involving hazardous materials. When gaining access, always try the simple approach first, such as checking all doors and windows for easy access. Check to see if anyone has keys. If you must forcibly gain access, several basic tools and techniques can be used.

A common mistake to avoid is forcibly gaining access or moving an ill or injured casualty unnecessarily. If you recognize a potentially life-threatening situation that requires a casualty to be moved, use one of the techniques described in this chapter. Use the safest and easiest method to rapidly move the casualty without causing injury to either yourself or the casualty.

In water emergencies, use the basics of reach, throw, or wade to rescue someone without endangering yourself. Enter the water only if you have been trained to do so and have the proper equipment.

## YOU ARE THE RESPONDER

*You are inspecting the work being done in a subway tunnel. Suddenly, you hear the sound of the ceiling giving way and the crash of metal scaffolding on which you saw two men standing. As you and others rush back to the scene, you notice that one of the workers is conscious but is in obvious pain and is holding his leg. The other worker, lying a short distance away, is unconscious. There is a possibility that the ceiling might give way again. Should these casualties be moved? Why or why not? If you decide to move them, how would you do so?*

# Multiple Casualty Incidents

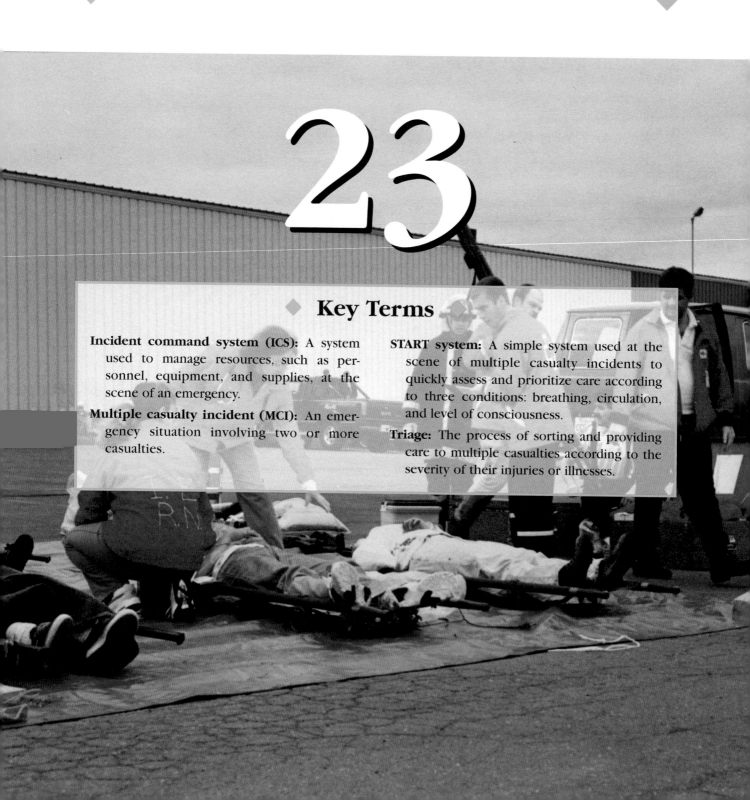

## 23

### ◆ Key Terms

**Incident command system (ICS):** A system used to manage resources, such as personnel, equipment, and supplies, at the scene of an emergency.

**Multiple casualty incident (MCI):** An emergency situation involving two or more casualties.

**START system:** A simple system used at the scene of multiple casualty incidents to quickly assess and prioritize care according to three conditions: breathing, circulation, and level of consciousness.

**Triage:** The process of sorting and providing care to multiple casualties according to the severity of their injuries or illnesses.

## ◆ For Review ◆

Before reading this chapter, you should have a basic understanding of your role as a first responder (Chapter 1), know the guidelines to follow to ensure your safety at an emergency scene (Chapter 2), and know how to assess a casualty's condition using a primary and a secondary survey (Chapter 5).

## ◆ INTRODUCTION

*In rush-hour traffic, the driver of a tractor trailer loses control of the vehicle on a rain-slick, four-lane highway. The rig crosses the centre line, "jackknifes," and slides into an embankment. Numerous cars and a loaded tour bus try frantically to avoid colliding with the tractor trailer. Two cars collide head on. The bus plunges over an embankment, coming to rest 5 metres (15 feet) below in a ditch. Minor collisions occur farther back from the scene. Many people are injured; some are probably dead.*

As a first responder, you are likely to be among the first trained individuals nearby or summoned to assist with a serious incident such as this. The task of trying to create order out of chaos will initially fall on you. To respond most effectively to an emergency with multiple casualties, you need a plan of action. This plan must enable you to rapidly determine what additional resources are needed and how best to use them. During a serious incident, it is not uncommon for you to be on the scene for 15 minutes before any other trained personnel arrive. It could be up to an hour before adequate resources are available to care for the large number of casualties.

An appropriate initial response can eliminate potential problems for arriving personnel and possibly save the lives of several injured casualties. To accomplish this, you must thoroughly understand your plan of action. Your plan must enable you to take charge. This includes making the scene safe for you and others to work, delegating responsibilities to others, managing available resources, identifying and caring for the casualties most in need of care, and relinquishing command as more highly trained personnel arrive.

## ◆ MULTIPLE CASUALTY INCIDENTS

As the term implies, a *multiple casualty incident (MCI)* refers to a situation involving two or more casualties (Fig. 23-1). You are most likely to encounter small MCIs involving injury to only a few casualties, such as a motor vehicle crash involving the driver and a passenger. But MCIs can also be large-scale events, such as those caused by natural or man made disasters. Examples include—

- ◆ Flood.
- ◆ Fire.
- ◆ Explosion.
- ◆ Structure collapse.
- ◆ Train derailment.
- ◆ Airliner crash.
- ◆ Hazardous materials incident.
- ◆ Earthquake.
- ◆ Tornado.
- ◆ Hurricane.

Incidents of this magnitude can result in hundreds or even thousands of injured or ill casualties. Whether small- or large-scale, multiple casualty incidents can strain the resources of a local community. Coping effectively with an MCI requires a plan that enables you to acquire and manage additional personnel, equipment, and supplies.

## Organizing Resources
### The Incident Command System

Providing appropriate help to one or more casualties in an emergency involves organization.

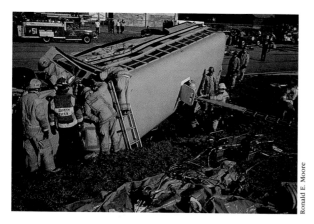

**Figure 23-1** A multiple casualty incident (MCI) involves two or more casualties.

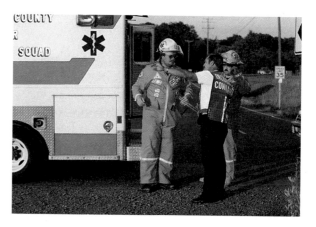

**Figure 23-2** The Incident Commander delegates responsibility as the need arises.

Different types of incidents vary in complexity. Multiple casualty incidents can strain the resources of the first responding personnel and require additional resources from other areas, some far away. To ensure that the various resources operate in an orderly, united fashion to accomplish a task, the incident command system was developed.

The ***incident command system (ICS)*** is a management system designed to be used for a wide variety of emergencies. It is especially useful in emergencies involving multiple casualties because of its ability to handle several emergency situations at the same time. It is a common system that can be easily understood by different agencies working together at the scene of an emergency.

Originally developed in California to manage the large numbers of fire fighters necessary for major brush and forest fires, the ICS has subsequently been modified for use in a variety of multiple casualty incidents. To understand the ICS, think of it as an organization. An organization is a group of people working together to achieve a common goal. To do this, the organization must clearly define who is in charge, the scope of authority and responsibility, the goal, and the objectives to accomplish the goal. This same approach applies to the ICS (Fig. 23-2). The advantages of the ICS for use in numerous situations include—

- ◆ Terms commonly understood by those taking part.
- ◆ One "boss" with the absolute authority to do what is necessary to accomplish the goal.
- ◆ One unified command structure with well-established divisions, all working to accomplish the same goal.
- ◆ An integrated communications system.
- ◆ Easily managed units normally consisting of not more than four people.

### Using the incident command system

A police officer is dispatched to a single motor vehicle collision. Since she is the first responder to arrive at the scene, she assumes the role of Incident Commander. She surveys the scene to determine the magnitude of the incident. She makes the scene safe for herself, bystanders, and any casualties. Once the scene is safe, she approaches the vehicle. The driver has already left the vehicle and is seated on the curb next to the vehicle. The officer determines that the driver is the only casualty and approximates the type of injuries. The officer notifies the dispatcher of the situation, requesting only an ambulance as an additional resource. She gathers information from the casualty while providing care until more advanced medical personnel arrive. Once the casualty is turned over to the arriving EMTs, the officer reassesses scene safety, checks to make sure nothing else is needed, finishes gathering information, and completes any paperwork.

In this situation, the resources needed were minimal. But what if the car had struck a utility pole and knocked down an electrical wire, the casualty had been trapped in a crushed vehicle, or there had been multiple casualties? As the Incident Commander, the police officer would have notified the dispatcher of the situation and requested additional resources. The power company would have been summoned for the downed wire. If a person was trapped in the vehicle, resources such as the fire department or specialized rescue squad personnel would have been sent to the scene.

As these personnel arrive, the police officer could continue to act as the Incident Commander, or command could be turned over to other more experienced personnel. These decisions are often based on the type of emergency and on local protocols. If the incident is beyond your scope, you should only act as Incident Commander until a more experienced person arrives. At this point, he or she will assume command.

At other times, you may be responding to a large-scale MCI because it requires additional personnel. Where you are placed and how your services are used will be based on your expertise and the needs at the time. This could include assisting medical personnel, aiding in crowd or traffic control, helping to maintain scene security, or helping to establish temporary shelter (Fig. 23-3). By using the ICS in numerous emergencies, the tasks of reaching, caring for, and transporting casualties are performed more effectively, thereby saving more lives. Since there are variations in the ICS throughout the country, you should become familiar with the ICS for your local community.

## Caring for the Ill or Injured

### Triage

In previous chapters, you learned how to conduct a systematic assessment of a casualty by doing a primary and a secondary survey. This

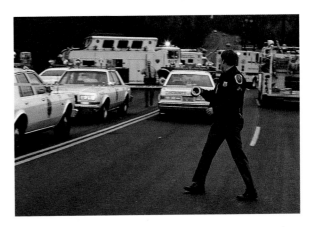

**Figure 23-3**  When you arrive on the scene, you may be asked to aid in crowd or traffic control.

enabled you to care for life-threatening emergencies before minor injuries. You will recall that the primary survey has three steps that involve checking the casualty's airway, breathing, and circulation. You will also recall that the secondary survey has three steps that include interviewing the casualty, checking vital signs, and doing a head-to-toe examination.

Though this approach is appropriate for one casualty, it is not effective when there are fewer rescuers than casualties. If you took the time to completely conduct each of these six steps and to correct all problems that you found, your entire time could be spent with only one casualty. A casualty who is unconscious and not breathing, simply because the tongue is blocking the airway, could be overlooked and die while your attention is given to caring for someone with a less severe injury, such as a broken arm.

In a multiple casualty incident, you must modify your technique for checking casualties. This requires you to understand your priorities. It also requires that you accept death and dying, because some casualties, such as those in cardiac arrest who would normally receive CPR and be high-priority casualties, will be beyond your ability to help in this situation.

To identify which casualties require urgent care in a multiple casualty incident, you use a process known as triage. *Triage* is an old French term that was first used to refer to the sorting and treatment of those injured in battle. Today, the triage process is used any time there are more casualties than rescuers. Its common definition is the sorting of casualties into categories according to the severity of their injuries or illnesses.

### The START system

Over the years, a number of systems have been used to triage casualties. Most, however, required you to "diagnose" the exact extent of injury or illness. This was often time consuming and resulted in delays in assessment and care for casualties in multiple casualty incidents. As a result, the *START system* was created. START stands for Simple Triage And Rapid Treatment. It is a simple way to quickly assess and prioritize casualties. The START system requires you to check only three items: breathing, circulation, and level of consciousness. As you check these items, you will classify casualties into one of three levels that reflect the severity of injury or illness and need for care. These levels are "immediate," "delayed," and "dead/non-salvageable."

Using the START system requires that the first rescuers on the scene clear the area of all those casualties with only minor problems. These are sometimes called the "walking wounded." If a casualty is able to walk from the site of the incident, allow him or her to do so (Fig. 23-4). Have these casualties walk to a designated area for evaluation by arriving medical personnel. This first action is critical to the success of START. It enables you to move people to safety, ensures higher-level medical care, and reduces the number of remaining casualties that you need to check.

Next, move quickly among the remaining casualties, assessing the severity of the problems. As you do so, you are attempting to classify each casualty into one of three categories for care.

The first of these categories is "immediate care." This categorization means that the casualty needs immediate transport to a medical facility. An example of an "immediate" casualty

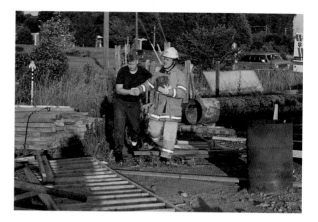

**Figure 23-4** Casualties who are able to move away from the scene on their own should walk to a designated area.

is one who requires his or her airway to be cleared to enable breathing to continue.

The second category is "delayed care." This category is assigned to a person who is breathing and has pulse and level of consciousness within normal limits but who may not be able to move because of a broken leg or back injury.

The final category is "dead/non-salvageable." This category is assigned to those individuals obviously dead. Casualties who are initially found not breathing and who fail to breathe after attempts are made to open and clear the airway are classified as dead/non-salvageable. This is also true for obvious mortal injury, such as decapitation.

As you classify each casualty into one of these three categories, you need to mark the casualty in some distinguishing manner so that rescuers coming behind you will be able to begin to care for and remove the most critical casualties first. This process of labelling casualties is easily done with commercial triage markers or multicolored tape, which should be fastened to the casualty in an easily noticeable area, such as around the wrist (Fig. 23-5). Colour codes are as follows:

- Immediate = red
- Delay = yellow or green
- Dead/non-salvageable = black or gray

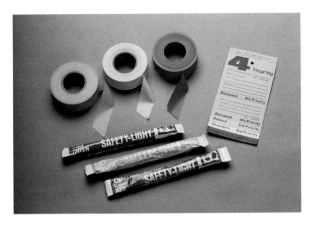

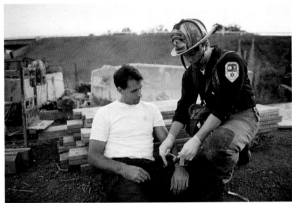

**Figure 23-5** Triage markers are used to label casualties.

To make this decision, take the following steps:

*Step one:* Check breathing. When you locate a casualty, begin by assessing whether he or she is breathing. If the casualty is not breathing, clear the mouth of any foreign object and make sure the airway is open. If the casualty does not begin breathing on his or her own, even with the airway open, the casualty is classified as "dead/non-salvageable." There is no need to check the pulse. Place a black or gray marker on the casualty and move on.

On the other hand, if the casualty does begin to breathe on his or her own when you open the airway, this casualty should be classified as needing "immediate" care. Any individual who needs help maintaining an open airway is a high priority. Position the casualty in a way that will maintain an open airway, place a red tag on the casualty, and move on to the next casualty. Once triage of all casualties is complete, you may be able to come back and assist with the care of the casualties.

If the casualty is breathing when you arrive, you must check the rate of the casualty's breathing. A casualty breathing more than 30 times a minute should be classified "immediate." A person breathing less than 30 times a minute should be further evaluated. This requires you to move to the next check—circulation.

*Step two:* Check circulation. The next step is to evaluate the breathing casualty's pulse. You do this by checking the radial pulse. You are only checking for *the presence* of the radial pulse. If you cannot find the radial pulse in either arm, then the casualty's blood pressure is substantially low. Control any severe bleeding by using direct pressure and elevation and applying a pressure bandage. Classify the casualty as one requiring "immediate" care and move on to the next casualty. If the pulse is present and no severe bleeding is evident, conduct the final check—level of consciousness.

*Step three:* Check level of consciousness. The final step is to assess the casualty's level of consciousness. At this point, you know the following about the casualty:

◆ Breathing is normal (less than 30 times per minute).
◆ Radial pulse is present. (Severe bleeding may or may not be present.)

This final check will serve to classify this casualty. You determine the casualty's level of consciousness by using the AVPU scale you learned in Chapter 5. You give a person who is alert and responds appropriately to verbal stimuli a final classification of "delayed." This person has some injury that prevents him or her from moving to safety, but his or her present condition is not life threatening. A casualty who remains unconscious, responds only to painful stimuli, or responds inappropriately to verbal stimuli is classified as "immediate."

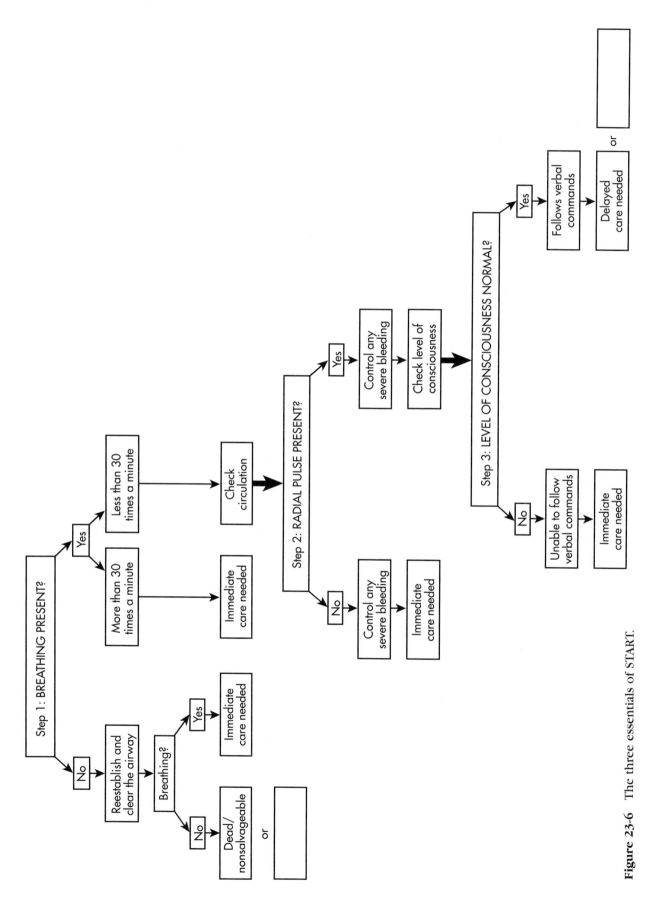

**Figure 23-6** The three essentials of START.

## Table 23-1    START Classification System

| Immediate (red) | Delayed (yellow/green) | Dead/non-salvageable (black/gray) |
|---|---|---|
| Breathing more than 30 times a minute | Breathing normal, radial pulse present, *and* level of consciousness normal | Not breathing |
| Breathing normal, but radial pulse absent | | |
| Breathing normal, radial pulse present, *but* level of consciousness abnormal | | |

By using the START system, you will be able to move quickly among casualties, assessing and classifying them (Fig. 23-6). Remember, your role is not to provide extensive care for the casualty. Instead, you are expected to get to as many casualties as possible. You should not at any time stop triaging casualties to begin CPR on one of them. This person is dead, and if you start CPR, you will need to continue. As a result, others who might have lived if you had done your job properly could now die as a result of delay. The likelihood that a trauma casualty in cardiac arrest will survive is extremely rare. Table 23-1 provides a simple overview of the START classification system.

## ◆ SUMMARY

Multiple casualty incidents (MCIs) can be small- or large-scale operations. They can range from two people injured in a motor vehicle collision to hundreds injured in the collapse of a structure. Coping effectively with the magnitude of the problem requires an organized approach.

The incident command system (ICS) provides this approach. The ICS provides for efficient use of resources, such as personnel, equipment, and supplies. When the ICS is used with an effective triage system such as START, the lives of many people can be saved because rescuers are able to reach, sort, and care for casualties in the most efficient manner.

### YOU ⯈ ARE THE RESPONDER

*Concrete has recently been poured on the uppermost floor of a three-level parking garage under construction. Suddenly, the floor buckles and a portion of the structure crashes down—floor after floor. Thirty workers are in the structure at the time of the collapse. Half of the workers escape injury. The remaining 15 are unaccounted for. Some are probably trapped or crushed under the debris. Others, however, jumped from the structure as it collapsed and are injured. You are the first to respond. Using the principles of the incident command system and triage, describe how you would handle this situation.*

# Glossary

**Abandonment:** Ending care of an ill or injured casualty without that casualty's consent or without ensuring that someone with equal or greater training will continue that care.

**Abdomen:** The part of the trunk below the ribs and above the pelvis.

**Abdominal cavity:** An area located in the trunk that contains the liver, pancreas, intestine, stomach, and spleen; not protected by any bones.

**Abdominal thrusts:** A technique for unblocking an obstructed airway by giving forceful pushes to the abdomen.

**Abrasion (ah BRA zhun):** A wound characterized by skin that has been scraped or rubbed away.

**Absorbed poison:** A poison that enters the body through the skin.

**Active listening:** A process that helps you more fully communicate with a casualty by focusing on what the casualty is saying.

**Adolescent:** A person between 13 and 18 years of age.

**Advanced cardiac life support (ACLS):** Techniques and treatments designed for use with casualties of cardiac emergencies.

**AIDS (acquired immune deficiency syndrome):** A condition caused by the human immunodeficiency virus (HIV).

**Airborne transmission:** The transmission of a disease by inhaling infected droplets that become airborne when an infected casualty coughs or sneezes.

**Airway:** The pathway for air from the mouth and nose to the lungs.

**Airway obstruction:** A blockage of the airway that prevents air from reaching a casualty's lungs.

**Alveoli (al VE oli):** Tiny air sacs in the lungs where gases and waste are exchanged between the lungs and the blood.

**Alzheimer's disease:** A progressive, degenerative disease that affects the brain; results in impaired memory, thinking, and behaviour.

**Amniotic (am ne OT ik) sac:** A fluid-filled sac that encloses, bathes, and protects the developing fetus; commonly called the bag of waters.

**Amputation:** The complete removal or severing of a body part.

**Anaphylactic (an ah fi LAK tik) shock:** A severe allergic reaction in which air passages may swell and restrict breathing; a form of shock.

**Anaphylaxis (an ah fi LAK sis):** see Anaphylactic shock.

**Anaphylaxis kit:** A container that holds the medication and any necessary equipment used to prevent or counteract anaphylactic shock.

**Anatomic splint:** A splint that uses an uninjured body part to immobilize an injured body part.

**Anatomical obstruction:** The blockage of the airway by an anatomical structure, such as the tongue.

**Aneurysm (AN u rizm):** A condition in which the wall of an artery or vein weakens, balloons out, and ruptures; usually caused by disease, trauma, or a natural weakness in the vessel wall.

**Angina (an JI nah) pectoris (pek TO ris):** Chest pain that comes and goes at different times, often brought on by physical exertion; commonly associated with cardiovascular disease.

**Angulated (AN gu la ted):** Sharply bent.

**Anterior:** Toward the front of the body.

**Antibiotics (an ti bi OT iks):** Medicines prescribed to help the body fight bacterial infections.

**Antibodies (AN ti bod ez):** Infection-fighting proteins released by white blood cells.

**Antivenin:** A material used to counteract the poisonous effects of snake, spider, or insect venom.

**Arm:** The entire upper extremity from the shoulder to the hand.

**Arteries (AR·ter ez):** The large blood vessels that carry oxygen-rich blood from the heart to all parts of the body.

**Arthritis (ar THRI tis):** An inflamed condition of the joints, causing pain and swelling and sometimes limiting motion.

**Ashen:** A grayish colour that darker skin becomes when it turns pale.

**Aspiration (as pi RA shun):** Taking blood, vomit, saliva, or other foreign material into the lungs.

**Assault:** Abuse, either physical or sexual, resulting in injury and often emotional crisis.

**Asthma:** A condition that narrows the air passages and makes breathing difficult.

**Asystole (ah SIS to le):** The stopping of all electrical activity in the heart.

**Atherosclerosis (ath er o skle RO sis):** A form of cardiovascular disease marked by a narrowing of the arteries in the heart and other parts of the body.

**Atria:** The upper chambers of the heart.

**Aura (AW rah):** An unusual sensation or feeling a casualty may experience before an epileptic seizure; may be a visual hallucination; a strange sound, taste, or smell; or an urgent need to get to safety.

**Auscultation (aws kul TA shun):** The process of using a blood pressure cuff and a stethoscope to listen for characteristic blood pressure sounds.

**Automatic external defibrillator (de FIB ri la tor) (AED):** An automatic device used to recognize a heart rhythm that requires a shock and either deliver the shock or prompt the rescuer to deliver it.

**Avulsion (ah VUL shun):** A wound in which a portion of the skin, and sometimes other soft tissue, is partially or completely torn away.

**Bacteria (bac TE re ah):** One-celled microorganisms that may cause infections.

**Bag-valve-mask (BVM) resuscitator:** A hand-held ventilation device, consisting of a self-inflating bag, a one-way valve, and a face mask, that can be used with or without supplemental oxygen.

**Bandage:** Material used to wrap or cover part of the body; commonly used to hold a dressing or splint in place.

**Bandage compress:** A thick gauze dressing attached to a gauze bandage; used to help control severe bleeding.

**Bile:** A yellow-green secretion of the liver that is stored in the gallbladder and is released to help the body digest and absorb fat.

**Biological death:** The irreversible damage caused by the death of brain cells.

**Birth canal:** The passageway from the uterus to the vaginal opening through which a baby passes during birth.

**Bladder:** An organ in the pelvis in which urine is stored until released from the body.

**Blood pressure (BP):** The force exerted against the blood vessel walls by blood as it travels throughout the body.

**Blood pressure cuff:** A device used to measure a person's blood pressure.

**Blood volume:** The total amount of blood circulating within the body.

**Body cavity:** A hollow place in the body that contains organs, glands, blood vessels, and nerves.

**Body substance isolation (BSI):** An infection control strategy that considers all body substances as potentially infectious.

**Body system:** A group of organs and other structures working together to carry out specific functions.

**Bone:** A dense, hard tissue that forms the skeleton.

**Brachial (BRA ke al) artery:** A large artery located in the upper arm.

**Brain:** The centre of the nervous system that controls all body functions.

**Breathing devices:** Devices used to help with ventilation.

**Breathing emergency:** A situation in which breathing is so impaired that life is threatened.

**Breech birth:** The delivery of a baby feet first or buttocks first.

**Bronchi (BRONG ki):** The air passages that lead from the trachea to the lungs.

**Burn:** An injury to the skin or other body tissues caused by heat, chemicals, electricity, or radiation.

**Capillaries (KAP i ler ez):** Tiny blood vessels linking arteries and veins that transfer oxygen and other nutrients from the blood to all body cells and remove waste products.

**Capillary refill:** An estimate of the amount of blood flowing through the capillary beds, such as those in the fingertips.

**Carbon dioxide:** A colourless, odourless gas; a waste product of respiration.

**Cardiac (KAR de ak) arrest:** A condition in which the heart has stopped or beats too irregularly or too weakly to pump blood effectively.

**Cardiac emergencies:** Sudden illnesses involving the heart.

**Cardiogenic (kar de o JEN ik) shock:** Shock caused by the heart failing to pump blood effectively.

**Cardiopulmonary (kar de o PUL mo ner e) resuscitation (re sus i TA shun) (CPR):** A technique that combines rescue breathing and chest compressions for a casualty whose breathing and heart have stopped.

**Cardiovascular (kar de o VAS ku lar) disease:** A disease of the heart and blood vessels; commonly known as heart disease.

**Carotid arteries:** Arteries located in the neck that supply blood to the head and neck.

**Cartilage (KAR ti lij):** An elastic tissue that acts as a shock absorber when a person is walking, running, or jumping.

**Case law:** A law based on judicial decisions (cases) rather than statutes, which are enacted by legislatures.

**Casualty:** Someone needing emergency medical care because of an injury or a sudden illness.

**Cells:** The basic units of all living tissue.

**Cervical collar:** A rigid device positioned around the neck to limit movement of the head and neck.

**Cervix (SER viks):** The upper part of the birth canal.

**Chemical burns:** Burns that are caused by caustic chemicals, such as strong acids or alkalies.

**Chest thrusts:** Forceful pushes on the chest; delivered to a casualty with an obstructed airway in an attempt to expel any foreign object blocking the airway.

**Chest:** The upper part of the trunk containing the heart, major blood vessels, and lungs.

**Child abuse:** The physical, psychological, or sexual assault of a child, resulting in injury or emotional trauma.

**Chocking:** The use of items, such as wooden blocks, placed against the wheels of a vehicle to help stabilize the vehicle.

**Cholesterol (ko LES ter ol):** A fatty substance made by the body and found in certain foods.

**Circulatory cycle:** The flow of blood in the body: oxygen-rich blood flows through arteries and oxygen-poor blood flows in the veins.

**Circulatory (SER ku lah tor e) system:** A group of organs and other structures that carry oxygen-rich blood and other nutrients throughout the body and remove waste.

**Cirrhosis (si RO sis):** A disease of the liver that hinders its function; commonly associated with alcohol abuse.

**Citizen responder:** Someone who recognizes an emergency and decides to help; the first link in the emergency medical services (EMS) system.

**Clavicle (KLAV i kl):** See collarbone.

**Clinical death:** The condition in which the heart stops beating and breathing stops.

**Closed fracture:** A fracture in which the skin is left unbroken.

**Closed wound:** A wound in which soft tissue damage occurs beneath the skin and the skin is not broken.

**Clothes drag:** An emergency move used for a casualty suspected of having a head or spinal injury; helps to keep the head and neck stabilized.

**Clotting:** The process by which blood thickens at a wound site to seal an opening in a blood vessel and stop bleeding.

**Collarbone:** A horizontal bone that connects with the sternum and the shoulder; also called the clavicle.

**Complete airway obstruction:** A completely blocked airway.

**Concussion:** A temporary impairment of brain function, usually without permanent damage to the brain.

**Confidentiality:** Protecting a casualty's privacy by not revealing any personal information you learn about the casualty except to law enforcement personnel or EMS personnel caring for the casualty.

**Consciousness:** The state of being aware of one's self and one's surroundings.

**Consent:** Permission to provide care given by an ill or injured casualty to a rescuer.

**Constricting band:** A band placed around an extremity to slow the flow of venom.

**Contraction:** The pumping action of the heart.

**Contractions:** The rhythmic tightening and relaxing of muscles in the uterus during labour.

**Coronary arteries:** Blood vessels that supply the heart muscle with oxygen-rich blood.

**Cranial cavity:** An area in the body that contains the brain and is protected by the skull.

**Cravat:** A triangular bandage folded to form a long, narrow strip.

**Critical burn:** Any burn that is potentially life threatening, disabling, or disfiguring; a burn requiring medical attention.

**Critical Incident Stress Debriefing (CISD):** A process by which emergency personnel are offered the support necessary to reduce job-related stress.

**Croup (kroop):** A viral infection that causes swelling of the tissues below the vocal cords; a common childhood illness.

**Crowning:** The time in labour when the baby's head is seen at the opening of the vagina.

**Cyanosis (si ah NO sis):** A blue discolouration of the skin and membranes of the mouth and eyes, resulting from a lack of oxygen in the blood.

**Decomposition:** The breaking down of the body's chemical composition after death.

**Defibrillation (de fib ri LA shun):** An electric shock administered to correct a life-threatening heart rhythm.

**Defibrillator (de FIB ri la tor):** A device that sends an electric shock through the chest to the heart.

**Demand valve resuscitator:** A device, attached to a face mask, that delivers oxygen. A nonrestricted valve automatically delivers oxygen to a breathing casualty. A restricted valve is triggered by a rescuer to deliver oxygen to a nonbreathing casualty.

**Dentures:** A set of false teeth.

**Depressants:** Substances that affect the central nervous system to slow physical and mental activity.

**Dermis (DER mis):** The deeper of the two layers of skin.

**Designer drugs:** Chemical variations of medically prescribed or illicit substances.

**Developmentally disabled:** A person with impaired mental function, resulting from injury or genetics.

**Diabetes (di ah BE tez) mellitus (mel I tus):** A condition in which the body does not produce enough insulin.

**Diabetic (di ah BET ik):** A person with the condition called diabetes mellitus, which causes the body to produce insufficient insulin.

**Diabetic coma:** A life-threatening emergency in which the body needs insulin.

**Diabetic emergency:** A situation in which a casualty becomes ill because of an imbalance of insulin or sugar.

**Diaphragm (DI ah fram):** A dome-shaped muscle that aids breathing and separates the chest from the abdomen.

**Diastolic (di as TOL ik):** The pressure in the arteries when the heart is at rest.

**Digestive system:** A group of organs and other structures that digests food and eliminates wastes.

**Direct contact transmission:** The transmission of a disease by touching an infected casualty's body fluids.

**Direct pressure:** The pressure applied on a wound to control bleeding.

**Disease transmission:** The passage of a disease from one person to another.

**Dislocation:** The displacement of a bone from its normal position at a joint.

**Disoriented:** A state of mental confusion; not knowing place, identity, or what happened.

**Distal:** Away from the trunk of the body.

**Dressing:** A pad placed directly over a wound to absorb blood and other body fluids and to prevent infection.

**Drowning:** Death by suffocation when submerged in water.

**Drug:** Any substances other than food intended to affect the functions of the body.

**Drug paraphernalia:** Equipment used to prepare and administer drugs.

**Duty to act:** A legal responsibility of some individuals to provide a reasonable standard of emergency care; may be required by case law, statute, or job description.

**Elastic bandage:** A stretchable bandage used to maintain continuous pressure on a body part.

**Elder abuse:** Any of four types of abuse: the infliction of pain or injury (physical abuse), mental anguish or suffering (psychological abuse), financial or material abuse, or unnecessary confinement or willful deprivation (neglect) by an elderly person's caretaker.

**Electrical burn:** A burn caused by an electrical source, such as an electrical appliance or lightning.

**Electrocardiogram (e lek tro KAR de o gram) (ECG):** The movement of the electrical impulses through the heart, shown as a tracing on a screen.

**Embolism (EM bo lizm):** A sudden blockage of a blood vessel by a traveling clot or other material, such as fat or air.

**Embryo (EM bre o):** The early stages of a developing ovum; characterized by the rapid growth and development of body systems.

**Emergency action principles (EAPs):** Six steps to guide your actions in any emergency.

**Emergency medical services (EMS) system:** A network of community resources and medical personnel that provides emergency care to victims of injury or sudden illness.

**Emergency medical technician (EMT):** Someone who has taken an approved Emergency Medical Technician training program; different levels of EMTs include paramedics at the highest level.

**Emergency move:** Moving a casualty before completing care; only performed if the casualty is in immediate danger.

**Emotional crisis:** A highly emotional state resulting from stress, often involving a significant event in a person's life, such as death of a loved one.

**Emphysema (em fi SE mah):** A disease in which the lungs lose their ability to exchange carbon dioxide and oxygen effectively.

**Endocrine (EN do krin) system:** A group of organs and other structures that regulates and coordinates the activities of other systems by producing chemicals that influence the activity of tissues.

**Epidermis (ep i DER mis):** The outer layer of skin.

**Epiglottis (ep i GLOT is):** The flap of tissue that covers the trachea to keep food and liquid out of the lungs.

**Epiglottitis:** A bacterial infection that causes a severe inflammation of the epiglottis.

**Epilepsy (EP i lep se):** A chronic condition characterized by seizures that vary in type and duration; usually can be controlled by medication.

**Esophagus (e SOF ah gus):** The tube leading from the mouth to the stomach.

**Exhale:** To breathe air out of the lungs.

**External bleeding:** Visible bleeding.

**Extremities:** The arms and legs, hands and feet.

**Extrication:** The freeing of someone or something from an entanglement or difficulty.

**Fainting:** A loss of consciousness resulting from a temporary reduction of blood flow to the brain.

**Febrile (FEB ril) seizure:** A seizure caused by an elevated body temperature.

**Femoral (FEM or al) arteries:** The large arteries that supply the legs with oxygen-rich blood.

**Femur (FE mur):** The thighbone.

**Fetus (FE tus):** The developing unborn offspring after the embryonic period.

**Fibula (FIB u lah):** One of the bones in the lower leg.

**Finger sweep:** A technique used to remove foreign material from a casualty's airway.

**First responder:** A person trained in emergency care who may be called on to provide such care as a routine part of his or her job; often the first trained professional to respond to emergencies.

**Flail chest:** An injury involving fractured ribs that do not move normally with the rest of the chest during breathing.

**Flowmeter:** A device used to regulate in litres per minute (lpm) the amount of oxygen administered to a casualty.

**Foot drag:** An emergency move used for casualties too large to carry or move otherwise; gives little protection to the casualties head and neck.

**Forearm:** The upper extremity from the elbow to the wrist.

**Fracture:** A break or disruption in bone tissue.

**Frostbite:** A serious condition in which body tissues freeze, most commonly in the fingers, toes, ears, and nose.

**Full-thickness burn:** A burn injury involving both layers of skin and underlying tissues; skin may be brown or charred, and underlying tissues may appear white.

**Gastric distention:** Air in the stomach.

**Genitalia:** The external reproductive organs.

**Genitals:** See genitalia.

**Genitourinary (jen i to U ri ner e) system:** A group of organs and other structures that eliminates waste and enables reproduction.

**Glands:** Organs that release fluid and other substances into the blood or on the skin.

**Good Samaritan laws:** Laws that protect people who willingly give emergency care while acting in good faith, without negligence, and within the scope of their training.

**Hallucinogens (hal lu SI no jenz):** Substances that affect mood, sensation, thought, emotion, and self-awareness; alter perceptions of time and space; and produce delusions.

**Haemmorrhage (HEM or ij):** A loss of a large amount of blood in a short time.

**Haemmorrhagic shock:** Shock caused by severe bleeding.

**Hazardous materials:** Substances that are harmful or toxic to the body; can be liquids, solids, or gases.

**Head-tilt/chin-lift:** A technique for opening the airway.

**Hearing impaired:** A nonspecific term applied to a person who is either deaf or partially deaf.

**Heart:** A fist-size muscular organ that pumps blood throughout the body.

**Heart attack:** A sudden illness involving the death of heart muscle tissue when it does not receive enough oxygen-rich blood; also called myocardial infarction (MI).

**Heat cramps:** Painful spasms of skeletal muscles following exercise or work in warm or moderate temperatures; usually involve the calf and abdominal muscles.

**Heat exhaustion:** A form of shock, often resulting from strenuous work or exercise in a hot environment.

**Heat stroke:** A life-threatening condition that develops when the body's cooling mechanisms are overwhelmed and body systems begin to fail.

**Heimlich maneuver:** A technique used to clear the airway of a choking victim; see abdominal thrusts.

**Hepatitis (hep ah TI tis):** A viral infection of the liver.

**Hepatitis A:** A type of hepatitis that is transmitted by contact with food or other products contaminated by the stool of an infected casualty; also called infectious hepatitis.

**Hepatitis B:** A type of hepatitis that is transmitted by sexual contact and blood-to-blood contact; also called serum hepatitis.

**Herpes (HER pez):** A viral infection that causes eruptions of the skin and mucous membranes.

**High efficiency particulate air-particulate respirator (HEPA-PR):** A protective breathing device containing a high efficiency air filter that prevents transmission of certain airborne infections.

**HIV (human immunodeficiency virus):** The virus that destroys the body's ability to fight infection. The resultant state is referred to as AIDS.

**Hormone:** A substance that circulates in body fluids and has a specific effect on cell activity.

**Humerus (HU mer us):** The bone of the upper arm.

**Hyperglycemia (hi per gli SE me ah):** A condition in which too much sugar is in the bloodstream.

**Hypertension (hi per TEN shun):** High blood pressure.

**Hyperventilation:** Breathing that is faster than normal.

**Hypoglycemia (hi po gli SE me ah):** A condition in which too little sugar is in the bloodstream.

**Hypothermia (hi po THER me ah):** A life-threatening condition in which the body's warming mechanisms fail to maintain normal body temperature and the entire body cools.

**Hypoxia (hi POK se ah):** A condition in which insufficient oxygen reaches the cells, resulting in cyanosis and in changes in consciousness and in breathing and heart rates.

**Immobilisation (im mo bi li ZA shun):** The use of a splint or other method to keep an injured body part from moving.

**Immobilise:** To use a splint or other method to keep an injured body part from moving.

**Immune system:** The body's group of responses for fighting disease.

**Immunization (im u ni ZA shun):** A specific substance containing weakened or killed pathogens that is introduced into the body to build resistance to specific infection.

**Impaled object:** An object remaining in a wound.

**Implied consent:** A legal concept assuming that casualties who are unconscious, or so severely injured or ill that they cannot respond, would consent to receive emergency care.

**Incident command system (ICS):** A system used to control and direct resources at the scene of an emergency; commonly used by fire and EMS personnel.

**Indirect contact transmission:** The transmission of a disease by touching a contaminated object.

**Infant:** A child up to 1 year of age.

**Infection:** A condition caused by disease-producing microorganisms, also called pathogens or germs, in the body.

**Infectious disease:** Disease capable of being transmitted from people, objects, animals, or insects.

**Inferior:** Toward the feet.

**Informed (actual) consent:** Permission the casualty, parent, or guardian gives the rescuer to provide care. This consent requires the rescuer to explain his or her level of training, what the rescuer thinks is wrong, and the care the rescuer intends to give.

**Ingested poison:** A poison that is swallowed.

**Inhalant:** A substance, such as a medication, that a person inhales to counteract or prevent a specific condition; a substance inhaled to produce an intoxicating effect.

**Inhale:** To breathe in.

**Inhaled poison:** A poison breathed into the lungs.

**Injected poison:** A poison that enters the body through a bite, sting, or syringe.

**In-line stabilization:** A technique used to minimize movement of a casualty's head and neck.

**Insulin (IN su lin):** A hormone that enables the body to use sugar for energy; frequently injected to treat diabetes.

**Insulin reaction:** A condition in which too much insulin is in the body.

**Integumentary (in teg u MEN tar e) system:** A group of organs and other structures that protects the body, retains fluids, and helps to prevent infection.

**Internal bleeding:** Bleeding inside the body.

**Joint:** A structure where two or more bones are joined.

**Kidney:** An organ that filters waste from the blood to form urine.

**Labour:** The birth process, beginning with the contraction of the uterus and the dilating of the cervix and ending with the birth of the baby.

**Laceration (las e RA shun):** A cut, usually from a sharp object; may have jagged or smooth edges.

**Larynx (LAR ingks):** A part of the airway connecting the pharynx with the trachea; commonly called the "voice box."

**Lateral:** Away from the midline.

**Leg:** The entire lower extremity from the pelvis to the foot.

**Level of consciousness (LOC):** A person's state of awareness, ranging from being fully alert to unconscious.

**Ligament (LIG ah ment):** A fibrous band that holds bones together at a joint.

**Lividity:** Following death, a large pooling of blood in the trunk resulting in discolouration.

**Living will:** A legal document stating that an individual does not wish to be resuscitated or further kept alive by mechanical means.

**Lower leg:** The lower extremity between the knee and the ankle.

**Lungs:** A pair of organs in the chest that provides the mechanism for taking oxygen in and removing carbon dioxide during breathing.

**Lyme disease:** An illness transmitted by a certain kind of infected tick.

**Mechanism of injury:** The event or forces that caused the casualty's injury.

**Mechanical obstruction:** The blockage of the airway by a foreign object, such as a small toy or food.

**Medial:** Toward the midline.

**Medication:** A drug given to prevent or correct the effects of a disease or condition or otherwise enhance mental or physical well being.

**Membranes:** A thin sheet of tissue that covers a structure or lines a cavity, such as the mouth or nose.

**Meningitis (men in JI tis):** An inflammation of the brain or spinal cord caused by a viral or bacterial infection.

**Mentally challenged:** A person who has an impairment of mental function that interferes with normal activity.

**Metabolism:** The process by which cells convert nutrients to energy.

**Microorganism (mi kro OR gah nizm):** A bacteria, virus, or other microscopic organism that may enter the body. Those that cause an infection or disease are called germs.

**Minor:** A person who has not reached full legal age.

**Multiple casualty incident (MCI):** An emergency situation involving two or more casualty.

**Muscle:** Tissue that lengthens and shortens to create movement.

**Multi-drug resistant TB:** A strain of tuberculosis that is resistant to certain drugs commonly used to treat tuberculosis.

**Musculoskeletal (mus ku lo SKEl e tal) system:** A group of tissues and other structures that supports the body, protects internal organs, allows movement, stores minerals, manufactures blood cells, and creates heat.

**Narcotics (nar KOT iks):** Powerful depressant substances used to relieve anxiety and pain.

**Nasal cannula:** A flexible tube used to administer oxygen through the nostrils to a breathing casualty.

**Near-drowning:** A situation in which a casualty who has been submerged in water survives.

**Negligence:** The failure to provide the level of care a person of similar training would provide, thereby causing injury or damage to another.

**Nerve:** A part of the nervous system that sends impulses to and from the brain and all other body parts.

**Nervous system:** A group of organs and other structures that regulates all body functions.

**Neurogenic (nu ro JEN ik) shock:** Shock caused by the failure of the nervous system to control the diameter of the blood vessels.

**Nonrebreathing mask:** A special mask combined with a reservoir bag, used to administer high concentrations of oxygen to a breathing casualty through a mask covering both the nose and mouth.

**Nonverbal communication:** Communication through body actions, such as assuming a non-threatening posture or using hand gestures.

**Normal sinus rhythm:** A regular heart rhythm that occurs within a normal rate and without unusual variations.

**Occlusive (o KLOO siv) dressing:** A dressing or bandage that seals a wound and protects it from the air.

**Open fracture:** A fracture that results when bone ends tear the skin and surrounding tissue or when an object penetrates the skin and breaks a bone.

**Open wound:** A wound resulting in a break in the skin's surface.

**Opportunistic infection:** An infection that strikes a casualty with a weakened immune system, such as that caused by AIDS.

**Organ:** A collection of similar tissues acting together to perform specific body functions.

**Oropharyngeal (o ro fer IN je al) airway:** A curved plastic tube inserted into the mouth and positioned at the back of the throat to keep the tongue from blocking the airway.

**Osteoporosis (os te o po RO sis):** The progressive weakening of bone.

**Overdose:** A situation in which a casualty takes enough of a substance that it has poisonous or fatal effects.

**Oxygen:** A tasteless, colourless, odourless gas necessary to sustain life.

**Oxygen cylinder:** A metal cylinder that contains 100 percent oxygen under high pressure.

**Oxygen delivery devices:** Devices of various types used to administer oxygen from a cylinder to either a breathing or non-breathing casualty.

**Pack-strap carry:** An emergency move that can be used on both conscious and unconscious casualties; leaves one hand free.

**Palpation (pal PA shun):** A technique requiring you to feel with your hand for the radial pulse when taking a person's blood pressure.

**Paralysis:** A loss of muscle control; a permanent loss of feeling and movement.

**Paramedics:** Highly specialized EMTs.

**Paraprofessionals:** Workers who are not members of a profession but who assist professionals.

**Partial airway obstruction:** An incomplete blockage of the airway.

**Partial-thickness burn:** A burn injury involving both layers of skin; characterized by red, wet skin and blisters.

**Patella (pah TEL ah):** The kneecap.

**Pathogen (PATH o jen):** A disease-causing agent; also called a microorganism or germ.

**Pelvic cavity:** The lowest part of the trunk that contains the bladder, rectum, and the reproductive organs in females.

**Pelvis:** The lower part of the trunk, containing the intestines, bladder, and female reproductive organs.

**Personal flotation device (PFD):** A buoyant device, such as a cushion or life jacket, designed to be held or worn to keep a person afloat.

**Personal protective equipment (PPE):** Specialized clothing or equipment worn for protection from a hazard.

**Pharynx (FAR ingks):** A part of the airway formed by the back of the nose and throat.

**Physical assault:** Abuse that may result in injury to the body.

**Physically challenged:** A person who suffers a serious injury that results in the loss of body function or one who is born with an impairment that interferes with normal activity.

**Physically disabled:** A person who is unable to move normally.

**Placard:** A sign or notice, a poster.

**Placenta (plah SEN tah):** An organ attached to the uterus and unborn child through which nutrients are delivered to the fetus; expelled after the delivery of the baby.

**Plasma:** The liquid part of blood.

**Platelets:** Disk-shaped structures in the blood that are made of cell fragments; help stop bleeding by forming blood clots at wound sites.

**Poison:** Any substance that causes injury, illness, or death when introduced into the body.

**Poison Centre (PC):** A specialized health centre that provides information in cases of poisoning or suspected poisoning.

**Posterior:** Toward the back.

**Pregnancy:** A condition in which the egg (ovum) of the female is fertilzed by the sperm of the male, forming an embryo.

**Preschooler:** A child 3, 4, or 5 years of age.

**Pressure bandage:** A bandage applied snugly to create pressure on a wound to aid in controlling bleeding.

**Pressure points:** Sites on the body where pressure can be applied to major arteries to slow the flow of blood to a body part.

**Pressure regulator:** A device attached to an oxygen cylinder to reduce cylinder pressure to a safe level for delivery of oxygen.

**Primary survey:** A check for conditions that are an immediate threat to a casualty's life.

**Prolapsed cord:** A complication of childbirth in which a loop of umbilical cord protrudes through the vagina before delivery of the baby.

**Protocols:** Standardized methods.

**Proximal:** Closer to the trunk of the body.

**Public safety personnel:** People employed in a governmental system who are required to respond to and assist with a medical emergency; includes police, fire fighters, and ambulance personnel.

**Pulse:** The beat felt in arteries with each contraction of the heart.

**Puncture:** A wound that results when the skin is pierced with a pointed object, such as a nail, a piece of glass, or a knife.

**Rabies:** A disease caused by a virus transmitted through the saliva of an infected animal.

**Radial pulse:** The pulse felt in the wrist.

**Radiation burn:** A burn caused by rays, energy, or electromagnetic waves.

**Rape:** A crime of violence or one committed under threat of violence involving a sexual attack.

**Refusal of care:** The declining of care by a casualty; a casualty has the right to refuse the care of anyone who responds to an emergency scene.

**Rehabilitation:** The restoration of a casualty of illness or injury to normal or near-normal health.

**Reproductive system:** A group of organs and other structures that enable sexual reproduction.

**Rescue breathing:** A technique of breathing for a nonbreathing casualty.

**Respiration (res pi RA shun):** The breathing process of the body that takes in oxygen and eliminates carbon dioxide.

**Respiratory arrest:** A condition in which breathing has stopped.

**Respiratory distress:** A condition in which breathing is difficult.

**Respiratory (re SPI rah to re or RES pah rah tor e) system:** A group of organs and other structures that bring air into the body and remove wastes through a process called breathing, or respiration.

**Resuscitation mask:** A pliable, dome-shaped device that can fit over a casualty's mouth and nose to aid in ventilation.

**Rib cage:** The cage of bones formed by the 12 pairs of ribs, the sternum, and the spine.

**Ribs:** Bones that attach to the spine and sternum and protect the heart and lungs.

**Rigid splint:** A splint made of boards, metal strips, and folded magazines or newspaper.

**Rigor mortis:** The rigid stiffening of heart and skeletal muscle after death.

**Risk factors:** Conditions or behaviours that increase the chance that a person will develop a disease.

**Roller bandage:** A bandage made of gauze or gauzelike material used to wrap around a dressing.

**Saturated fat:** Fat derived from animal products; a solid at room temperature.

**Scapula (SKAP u lah):** See shoulder blade.

**School-age:** A child between 6 and 12 years of age.

**Secondary survey:** A check for injuries or conditions that could become life threatening if not cared for.

**Seizure (SE zhur):** A disorder in the brain's electrical activity, marked by loss of consciousness and often uncontrollable muscle movement.

**Sexual assault:** Forcing another person to take part in a sexual act.

**Shock:** The failure of the circulatory system to provide adequate oxygen-rich blood to all parts of the body.

**Shoulder blade:** A large, flat, triangular bone at the back of the shoulder in the upper part of the back; also called the scapula.

**Signs:** Any observable evidence of injury or illness, such as bleeding or an unusually pale skin colour.

**Skeletal muscles:** Muscles that attach to bones.

**Skeleton:** The 206 bones of the body that protect vital organs and other soft tissue.

**Skin:** A tough, supple membrane that covers the entire surface of the body.

**Sling:** A bandage used to hold and support an injured part of the body; often used to support an injured arm.

**Soft tissues:** Body structures that include the layers of skin, fat, and muscles.

**Spinal cavity:** An area in the body that contains the spinal cord and is protected by the bones of the spine.

**Spinal column:** The column of vertebrae extending from the base of the skull to the tip of the tailbone (coccyx).

**Spinal cord:** A bundle of nerves extending from the base of the skull to the lower back; protected by the spinal column.

**Spine:** A series of bones (vertebrae) that surrounds and protects the spinal cord; also called the backbone.

**Spleen:** An organ in the abdomen; one function is to store blood.

**Splint:** A device used to immobilize body parts; to support or immobilize a body part using a device or part of the body.

**Spontaneous abortion:** The spontaneous termination of pregnancy before the fetus is born.

**Sprain:** The excessive stretching and tearing of ligaments and other soft tissue structures at a joint.

**Standard of care:** The minimal standard and quality of care expected of an emergency care provider.

**START system:** A triage system based on assessment of three conditions: breathing, circulation, and level of consciousness. The name stands for Simple Triage And Rapid Treatment.

**Statute:** A written law; a law enacted by a legislature.

**Sternum (STER num):** The long, flat bone in the middle of the front of the rib cage; also called the breastbone.

**Stethoscope (STETH o skop):** An instrument used to hear heart and lung sounds and to determine the systolic and diastolic blood pressure.

**Stimulants:** Substances that affect the central nervous system to speed up physical and mental activity.

**Stimuli (STIM u li):** Anything that rouses or excites an organism or body part to respond.

**Stoma:** An opening in the front of the neck through which a person whose larynx has been removed breathes.

**Stomach:** One of the main organs of digestion, located in the abdomen.

**Strain:** The excessive stretching and tearing of muscles and tendons.

**Stroke:** A disruption of blood flow to a part of the brain that causes permanent damage; also called a cerebrovascular accident (CVA).

**Substance abuse:** The deliberate, persistent, excessive use of a substance without regard to health concerns or accepted medical practises.

**Substance misuse:** The use of a substance for unintended purposes or for intended purposes but in improper amounts or doses.

**Sucking chest wound:** A type of penetrating chest injury in which a sucking sound is heard with each breath a casualty takes due to air freely passing in and out of the chest cavity.

**Suctioning:** The process of removing matter, such as saliva, vomitus, or blood, from a casualty's mouth and throat by means of a mechanical or manual device.

**Suction tip:** A rigid or flexible tubing attached to the end of a suction device and placed in the mouth or throat of a casualty to remove foreign matter.

**Sudden death:** The occurrence of cardiac arrest without any prior sign of heart attack.

**Sudden infant death syndrome (SIDS):** The sudden death of a seemingly normal, healthy infant that occurs during the infant's sleep without evidence of disease.

**Suicide:** Self-inflicted death.

**Superficial burn:** A burn involving only the top layer of skin, characterized by red, dry skin.

**Superior:** Toward the head.

**Supplemental oxygen:** Additional oxygen provided a casualty.

**Survival floating:** A face-down floating technique that enables a casualty in warm water to conserve energy while waiting for rescue.

**Symptoms:** Something the casualty tells you about his or her condition, such as, "my head hurts," or "I am dizzy."

**Systolic (sis TOL ic):** The pressure in the arteries when the heart is contracting.

**Tendon (TEN don):** A fibrous band that attaches muscle to bone.

**Thigh:** The lower extremity between the pelvis and the knee.

**Thoracic (tho RAS ik) cavity:** An area in the body that contains the heart and lungs and is protected by the rib cage and upper portion of the spine.

**Thrombus (THROM bus):** A collection of blood components that forms in the heart or vessels, obstructing blood flow.

**Tibia (TIB e ah):** One of the bones in the lower leg.

**Tissue:** A collection of similar cells acting together to perform specific body functions.

**Toddler:** A child 1 or 2 years of age.

**Tourniquet (TOOR ni ket):** A tight band placed around an arm or leg to constrict blood vessels to stop the flow of blood to a wound.

**Trachea (TRA ke ah):** A tube leading from the upper airway to the lungs; also called the windpipe.

**Traction (TRAK shun) splint:** A mechanical device that reduces the deformity of a leg fracture by stretching the muscles to prevent the leg from shortening.

**Transient (TRANZ e ent) ischemic (is KE mik) attack (TIA):** A temporary disruption of blood flow to the brain; sometimes called a mini-stroke.

**Trauma:** Physical injury caused by shock, pressure, or violence.

**Triage:** The process of sorting and providing care to multiple victims according to the severity of their injuries or illnesses.

**Triangular bandage:** A bandage that can be used as a sling or to hold a dressing or splint in place.

**Triple airway maneuver:** A three-step technique used by a rescuer to maintain an open airway while using a resuscitation mask to perform rescue breathing.

**Trunk:** The part of the body containing the chest, abdomen, and pelvis.

**Tuberculosis (tu ber ku LO sis) (TB):** A respiratory disease caused by a bacteria.

**Two-person seat carry:** A method for moving a casualty that requires two rescuers; should not be used on a casualty with suspected head or spinal injury.

**Umbilical (um BIL i kal) cord:** A flexible structure that attaches the placenta to the unborn child, allowing for the passage of blood, nutrients, and waste.

**Universal dressing:** A large dressing used to cover large wounds or multiple wounds in one area.

**Universal precautions:** Safety measures taken to prevent occupational-risk exposure to blood or other body fluids containing visible blood.

**Upper arm:** The upper extremity from the shoulder to the elbow.

**Urinary system:** A group of organs and other structures that eliminates waste products from the blood.

**Uterus (U ter us):** A pear-shaped organ in a woman's pelvis in which an embryo is formed and develops into a baby.

**Vaccine:** A medical substance containing killed or weakened microorganisms that is introduced into the body to prevent, kill, or treat a disease.

**Vagina (vah JI nah):** The lower part of the birth canal through which the baby passes during birth.

**Vector transmission:** The transmission of a disease by an animal or insect bite through exposure to blood or other body fluids.

**Veins:** Blood vessels that carry oxygen-poor blood from all parts of the body to the heart.

**Ventilation:** The process of providing oxygen to the lungs.

**Ventricles (VEN tri kelz):** The two lower chambers of the heart.

**Ventricular (ven TRIK u lar) fibrillation (fi bri LA shun) (V-fib):** A state of totally disorganized electrical activity in the heart, resulting in the quivering (fibrillation) of the ventricles.

**Ventricular tachycardia (tak e KAR de ah):** A heart rate so fast that the heart is unable to pump blood properly.

**Vertebrae (VER te bra):** The 33 bones of the spinal column.

**Virus (VI rus):** A disease-causing agent, or pathogen, that requires another organism to live and reproduce.

**Visually impaired:** A nonspecific term applied to a person who is either blind or partially blind.

**Vital organs:** Organs, such as the brain, heart, and lungs, whose functions are essential to life.

**Vital signs:** Important information about the casualty's condition, obtained by checking level of consciousness, pulse, breathing, skin characteristics, and blood pressure.

**Walking assist:** A basic emergency move used with casualties who need assistance to walk to safety.

**Withdrawal:** A condition produced when a person stops using or abusing a substance to which he or she is addicted.

**Wound:** An injury to the soft tissues.

**Xiphoid (ZI foid):** An arrow-shaped piece of hard tissue at the lowest point of the sternum.

# Index